Problem Solving in
Diabetes

LEE KENNEDY
James Cook University, Queensland, Australia

ISKANDAR IDRIS
Sherwood Forest Hospitals, Sutton-in-Ashfield, UK

ANASTASIOS GAZIS
Queen's Medical Centre University Hospital, Nottingham, UK

CLINICAL PUBLISHING

OXFORD

CLINICAL PUBLISHING

An imprint of Atlas Medical Publishing Ltd

Oxford Centre for Innovation
Mill Street, Oxford OX2 0JX, UK

T: +44 1865 811116
F: +44 1865 251550
W: www.clinicalpublishing.co.uk

Distributed by:
Marston Book Services Ltd
PO Box 269, Abingdon
Oxon OX14 4YN, UK

T: +44 1235 465500
F: +44 1235 465555
E: trade.orders@marston.co.uk

A catalogue record for this book is available from the British Library

ISBN 1 904392 61 X

The publisher makes no representation, express or implied, that the
dosages in this book are correct. Readers must therefore always check
the product information and clinical procedures with the most
up–to–date published product information and data sheets provided by
the manufacturers and the most recent codes of conduct and safety
regulations. The authors and the publisher do not accept any liability
for any errors in the text or for the misuse or misapplication of material
in this work

Project manager:
Series design by Pete Russell, Faringdon, Oxon
Typeset by Pete Russell, Faringdon, Oxon
Printed by TG Hostench S.A., Barcelona

Problem Solving in Diabetes

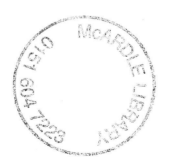

Contents

Abbreviations vii

SECTION 01 **Prevention and Diagnosis** 1

1 Preventing type 1 diabetes 1
2 Preventing type 2 diabetes 5
3 Diabetes risk after the menopause 9
4 Genetic diabetes syndromes (MODY) 13
5 Screening and impaired glucose tolerance 17
6 Type A/B diabetes and insulin resistance 21

SECTION 02 **Acute Diabetes** 25

7 Diabetic ketoacidosis 25
8 Hyperosmolar hyperglycaemic state 30
9 Recurrent hypoglycaemia 34
10 Diabetes and acute myocardial infarction 40
11 Diabetes and acute stroke 43
12 Diabetes and critical limb ischaemia 47
13 Perioperative management of diabetes 51
14 The hot foot 55

SECTION 03 **Managing Diabetes** 61

15 Insulin pumps 61
16 Type 1 diabetes and exercise 65
17 Adolescent diabetes 69
18 Low-carbohydrate diets 72
19 Treatments that stimulate insulin production 77
20 Treatments that improve insulin resistance 81
21 Diabetes and enteral feeding 85
22 Obesity and diabetes 89
23 Diabetes in the elderly 93

SECTION 04 **Reproductive Complications** 99

24 Polycystic ovarian syndrome 99
25 Gestational diabetes 103
26 Type 1 diabetes and pregnancy 107

27   Erectile dysfunction 111
28   Pre-eclampsia 115

SECTION 05 Cardiovascular Risk Factors in Diabetes 121

29   Smoking cessation 121
30   Hypertriglyceridaemia 125
31   Hyperlipidaemia in type 1 diabetes 129
32   Hyperlipidaemia in type 2 diabetes 133
33   Aspirin use in diabetes 137
34   Hypertension—uncomplicated 140
35   Hypertension—hard to control 143

SECTION 06 Microvascular Complications 149

36   Painful neuropathy 149
37   Microalbuminuria 154
38   ACE inhibitor treatment 159
39   Advancing renal failure 163
40   Background retinopathy 167
41   Proliferative and pre-proliferative retinopathy 171
42   Macular disease 175
43   Autonomic neuropathy 178
44   The Charcot foot 182

SECTION 07 Macrovascular and Other Complications 187

45   Angina in patients with type 2 diabetes 187
46   Advances in management of peripheral arterial disease 191
47   Renal artery stenosis 195
48   Foot ulceration 199
49   Transient ischaemic attack 203

SECTION 08 Diabetes in Special Groups of Patients 207

50   Diabetes and respiratory disease 207
51   Diabetes and cystic fibrosis 212
52   Diabetes and dialysis 216
53   Diabetes and coeliac disease 220

General index 225

Abbreviations

4S Scandinavian Simvastatin Survival Study

ABCD trial Appropriate Blood Pressure Control in Diabetes Trial

ABPI Ankle–brachial pressure index

ABPM Ambulatory blood pressure monitoring

ACAS Asymptomatic Carotid Atherosclerosis Study

ACE Angiotensin-converting enzyme

ACR Albumin–creatinine ratio

ACHOIS trial Australian Carbohydrate Intolerance Study in Pregnant Women

AER Albumin excretion rate

AHI Apnoea–Hypopnea Index

ALLHAT Antihypertensive and Lipid-Lowering Treatment to Prevent Heart Attack Trial

AMD Age-related macular degeneration

ANG-1 and ANG-2 Angiopoetin

APT Anti-Platelet Trialists

ARB Angiotensin receptor blocker

ASTRAL trial Angioplasty and Stent for Renal Artery Lesions trial

BARI trial Bypass Angioplasty Revascularization Investigation

BMI Body mass index

BP Blood pressure

CABG Coronary artery bypass grafting

CALM study Candesartan And Lisinopril Microalbuminuria study

CAPD Continuous ambulatory peritoneal dialysis

CAPRIE study Clopidogrel versus Aspirin in Patients at Risk of Ischaemic Events study

CARDS Collaborative Atorvastatin Diabetes Study

CARE study Cholesterol and Recurrent Events study

CAS Carotid artery stenosis

CETP Cholesteryl ester transfer protein

CF Cystic fibrosis

CFRD Cystic fibrosis-related diabetes

CHD Coronary heart disease

CHHIPS Controlling Hypertension and Hypotension Immediately Post-Stroke trial

CI Confidence interval

CK Creatine kinase

CPAP Continuous positive airway pressure

CSII Continuous subcutaneous infusion of insulin

CSMO Clinically significant macular oedema

CT Computed tomography

CWS Cotton-wool spot

DAN Diabetic autonomic neuropathy

DCCT Diabetes Control and Complications Trial

DIGAMI Diabetes and Insulin-Glucose Infusion in Acute Myocardial Infarction study

DIRECT DIabetic Retinopathy Candesartan Trial

DKA Diabetic ketoacidosis

DMa Diabetic maculopathy

DME study Diabetic Macular Edema study

DPN Distal sensory peripheral neuropathy

DPP Diabetes Prevention Program

DPP-IV Dipeptidyl peptidase IV

DPS Diabetes Prevention Study

DRS Diabetic Retinopathy Study

ECG Electrocardiogram

ECST European Carotid Surgery Trial

EDIC Epidemiology of Diabetes Interventions and Complications

ELISA Enzyme-linked immunosorbent assay

ENDIT European Nicotinamide Diabetes Intervention Trial

ETDRS Early Treatment Diabetic Retinopathy Study

ETF Enteral tube feeding

EUCLID study EURODIAB Controlled Trial of Lisinopril in Insulin-Dependent Diabetes Mellitus

FEV(1) Forced expiratory volume in one second

FOOD Feed or ordinary diet trial

FSH   Follicle-stimulating hormone

GABA   Gamma-aminobutyric acid

G-CSF   Granulocyte–colony stimulating factor

GDM   Gestational diabetes mellitus

GFD   Gluten-free diet

GFR   Glomerular filtration rate

GI   Glycaemic index

GIK   Glucose insulin potassium

GIST   Glucose Insulin in Stroke Trial

GLP-1   Glucagon-like peptide-1

HAAF   Hypoglycaemia associated autonomic failure

HAIR-AN syndrome   HyperAndrogenism, Insulin Resistance and Acanthosis Nigricans

HbA1c   Glycosylated haemoglobin

HDL   High-density lipoprotein

HELLP syndrome   Haemolysis, Elevated Liver enzymes, Low Platelets

HERS   Hormone Estrogen-Progestin Replacement Study

HHS   Hyperosmolar hyperglycaemic state

HLA   Human leucocyte antigen

HOPE   Heart Outcomes Protection Evaluation study

HOT study   Hypertension Optimal Treatment study

HPS   Heart Protection Study

HRT   Hormone replacement therapy

ICU   Intensive care unit

IFG   Impaired fasting glucose

IGF   Insulin-like growth factor

IgG   Immunoglobulin G

IGT   Impaired glucose tolerance

IHD   Ischaemic heart disease

IMT   Intima–media thickness

INR   International normalized ratio

IRS   Insulin resistance state

IRMA   Intraretinal microvascular abnormality

ISDN   Isosorbide dinitrate

IV   Intravenous

IVF   in vitro fertilization

LAD   Left anterior descending

LDH   Lactate dehydrogenase

LDL   Low-density lipoprotein

LIFE study   Losartan Intervention For Endpoint reduction in hypertension

LIPID study   Long-term Intervention with Pravastatin in Ischaemic Disease study

LH   Leuteinizing hormone

MA   Microaneurysm

MDI   Multiple daily injections

MDRD study   Modification of Diet in Renal Disease Study

MIDD   Maternally inherited diabetes and deafness

MO   Macular oedema

MODY   Maturity-onset diabetes of youth

MRA   Magnetic resonance angiography

MRFIT   Multiple Risk Factor Intervention Trial

MRI   Magnetic resonance imaging

MRSA   Methicillin-resistant *Staphylococcus aureus*

NAOIN   Non-arteritic optic ischaemic neuropathy

NASCET   North American Symptomatic Carotid Endarterectomy Trial

NGF   Nerve growth factor

NHANES   National Health and Nutrition Evaluation Study

NMR   Nuclear magnetic resonance

NO   Nitric oxide

NTD   Neural tube defects

NRT   Nicotine replacement therapy

OAD   Oral antidiabetic agent

oGTT   Oral glucose tolerance test

OSA   Obstructive sleep apnoea

PAD   Peripheral arterial disease

PARP   Poly-ADP-ribose polymerase

PCI   Percutaneous coronary intervention

PCOS   Polycystic ovarian syndrome

PDE   Phosphodiesterase

PDGF   Platelet-derived growth factor

PEDF   Pigment Epithelial-Derived Factor

PEG   Percutaneous endoscopic gastrostomy

PKC   Protein kinase C

PPAR   Peroxisome proliferator-activated receptor

PPP   Primary Prevention Project

PROGRESS   Perindopril PROtection aGainst Recurrent Stroke Study

RAS   Renin–angiotensin system

RANKL   Receptor Activator of Nuclear factor Kappa B Ligand

RArtS Renal artery stenosis

RIO Rimonabant In Obesity trial

rTPA Recombinant tissue plasminogen activator

RR Relative risk

SDB Sleep-disordered breathing

SHBG Sex-hormone binding globulin

SR Sustained release

STOP-NIDDM Study to Prevent Non-Insulin-Dependent Diabetes Mellitus

SHHS Sleep Heart Health Study

SSRI Selective serotonin reuptake inhibitor

SUR Sulphonylurea receptor

SWAN Study of Women's health Across the Nation

T1DM Type 1 diabetes

TCC Total contact casting

TIA Transient ischaemic attack

TNT study Treating to New Target study

UAE Urinary albumin excretion

UKPDS United Kingdom Prospective Diabetes Study

VAT Visceral adipose tissue

VA-HIT Veterans Affairs High-Density Lipoprotein Intervention Trial

VEGF Vascular endothelial growth factor

VLDL Very-low-density lipoprotein

VO_2max Maximal oxygen uptake

WHI Women's Health Initiative

WOSCOPS West of Scotland Coronary Prevention Study

XENDOS study XENical in the prevention of Diabetes in Obese Subjects study

Prevention and Diagnosis

1   Preventing type 1 diabetes
2   Preventing type 2 diabetes
3   Diabetes risk after the menopause
4   Genetic diabetes syndromes (MODY)
5   Screening and impaired glucose tolerance
6   Type A/B diabetes and insulin resistance

PROBLEM

1 Preventing Type 1 Diabetes

Case History

The parent of a 4-year-old boy with type 1 diabetes consults you wanting to know if there is anything he can do to prevent a future child developing the condition. He already has an 8-year-old daughter with diabetes and there is a strong family history of autoimmune thyroid disease on both his and his wife's side of the family. They are contemplating having a third child.

Is there any evidence that type 1 diabetes is preventable?

Is there any general advice the parents can usefully follow?

Can we predict the onset of type 1 diabetes?

Background

Preventing or curing type 1 diabetes is one of the holy grails for those who research autoimmune disease or treat patients with diabetes. The disease typically presents in childhood, currently necessitates lifelong use of insulin injections and exposes the individual to increased risk of vascular complications. The risk of type 1 diabetes in the general population is about 1 in 300, and this is increased up to 20-fold in first-degree relatives. Genetic markers do not provide an accurate prediction of diabetes, with only 5% of those with susceptibility markers actually developing the disease. However, the fact that the disease has a long latent period and that the pre-diabetic phase can be identified by measuring islet cell antibodies or by assessing beta cell function yields an opportunity for preventative therapy. The results of trials using non-specific immunosuppression in the 1980s were disappointing with only temporary improvements in insulin production demonstrated.

Type 1 diabetes in children became much more common in the course of the 20th century.[1] In fact, available evidence suggests that the disease was quite uncommon, although generally fatal, in children during the 19th century. This, along with the geographical variation in the prevalence of childhood diabetes that is not accounted for by variations in the prevalence of susceptible genotypes, strongly suggests that environmental factors are important.[2] The wide variation in incidence rates applies much more to childhood than to adult type 1 diabetes.[3] It is not surprising that there has been intensive research into environmental triggers for diabetes that might be modified, or into safe and effective nutritional or immunological manipulations that might decrease risk of developing the disease (Figure 1.1). Recent evidence suggests that most parents of children at risk of type 1 diabetes will attempt preventative measures,[4] and it is increasingly important for health professionals to be able to enter into a balanced discussion with parents and would-be parents.

Both macronutrient and micronutrient components of the diet have received attention.[5] A protective effect of breast-feeding has been proposed, but not confirmed in all

Factors Predisposing To Type 1 Diabetes	Level of Evidence
Genetic (including HLA)	***
Non-breast-fed	*
Early exposure to cows' milk	*
Low vitamin D status	**
Viral infection	*
Rapid weight gain in childhood	*

The Following Do Not Appear To Modify Risk

Childhood vaccination
Treatment with nicotinamide
Oral insulin therapy

***	Strong evidence supported by multiple well-conducted and randomized clinical studies
**	Reasonable evidence supported by clinical studies (not randomized)
*	Some evidence supported by observational studies and expert opinion

Fig.1.1 Factors predisposing to type 1 diabetes. HLA = human leucocyte antigen.

studies. Breast-feeding may afford protection through early oral exposure to human milk (inducing tolerance to insulin; see below), through protection against infectious agents, and by decreasing the risk of excessive weight gain in infancy. The latter is also probably a trigger for diabetes during adolescence. On the other hand, early exposure to cows' milk may increase risk through exposure to bovine insulin or β-casein, the latter being a known immunomodulatory protein contained in cows' milk. Bottle-feeding can also be associated with excessive weight gain. Amongst micronutrient components of the diet, nitroso compounds (related to streptozotocin), nitrates and nitrites, all used as preservatives in meat products, have been considered. Variations in vitamin D status may be another reason for the geographical variation in the incidence of type 1 diabetes. Vitamin D has important regulatory effects on the immune system. A protective effect of cod liver oil (a source of both vitamin D and long-chain n-3 fatty acids, which are also anti-inflammatory) was shown against childhood diabetes in the recent study reported by the Norwegian Childhood Diabetes Study Group.[6]

Certain infectious agents, including enteroviruses, have been associated with development of diabetes in animal models and in rare cases of human diabetes. This has led to worries that childhood vaccination, particularly with live attenuated vaccines, may be a risk factor for type 1 diabetes. A Danish study, along with other recent evidence, has gone a long way to dispel worries on this score; Hviid and colleagues[7] studied a cohort including all Danish children born between 1990 and 2000, and found no evidence of any association between childhood vaccinations and diabetes. On the contrary, the vaccines may be protective by limiting the effect of potentially diabetogenic infections, particularly rubella.

Recent Developments

1   Vitamin B$_3$ (niacin) consists of nicotinic acid and nicotinamide. The latter is tolerated in high doses, and has been shown to decrease the incidence of diabetes in streptozotocin-treated animals, and in non-obese diabetic mice. Some early preclinical studies showed promise for the agent. The vitamin inhibits poly-ADP-ribose polymerase (PARP), an enzyme involved in DNA repair. Activation of PARP leads to depletion of intracellular nicotinamide adenine dinucleotide. This depletion of cellular energy stores may predispose to cell damage, including in the pancreatic beta cell. The European Nicotinamide Diabetes Intervention Trial (ENDIT)[8] was a randomized, double-blind, placebo-controlled trial in which 552 islet cell antibody-positive first-degree relatives of patients with diabetes took either nicotinamide or placebo. There was no difference in the incidence of diabetes during the five years of the trial (82 vs 77 cases, respectively).

2   Autoimmunity directed at insulin epitopes is one of the critical driving forces in the pathogenesis of type 1 diabetes. In animal models, exposure to mucosal insulin induces tolerance and thus decreases risk of diabetes. This mechanism is of particular interest because of the recent developments of insulin formulations which are active after oral or nasal administration. The Diabetes Prevention Trial-Type 1 reported recently.[9] In this trial, a large number of first- and second-degree relatives of patients with diabetes were screened for pre-diabetes. Those found to be positive were ran-

domized to receive either oral insulin or placebo. Again, there was no difference in the incidence of new diabetes between the control and the treatment groups.

3 The prospects of gene therapy for diabetes are improving rapidly. Approaches to introduce a functioning insulin-producing mechanism in glucose-responsive cells have been considered. The genetic susceptibility to diabetes is mainly through class II histocompatibility alleles. Recent experiments in non-obese diabetic mice have been carried out to replace diabetes-prone genes with those that are protective.[10]

Conclusion

There is not, currently, any way to accurately predict which individuals are going to get diabetes, or to prevent its occurrence. Family history is a major risk factor, increasing susceptibility by up to 20-fold, and there might be a slight bias towards males developing diabetes. Epidemiological data strongly support a role for environmental influences, especially for childhood diabetes. There is no evidence currently to support specific preventative measures. Breast-feeding should be promoted for its possible role in preventing type 1 diabetes, as well as its other health benefits. Efforts to limit excessive weight gain in infancy and adolescence should be promoted, as high body weight at these times may favour development of type 1 diabetes. Among the other nutritional factors, the best evidence is for a protective effect of vitamin D and supplementation should be considered (perhaps as cod liver oil) in areas where sunlight exposure is low. Finally, parents should be encouraged to have their children vaccinated as per normal childhood schedules— there is no evidence that vaccination predisposes to diabetes and it may be that, by decreasing infection with some agents, it actually protects.

Further Reading

1 Gale EAM. The rise of childhood type 1 diabetes in the 20th century. *Diabetes* 2002; **51**: 3353–61.

2 Kukko M, Virtanen SM, Toivonen A, Simmell S, Korhonen S, Ilonen J, Simel O, Knip M. Geographical variation in risk HLA-DQB1 genotypes for type 1 diabetes and signs of beta-cell autoimmunity in a high-incidence country. *Diabetes Care* 2004; **27**: 676–81.

3 Kyvik KO, Nystrom L, Gorus F, Songini M, Oestman J, Castell C, Green A, Guyrus E, Ionescu-Tirgoviste C, McKinney PA, Michalkova D, Ostrauskas R, Raymond NT. The epidemiology of Type 1 diabetes mellitus is not the same in young adults as in children. *Diabetologia* 2004; **47**: 377–84.

4 Baughcum AE, Johnson SB, Carmichael SK, Lewin AB, She JX, Schatz DA. Maternal efforts to prevent type 1 diabetes in at-risk children. *Diabetes Care* 2005; **28**: 916–21.

5 Virtanen SM, Knip M. Nutritional risk predictors of beta cell autoimmunity and type 1 diabetes at a young age. *Am J Clin Nutr* 2003; **78**: 1053–67.

6 Stene LC, Joner G, Norwegian Childhood Diabetes Study Group. Use of cod liver oil during the first year of life is associated with lower risk of childhood-onset type 1 diabetes: a large, population-based, case-control study. *Am J Clin Nutr* 2003; **78**: 1128–34.

7 Hviid A, Stellfeld M, Wohlfahrt J, Melbye M. Childhood vaccination and type 1 diabetes. *N Engl J Med* 2004; **350**: 1398–1404.

8 Gale EA, Bingley PJ, Emmett CL, Collier T. European Nicotinamide Diabetes Intervention Trial (ENDIT): a randomised controlled trial of intervention before the onset of type 1 diabetes. *Lancet* 2004; **363**: 925–31.

9 Skyler JS, Krischer JP, Wolfsdorf J, Cowie C, Palmer JP, Greenbaum C, Cuthbertson D, Rafkin-Mervis LE, Chase HP, Leschek E. Effects of oral insulin in relatives of patients with type 1 diabetes: The Diabetes Prevention Trial-Type 1. *Diabetes Care* 2005; **28**: 1068–76.

10 Tian C, Bagley J, Cretin N, Seth N, Wucherpfennig KW, Iacomini J. Prevention of type 1 diabetes by gene therapy. *J Clin Invest* 2004; **114**: 969–78.

2 Preventing Type 2 Diabetes

Case History

You are consulted by a 43-year-old man who has a strong family history of diabetes. He is concerned because his father developed diabetes at the age of 56 and has recently (aged 60 years) had a lower limb amputation. Your patient is generally in good health. He has a body mass index of 28 kg/m² and takes very little exercise as he has a busy job and a young family. He smokes 20 cigarettes per day, and has been noted to be mildly hypertensive although not requiring treatment at present.

How would you advise him?

Are we able to prevent development of type 2 diabetes?

Is there a role for drug therapy?

Background

Once the condition is established, it is extremely difficult to maintain tight control of blood glucose and other vascular risk factors in patients with type 2 diabetes. A number of very important studies have been published in the past three years demonstrating the potential for lifestyle interventions and drugs to either prevent diabetes, or at least to delay its onset. These studies, along with the acknowledged costs of managing patients with type 2 diabetes, have heightened awareness of the value of preventative measures.

The best-known of the prevention studies is the Diabetes Prevention Program (DPP), carried out in 27 North American centres.[1] In this study, 3234 non-diabetic patients with impaired glucose tolerance were randomly assigned to placebo, metformin (850 mg twice daily) or lifestyle intervention. The latter consisted of dietary advice plus at least 150 minutes of physical activity per week. After 2.8 years of follow-up, the incidence of diabetes was 11.0, 7.8 and 4.8 cases per 100 patient-years in the placebo, metformin and lifestyle groups, respectively. Metformin reduced the incidence of new diabetes by 31%, while lifestyle intervention reduced it by 58%. Some of the benefit associated with metformin use is lost after the drug is stopped. However, a recent washout study using the DPP cohort confirms that much of the benefit persists.[2] A very recent cost–benefit analysis of this study confirmed that both interventions were cost effective.[3] However, lifestyle intervention was much more cost effective with a cost, relative to placebo, of $1100 per quality-adjusted life-year, compared with $31 300 for metformin.

The benefit of lifestyle intervention was confirmed in the Finnish Diabetes Prevention Study (DPS).[4] Usual diabetes care was compared with a lifestyle intervention programme in 522 overweight, middle-aged subjects with impaired glucose tolerance. The lifestyle intervention group experienced greater weight loss and improved glycaemic and lipid parameters. The STOP-NIDDM trial[5] (Study to Prevent Non-Insulin-Dependent Diabetes Mellitus) randomized 714 patients with impaired glucose tolerance to either placebo or acarbose, and followed them up for over three years. Forty-two per cent of patients in the placebo wing and 32% of patients taking acarbose developed diabetes. The decrease in new diabetes was highly significant, although the study has been criticized because of possible bias due to the large proportion of patients that did not complete their treatment regime. There is further evidence that drug treatment can prevent, or delay the onset of, diabetes from small studies using either sulphonylureas or the thiazolidinedione drug, troglitazone.[6]

One in five of the population in most developed countries is now obese, and this is the major factor underlying the global increase in diabetes prevalence in recent years. It is not surprising, therefore, that obesity has become an increasing focus for treatment and prevention of diabetes and cardiovascular disease. In the XENDOS study (XENical in the prevention of Diabetes in Obese Subjects), 3305 patients were treated with lifestyle intervention and randomized either to placebo or to treatment with the gastrointestinal lipase inhibitor, orlistat.[7] After four years' treatment, diabetes had developed in 9.0% of placebo patients and in 6.2% of orlistat-treated patients. Patients treated with orlistat also lost more weight and had improved lipid profiles. Again, and as with many long-term studies in this area, a relatively large proportion of patients did not complete the study.

In summary, a number of recent studies confirm that both lifestyle interventions and drug treatments can reduce the incidence of new diagnoses of diabetes, and also improve some of the associated cardiovascular risk factors (Figure 2.1). Lifestyle intervention is clearly preferable, particularly if changes can be sustained long-term. Diet and exercise can also be cost-effective interventions. For those who do not succeed with lifestyle management, drug treatment appears to be both a safe and an effective option.

Recent Developments

1   Other drug groups used in the prevention of cardiovascular disease may affect the development of diabetes.[6] Blockade of the renin–angiotensin system has now been shown in several studies, including the Heart Outcomes Protection Evaluation (HOPE) study, to modestly decrease incidence of diabetes. Lipid-lowering drugs may have a similar effect, perhaps by decreasing insulin resistance. For some patients, vig-

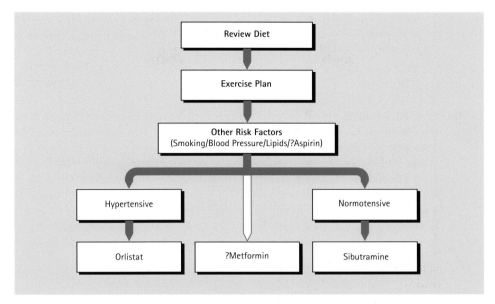

Fig. 2.1 Figure shows suggested scheme for prevention of type 2 diabetes using lifestyle interventions and anti-obesity drugs

orous treatment of cardiovascular risk factors may be the best line of attack, and decreased risk of diabetes an important secondary benefit of treatment.

2   Individuals at high risk of vascular disease should have vigorous management of their multiple risk factors wherever possible. One of the largest randomized trials of lifestyle intervention conducted is the Multiple Risk Factor Intervention Trial (MRFIT). Recent data[8] from nearly 13 000 men followed for up to seven years show, again, that diet and exercise can prevent diabetes. However, there were interesting differences between smokers and non-smokers; with lifestyle intervention, diabetes incidence was 18% lower in non-smokers but 26% higher in smokers. The exact reasons for this are not clear but use of antihypertensive drugs in smokers and weight gain associated with attempts to quit smoking are possible confounding factors.

3   The role of exercise in improving glucose tolerance is now well established. Traditionally, vigorous aerobic exercise was recommended but was often unpalatable or unachievable for overweight and untrained subjects. Now, almost any type of exercise—depending on the patient's preferences and capabilities—is regarded as beneficial. Recent data from the Finnish Diabetes Prevention Study have confirmed the link between leisure-time physical activity and reduced risk of diabetes.[9] Even low-intensity and walking activity were associated with improved glucose tolerance.

4   There is currently great focus on the effects of diets with differing macronutrient contents. Diets that are low glycaemic index, high in fibre and rich in wholegrain foodstuffs can improve glucose tolerance and diminish the risk of developing diabetes. These findings have been confirmed in a number of substantial studies published in the past two years. In one recent study involving over 36 000 Australian

men,[10] consumption of a low glycaemic diet correlated strongly with a decreased risk of diabetes. Also, and in keeping with other studies, low dietary magnesium intake was also associated with increased risk of diabetes.

Conclusion

Given the difficulty experienced in reducing the risk associated with type 2 diabetes once the condition has developed, it seems imperative to try to prevent the condition whenever the opportunity arises. Although the above patient is fit and healthy at present, he is at risk in the future of developing type 2 diabetes. Initial management should be with dietary advice from a registered dietician and the patient should be advised about the benefits of exercise. Even a modest increase in low-intensity activity might be of benefit. He should have a thorough assessment of his overall cardiovascular risk and, if necessary, receive treatment for poorly controlled risk factors. Given that he is healthy and young, he should be strongly advised to keep his weight down and to engage in regular physical activity. Once he commences drug therapy, he is likely to take it for life. He should be advised to stop smoking and offered smoking cessation support if needed. This will reduce his risk of cardiovascular events and may also decrease his risk of diabetes. His glycaemic status should be assessed by fasting blood glucose and, preferably, also with a random or postprandial measurement. Drug therapy—for example with metformin—could be considered if he has impaired glucose tolerance. The benefit is not likely to be as great as that with diet and exercise, and this should be repeatedly emphasized to the patient.

Further Reading

1 Knowler WC, Barrett-Connor E, Fowler SE, Hamman RF, Lachin JM, Walker EA, Nathan DM. Reduction in the incidence of type 2 diabetes with lifestyle intervention or metformin. *N Engl J Med* 2002; **346**: 393–403.

2 Diabetes Prevention Program Research Group. Effects of withdrawal from metformin on the development of diabetes in the diabetes prevention program. *Diabetes Care* 2003; **26**: 977–80.

3 Herman WH, Hoerger TJ, Brandle M, Hicks K, Sorensen S, Zhang P, Hamman RF, Ackermann RT, Engelgau MM, Ratner RE. The cost-effectiveness of lifestyle modification or metformin in preventing type 2 diabetes in adults with impaired glucose tolerance. *Ann Intern Med* 2005; **142**: 323–32.

4 Lindström J, Louheranta A, Mannelin M, Rastas M, Salminen V, Eriksson J, Uusitupa M, Tuomilehto J. The Finnish Diabetes Prevention Study (DPS): Lifestyle intervention and 3-year results on diet and physical activity. *Diabetes Care* 2003; **26**: 3230–6.

5 Chiasson JL, Josse RG, Gomis R, Hanefeld M, Karasik A, Laakso M. Acarbose for prevention of type 2 diabetes mellitus: the STOP-NIDDM randomised trial. *Lancet* 2002; **359**: 2072–7.

6 Padwal R, Majumdar SR, Johnson JA, Varney J, McAlister FA. A systematic review of drug therapy to delay or prevent type 2 diabetes. *Diabetes Care* 2005; **28**: 736–44.

7 Torgerson JS, Hauptman J, Boldrin MN, Sjöströöm L. XENical in the prevention of diabetes in obese subjects (XENDOS) study: a randomized study of orlistat as an adjunct to lifestyle changes for the prevention of type 2 diabetes in obese patients. *Diabetes Care* 2004; **27**: 155–61.

8 Davey Smith G, Bracha Y, Svendsen KH, Neaton JD, Haffner SM, Kuller LH. Incidence of type 2 diabetes in the randomized multiple risk factor intervention trial. *Ann Intern Med* 2005; **142**: 313–22.

9 Laaksonen DE, Lindström J, Lakka TA, Eriksson JG, Niskanen L, Wikström K, Aunola S, Keinänen-Kiukaanniemi S, Laakso M, Valle TT, Ilanne-Parikka P, Louheranta A, Hämäläinen H, Rastas M, Salminen V, Cepaitis Z, Hakumäki M, Kaikkonen H, Härkönen P, Sundvall J, Tuomilehto J, Uusitupa M. Physical activity in the prevention of type 2 diabetes: the Finnish diabetes prevention study. *Diabetes* 2005; **54**: 158–65.

10 Hodge AM, English DR, O'Dea K, Giles GG. Glycemic index and dietary fiber and the risk of type 2 diabetes. *Diabetes Care* 2004; **27**: 2701–6.

PROBLEM

3   Diabetes Risk after the Menopause

Case History

A 54-year-old Afro-Caribbean woman is referred to you. She is two years post-menopausal and type 2 diabetes was diagnosed eight months ago. Despite having visited the dietician three times since then, her body mass index remains high at 30 kg/m². She takes atenolol 50 mg/day for hypertension, which is well controlled. Diabetes is treated by diet alone, and her glycosylated haemoglobin (HbA1c) is reasonable at 7.1%. Fasting cholesterol is 5.8 mmol/l and triglycerides 2.5 mmol/l. She has a strong family history of type 2 diabetes.

How would you manage her diabetes and hypertension?

Is her age and menopausal status relevant to her management?

Is her racial background important?

She wants to know whether she should consider hormone replacement therapy

Background

Compared with men, women are relatively protected from cardiovascular disease except when they are post-menopausal or they have diabetes. Sex steroids have important roles in regulating lipid metabolism, endothelial function, blood vessel tone and other aspects of vascular function. Menopause is associated with a relatively abrupt decrease in circulating oestrogen. There is no comparable process in men. Since the general population is aging, and women spend an increasing proportion of their life in an oestrogen-deficient state in which they are at risk of atherosclerotic disorders, management of cardiovascular risk in the peri- and post-menopausal periods is of particular importance.

The period of declining ovarian function leading up to the menopause, the peri-menopause, is associated with declining sex steroid levels and important alterations in body composition. Thus total and visceral adiposity increase, and bone mineral density decreases. The change in fat mass and distribution may relate to decreased lipolysis and increased activity of lipoprotein lipase. Weight gain around the menopause is greater in women from more deprived socio-economic backgrounds and in those who do not smoke, do not exercise regularly and have never used HRT. In a prospective 9-year study of women during the menopausal transition, Guthrie et al.[1] demonstrated that mood changes and decreased quality of life appeared to contribute to the changes in body composition and cardiovascular risk profile around the menopause.

HRT is not currently recommended for prevention of cardiovascular disease. Although benefits in risk-markers have been documented, there is debate about which oestrogen, which progestogen, or which combination, and which route of administration. Set against the possibility of a marginal benefit in cardiovascular disease prevention, there is un-doubtedly increased risk of thromboembolic events and breast cancer. Moreover, two important trials—the Women's Health Initiative (WHI) and the Hormone Estrogen-Progestin Replacement Study (HERS)—actually reported increased cardiac events in the short term. A recent large, Swedish study[2] appears to confirm that oestrogen use can improve cardiovascular risk profile and there are now several lines of evidence that either oral or transdermal oestrogen may improve insulin sensitivity and slow the progress of the metabolic syndrome, thus retarding development of diabetes in those at risk.[3]

The impact of diabetes on cardiovascular risk is higher for women than it is for men. In a recent Finnish study,[4] the event rate per 1000 patient-years was 11.6 for non-diabetic men and 1.8 for non-diabetic women, while comparable event rates for males and females with diabetes were 36.3 and 31.6, respectively. In the recent Study of Women's health Across the Nation (SWAN),[5] differences between insulin sensitivity and beta cell function were compared in groups of pre- or peri-menopausal women from differing racial backgrounds. Insulin sensitivity was lower in African-Americans compared with other racial groups, while beta cell function was relatively preserved in this group. Thus measures to improve insulin sensitivity, including weight loss, should be the approach of choice in this group.

Recent Developments

1   Increased abdominal obesity in women is linked with insulin resistance and with markers of inflammation that predispose to ischaemic heart disease and other com-plications of obesity (Figure 3.1).[6] Although visceral obesity does not account for all of the increased risk associated with the post-menopausal state, it is an important therapeutic target, and regular exercise goes a long way to ameliorate the fat accumu-lation and accompanying risk factors.[7]

2   Attempts to improve health and deal with cardiovascular risk factors should not wait until the menopause. Recent data from the Nurses Health Study[8] demonstrate that

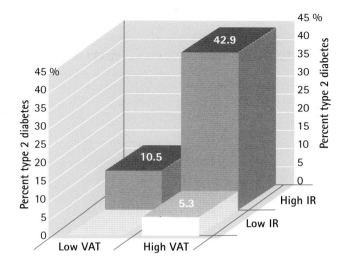

Fig. 3.1 Contributions of visceral adipose tissue (VAT) and insulin resistance (IR) to risk of diabetes. Post-menopausal women were screened for diabetes using an oral glucose tolerance test. Diabetes was particularly prevalent in women who had both increased visceral adipose tissue and insulin resistance. *$P<0.0001$. *Source*: Piché *et al.* 2005.[6]

increasing obesity in the pre-menopause is associated with increased levels of inflammatory markers (tumour necrosis factor-receptor, interleukin-6 and C-reactive protein), and these markers are predictive of the development of diabetes.

3   Micronutrient status also changes around the time of the menopause and there is considerable evidence now that some of these changes may relate to risk of diabetes and cardiovascular disease. Thus, decreased magnesium levels are more common after the menopause, and predispose to insulin resistance and the metabolic syndrome.[9] Increased iron stores are associated with increased cardiovascular risk factors,[10] and this may be a factor in the peri-menopausal period for many women.[11]

Conclusion

This woman is at increased risk on the grounds of age, ethnicity, menopausal status and the fact that she has diabetes. She should try hard with diet and exercise to manage her weight and glycaemic control (Figure 3.2). Given her imperfect glycaemic control at present, she might consider metformin to help preserve her beta cell function long term. Her hypertension is well controlled but atenolol might not be the ideal agent given her weight and imperfect glycaemic control. An angiotensin-converting enzyme inhibitor or angiotensin II receptor blocker might be preferable. HRT is not routinely recommended for cardiovascular disease prevention but patient choice is important, and she may consider this if she is experiencing menopausal symptoms. She may benefit from aspirin treatment (see Chapter 33).

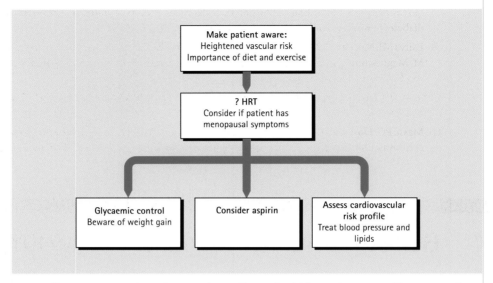

Fig. 3.2 Figure suggests a scheme for managing cardiovascular risk in a patient approaching, or soon after, the menopause. HRT = hormone replacement therapy.

Further Reading

1 Guthrie JR, Dennerstein L, Taffe JR, Lehert P, Burger HG. The menopausal transition: a 9-year prospective population-based study. The Melbourne Women's Midlife Health Project. *Climacteric* 2004; **7**: 375–89.

2 Shakir YA, Samsioe G, Nyberg P, Lidfeldt J, Nerbrand C. Cardiovascular risk factors in middle-aged women and the association with use of hormone therapy: results from a population-based study of Swedish women. The Women's Health in the Lund Area (WHILA) Study. *Climacteric* 2004; **7**: 274–83.

3 Rossi R, Origliani G, Modena MG. Transdermal 17-beta-estradiol and risk of developing type 2 diabetes in a population of healthy, nonobese postmenopausal women. *Diabetes Care* 2004; **27**: 645–9.

4 Juutilainen A, Kortelainen S, Lehto S, Rönnemaa T, Pyörälä K, Laakso M. Gender difference in the impact of type 2 diabetes on coronary heart disease risk. *Diabetes Care* 2004; **27**: 2898–904.

5 Torrens JI, Skurnick J, Davidow AL, Korenman SG, Santoro N, Soto-Greene M, Lasser N, Weiss G. Ethnic differences in insulin sensitivity and beta-cell function in premenopausal or early perimenopausal women without diabetes: the Study of Women's health Across the Nation (SWAN). *Diabetes Care* 2004; **27**: 354–61.

6 Piché ME, Weisnagel SJ, Corneau L, Nadeau A, Bergeron J, Lemieux S. Contribution of abdominal visceral obesity and insulin resistance to the cardiovascular risk profile of postmenopausal women. *Diabetes* 2005; **54**: 770–7.

7 Holcomb CA, Heim DL, Loughin TM. Physical activity minimizes the association of body fatness with abdominal obesity in white, premenopausal women: results from the Third National Health and Nutrition Examination Survey. *J Am Diet Assoc* 2004; **104**: 1859–62.

8   Hu FB, Meigs JB, Li TY, Rifai N, Manson JE. Inflammatory markers and risk of developing type 2 diabetes in women. *Diabetes* 2004; **53**: 693–700.

9   Laires MJ, Moreira H, Monteiro CP, Sandinha L, Limao F, Veiga L, Goncalves A, Ferreira A, Bicho M. Magnesium, insulin resistance and body composition in healthy postmenopausal women. *J Am Coll Nutr* 2004; **23**: 510S–513S.

10 Jehn M, Clark JM, Guallar E. Serum ferritin and risk of the metabolic syndrome in U.S. adults. *Diabetes Care* 2004; **27**: 2422–8.

11 Masse PG, Dosy J, Cole DEC, Evroski J, Allard J, D'Astous M. Is serum ferritin an additional cardiovascular risk factor for all postmenopausal women? *Ann Nutr Metab* 2004; **48**: 381–9.

PROBLEM

4   Genetic Diabetes Syndromes (MODY)

Case History

A 24-year-old woman attends your clinic for annual diabetes review. She was diagnosed with diabetes at the age of 18 years. She is not overweight. She checks her blood sugar two days per week and fasting values are always below 7.0 mmol/l and her glycosylated haemoglobin (HbA1c) is 5.8%. She takes gliclazide 80 mg/day. Checking her eyes, you find that she has moderate diabetic retinopathy. Her blood pressure is 138/92 mmHg. She has a brother who was diagnosed with diabetes at the age of 18 and commenced on insulin.

What type of diabetes does she have?

How would you manage her?

What is her prognosis regarding diabetic complications?

Background

Maturity-onset diabetes of youth (MODY) is an unusual cause of diabetes, and accounts for 1–2% of all cases of diabetes. The fact that the diagnosis is seldom made in clinical practice almost certainly reflects the fact that there is no simple clinical test for the syndrome and it is, therefore, under-diagnosed. It is important to recognize MODY for a number of reasons: the syndrome is usually diagnosed in adolescence or early adulthood and patients may thus have diabetes for a substantial portion of their life; there is an appreciable risk of diabetic complications even though the degree of hyperglycaemia may be mild; the approach to treatment is different to that to either type 1 or type 2 diabetes; and other family members are usually affected. Diabetes usually develops before the age of 25 years, subsequent generations of the family are affected and there is usually no family history suggestive of type 1 or type 2 diabetes (e.g. organ-specific autoimmunity or obesity). The crude prevalence of MODY in the United Kingdom is around 0.2 per 100 000 of the population under 16 years.[1] This is slightly less than the prevalence of type 2 diabetes in children, although type 2 diabetes is much more common in children and young adults in populations with high-risk ethnic backgrounds.

MODY is due to one of a number of identified genetic defects inherited in an autosomal dominant fashion, but usually with incomplete penetrance. Common to each is a defect in the ability of the pancreatic beta cell to produce insulin in response to glucose. The spectrum of MODY syndromes and their relative prevalence in the United Kingdom are shown in Table 4.1[2] By far the commonest syndrome is MODY 3, which occurs due to mutations in the gene for the transcription factor hepatic nuclear factor-1α. This accounts for around 70% of cases of MODY and has a mean age of diagnosis of around 20 years. The next most common syndrome is MODY 2, attributable to a defect in the glucokinase gene. This enzyme is not only involved in the flux of glucose into intermediary metabolism but is also critical to the ability of the beta cell to sense the prevailing level of glucose. The abnormality in blood glucose is relatively mild in MODY 2, and the risk of vascular complications is correspondingly lower than in the other types of MODY. Other identified types of MODY are quite rare. MODY 4, occurring due to defects in the insulin promoter factor-1 gene, is very rare and usually presents at a later age than other types of MODY. About 12% of cases are due to defects other than those identified as MODY 1 to 5.

There is no specific treatment for the MODY syndromes, and no long-term trial evidence to document the benefits of treatment. However, patients with MODY are generally at risk from microvascular complications, even though they are often not markedly hyperglycaemic. This presumably relates to the early onset of the disease. As with other types of diabetes, attention to lifestyle factors (diet, body weight and exercise) will improve glucose tolerance and thus reduce risk of complications. Because MODY is rare, there is little published information regarding its treatment and certainly no randomized, long-term trials with outcome data. In a small, randomized, crossover trial, Pearson et al.[3] compared the

Table 4.1 Relative Frequency of MODY Syndromes			
MODY Type	Gene Responsible	% of Cases	Likelihood of Complications
1	Hepatic nuclear factor-4α (HNF-4α)	3	++
2	Glucokinase	14	±
3	Hepatic nuclear factor-1α (HNF-1α)	70	++
4	Insulin promoter factor-1 (IPF-1)	Rare	±
5	Hepatic nuclear factor-1β (HNF-1β)	4	++
X	Gene not identified	12	+

++ High risk of complications
+ Moderate risk of complications
± Low risk of vascular complications

effects of gliclazide and metformin in a group of patients with MODY 3. The sulphony-lurea, gliclazide, was over five times more potent than metformin in lowering blood glucose. This is in keeping with a condition that is predominantly caused by a defect in insulin production by the beta cell. Thus, insulin secretagogues are the drugs of first choice although other drugs, including metformin, can be used if first-line treatment fails or if the patient is intolerant of sulphonylurea. Care should be taken with the sulphonylureas as, in MODY 3 patients, there is impaired hepatic uptake and clearance of the drugs leading to an increased susceptibility to hypoglycaemia.[4] Where the patient is susceptible to hypoglycaemia, the drug of choice should be a short-acting insulin secretagogue. There are no systematic published data on either nateglinide or repaglinide but, intuitively, these should be suitable treatments. Also, in MODY 3 there may be a decreased renal threshold for glucose, making urinalysis an unsuitable means of monitoring the condition. Because the patients are usually diagnosed young, and are susceptible to complications, the aim should be for as near-normal glycaemic control as possible. Given the lack of specific drugs, the threshold for considering insulin therapy should be relatively low.

Recent Developments

1   Type 1 diabetes prevalence varies widely and is increasing. Although type 1 diabetes remains the most common type of diabetes affecting children and young adults, other forms of diabetes are increasingly being recognized in clinical practice. Diabetes, often in association with deafness and other neurological abnormalities, may arise from defects in the mitochondrial genome and is inherited maternally (MIDD—maternally inherited diabetes and deafness).[5] Patients with mitochondrial diabetes syndromes are increasingly being recognized in specialist neurology or diabetes clinics. Patients with apparent type 1 diabetes—ketosis prone and insulin dependent—but with fluctuating insulin requirements and no evidence of islet cell autoimmune markers (type 1B diabetes) are common in some high-risk populations.[6] The pathogenesis of this type of diabetes is poorly understood at present.

2   One in eight patients with MODY does not have an abnormality in one of the five genes responsible for the identified MODY syndromes. Further study of such patients is leading to identification of new susceptibility loci.[7] Such studies will not only benefit families with rarer forms of MODY but may also lead to the identification of new candidate genes for type 2 diabetes.

Conclusion

The patient described above is unusual in that she had diabetes diagnosed at an early age and her glycaemic control is good, yet at the age of 24 she is already developing microvascular complications of diabetes. This, and her family history of diabetes, should make you think that she may have one of the MODY syndromes (Figure 4.1). This diagnosis is difficult to fully substantiate unless genotyping studies are undertaken in a specialist laboratory. Assuming that she does have MODY, it is incumbent upon the physician to ensure that diabetes control is as tight as possible, as there is a significant risk of complications, even though the level of glycaemic control may appear reasonable. If lifestyle modification fails, the drug of first choice would be a short-acting insulin secretagogue. As with other diabetic patients, advancing age, increasing insulin resistance and chronic hyperglycaemia may all contribute to progressive treatment failure and many MODY patients will eventually require insulin treatment.

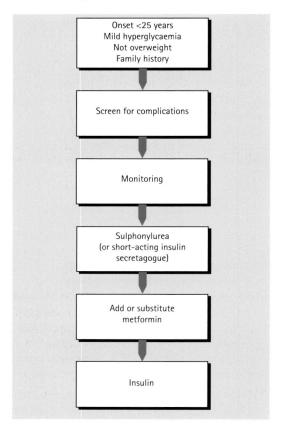

Fig. 4.1 Diagnosis and management of a patient with suspected MODY.

Further Reading

1 Ehtisham S, Hattersley AT, Dunger DB, Barrett TG. First UK survey of paediatric type 2 diabetes and MODY. *Arch Dis Child* 2004; **89**: 526–9.

2 Frayling TM, Evans JC, Bulman MP, Pearson E, Allen L, Owen K, Bingham C, Hannemann M, Shepherd M, Ellard S, Hattersley AT. Beta-cell genes and diabetes: molecular and clinical characterization of mutations in transcription factors. *Diabetes* 2001; **50** (Suppl 1): S94–100.

3 Pearson ER, Starkey BJ, Powell RJ, Gribble FM, Clark PM, Hattersley AT. Genetic cause of hyperglycaemia and response to treatment in diabetes. *Lancet* 2003; **362**: 1275–81.

4 Boileau P, Wolfrum C, Shih DQ, Yang TA, Wolkoff AW, Stoffel M. Decreased glibenclamide uptake in hepatocytes of hepatocyte nuclear factor-1alpha-deficient mice: a mechanism for hypersensitivity to sulfonylurea therapy in patients with maturity-onset diabetes of the young, type 3 (MODY3). *Diabetes* 2002; **51** (Suppl 3): S343–8.

5 Maassen JA. Mitochondrial diabetes: pathophysiology, clinical presentation, and genetic analysis. *Am J Med Genet* 2002; **115**: 66–70.

6 Aguilera E, Casamitjana R, Ercilla G, Oriola J, Gomis R, Conget I. Adult-onset atypical (type 1) diabetes: additional insights and differences with type 1A diabetes in a European Mediterranean population. *Diabetes Care* 2004; **27**: 1108–14.

7 Frayling TM, Lindgren CM, Chevre JC, Menzel S, Wishart M, Benmezroua Y, Brown A, Evans JC, Rao PS, Dina C, Lecoeur C, Kanninen T, Almgren P, Bulman MP, Wang Y, Mills J, Wright-Pascoe R, Mahtani MM, Prisco F, Costa A, Cognet I, Hansen T, Pedersen O, Ellard S, Tuomi T, Groop LC, Froguel P, Hattersley AT, Vaxillaire M. A genome-wide scan in families with maturity-onset diabetes of the young: evidence for further genetic heterogeneity. *Diabetes* 2003; **52**: 872–81.

PROBLEM

5 Screening and Impaired Glucose Tolerance

Case History

A 48-year-old manual worker was found to have glycosuria at a routine medical carried out for insurance purposes. He has been seen by a practice nurse who checked his blood glucose using a fingerprick test. The result was 9.0 mmol/l. His general health is very good, and he has no family history of note.

How would you proceed from here?

What do you think of using urine tests or fingerprick blood tests to screen for diabetes?

Is population screening for diabetes now warranted?

If he has impaired glucose tolerance, what are the implications for his future health?

Background

The diagnostic criteria in current usage (Figure 5.1) are summarized as follows:
Diabetes (one of the following):

● Random venous plasma glucose ≥11.1 mmol/l in the presence of symptoms

● Fasting plasma glucose ≥7.0 mmol/l

● Two-hour plasma glucose ≥11.1 mmol/l after a 75 gram oral glucose load

● In the absence of symptoms, confirmatory glucose measurements should be made on two separate days

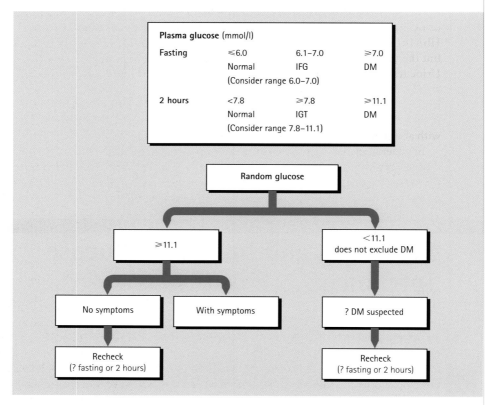

Fig. 5.1 Diagnostic criteria for IFG, IGT and diabetes mellitus (DM).

Impaired glucose tolerance (IGT):

● Fasting plasma glucose <7.0 mmol/l

● Two-hour value on oral glucose tolerance test (oGTT) ≥7.8 mmol/l but <11.1 mmol/l

Impaired fasting glucose (IFG):

● Fasting plasma glucose ≥6.1 mmol/l but <7.0 mmol/l

IFG and IGT are states where carbohydrate tolerance is decreased compared with normal and associated with increased risk of progression to diabetes and increased cardiovascular risk. The values of 7.8 mmol/l and 11.1 mmol/l seem very precise, and correspond to 140 mg/dl and 200 mg/dl, respectively. These can be regarded as optimal thresholds for diagnosing states of carbohydrate intolerance but it should be recognized that risk of macrovascular complications increases continuously with increasing plasma glucose. There is no generalized agreement about screening policies for diabetes. Opportunistic screening of high-risk individuals, including all subjects over 45 years, at two-yearly intervals is normal practice. Screening modes include fasting glucose, random glucose, oGTT, and glycosylated haemoglobin (HbA1c) measurement. Routine glucose measurements are the most convenient in day-to-day practice but may need to be followed by repeat tests or oGTT in subjects who are either not symptomatic or have values below 11.1 mmol/l. HbA1c can be useful as part of a screening strategy to identify those likely to have diabetes, but the various states outlined above are defined on the basis of glucose measurements.[1] Urine testing is not recommended for population screening of diabetes, but stick testing also identifies proteinuria and haematuria and is thus useful in screening in general medical examinations. Recent data from the Diabetes Prevention Program Group[2] confirm that capillary blood glucose measurements are suitable for screening so long as patients with abnormal results are followed-up with appropriate laboratory tests.

In general, insulin resistance is the forerunner to states of carbohydrate intolerance in most cases. Progressive carbohydrate intolerance (IFG, IGT) arises from relative failure of the beta cell against the background of insulin resistance. The decreased insulin secretion in the face of hyperglycaemia appears to progress faster than was previously believed.[3] This is confirmed by results from the Baltimore Longitudinal Study of Aging[4] where the cumulative 5- and 10-year incidence of diabetes was 21.0% and 37.4%, respectively, for those with IGT at baseline. Other data from this study confirm the strong association between IGT and cardiovascular risk factors. The relationship between IFG and cardiovascular risk is much weaker. These data reaffirm the need for intensive management of subjects with pre-diabetic states.

The metabolic syndrome, now present in one in four adults in the United States (US), is a powerful predictor of morbidity and mortality. The most common cause of death amongst individuals with metabolic syndrome is cardiovascular disease. The importance of metabolic syndrome as a predictor of cardiovascular death has been confirmed in two recent large cohort studies from Italy[5] and Canada.[6] These and other studies are changing the view of the management of patients with pre-diabetic states from a 'wait and see' approach to vigorous lifestyle management where this is tolerated. For patients who cannot reduce weight, improve diet and take regular exercise, pharmacological management of hyperglycaemia, dyslipidaemia and hypertension should be considered.

Recent Developments

1 The Finnish Diabetes Prevention Study[7] and the US Diabetes Prevention Program[8] have both demonstrated that intensive lifestyle modification, including exercise, decreases the incidence of new diabetes in subjects at risk. Furthermore, the associated cardiovascular risk factors are also improved, and the interventions are cost effective.

2 Genetic studies arising from the above lifestyle modification trials are beginning to reveal some of the mechanisms that may underlie progression of carbohydrate intolerance. Thus, certain polymorphisms in the genes for the pro-inflammatory cytokines tumour necrosis factor-α and interleukin-6 are associated with progression,[9] as are polymorphisms in the gene for adiponectin.[10]

3 Microvascular disease has been traditionally regarded as the hallmark of the diabetic state. However, there is now considerable evidence that microvascular changes are highly prevalent in patients with IGT.[11] This association may underlie the high prevalence of renal disease in some populations that are also very prone to diabetes, and

again underlines the need for active management of patients who are discovered to have abnormal carbohydrate tolerance.

Conclusion

The above patient appears to have IGT, although this needs to be confirmed using laboratory measures of venous plasma glucose. While the oGTT is not routinely used for screening, there is a strong argument for an oGTT in a patient who is discovered to have abnormal glucose tolerance. With existing evidence, a precise classification of abnormalities of carbohydrate tolerance provides a rationale for the approach to therapy. Finger-prick blood tests are fine for identifying patients at risk, but urine tests are not recommended. IGT is part of the metabolic syndrome and this diagnosis carries with it a high risk of future diabetes and cardiovascular disease. The approach to the above patient should include diet and exercise advice, along with screening for other cardiovascular risk factors. Although population screening for diabetes is not carried out at present, opportunistic encounters with all patients at risk, including anyone over 45 years old, should be used to screen for hyperglycaemia.

Further Reading

1 Icks A, Haastert B, Gandjour A, John J, Lowel H, Holle R, Giani G, Rathmann W. Cost-effectiveness analysis of different screening procedures for type 2 diabetes: the KORA Survey 2000. *Diabetes Care* 2004; **27**: 2120–8.

2 The Diabetes Prevention Program Research Group. Strategies to identify adults at high risk for type 2 diabetes: the Diabetes Prevention Program. *Diabetes Care* 2005; **28**: 138–44.

3 Ferrannini E, Nannipieri M, Williams K, Gonzales C, Haffner SM, Stern MP. Mode of onset of type 2 diabetes from normal or impaired glucose tolerance. *Diabetes* 2004; **53**: 160–5.

4 Meigs JB, Muller DC, Nathan DM, Blake DR, Andres R. The natural history of progression from normal glucose tolerance to type 2 diabetes in the Baltimore Longitudinal Study of Aging. *Diabetes* 2003; **52**: 1475–84.

5 Bruno G, Merletti F, Biggeri A, Bargero G, Ferrero S, Runzo C, Prina Cerai S, Pagano G, Cavallo-Perin P. Metabolic syndrome as a predictor of all-cause and cardiovascular mortality in type 2 diabetes: the Casale Monferrato Study. *Diabetes Care* 2004; **27**: 2689–94.

6 Katzmarzyk PT, Church TS, Janssen I, Ross R, Blair SN. Metabolic syndrome, obesity, and mortality: impact of cardiorespiratory fitness. *Diabetes Care* 2005; **28**: 391–7.

7 Laaksonen DE, Lindström J, Lakka TA, Eriksson JG, Niskanen L, Wikström K, Aunola S, Keinänen-Kiukaanniemi S, Laakso M, Valle TT, Ilanne-Parikka P, Louheranta A, Hämäläinen H, Rastas M, Salminen V, Cepaitis Z, Hakumäki M, Kaikkonen H, Härkönen P, Sundvall J, Tuomilehto J, Uusitupa M. Physical activity in the prevention of type 2 diabetes: the Finnish diabetes prevention study. *Diabetes* 2005; **54**: 158–65.

8 Haffner S, Temprosa M, Crandall J, Fowler S, Goldberg R, Horton E, Marcovina S, Mather K, Orchard T, Ratner R, Barrett-Connor E. Intensive lifestyle intervention or metformin on inflammation and coagulation in participants with impaired glucose tolerance. *Diabetes* 2005; **54**: 1566–72.

9 Kubaszek A, Pihlajamäki J, Komarovski V, Lindi V, Lindström J, Eriksson J, Valle TT, Hämäläinen H, Ilanne-Parikka P, Keinänen-Kiukaanniemi S, Tuomilehto J, Uusitupa M, Laakso M. Promoter polymorphisms of the TNF-alpha (G-308A) and IL-6 (C-174G) genes predict the conversion from impaired glucose tolerance to type 2 diabetes: the Finnish Diabetes Prevention Study. *Diabetes* 2003; **52**: 1872–76.

10 Zacharova J, Chiasson JL, Laakso M. The common polymorphisms (single nucleotide polymorphism (SNP) +45 and SNP +276) of the adiponectin gene predict the conversion from impaired glucose tolerance to type 2 diabetes: the STOP-NIDDM trial. *Diabetes* 2005; **54**: 893–9.

11 Singleton JR, Smith AG, Russell JW, Feldman EL. Microvascular complications of impaired glucose tolerance. *Diabetes* 2003; **52**: 2867–73.

6 Type A/B Diabetes and Insulin Resistance

Case History

A motivated 42-year-old man, body mass index (BMI) 24.8 kg/m², with type 2 diabetes complained of persistent symptomatic hyperglycaemia despite taking a total of 400 units of insulin a day. Urinalysis revealed no ketonuria. Clinical examination showed no evidence of lipohypertrophy. Past medical history includes pemphigus vulgaris for which he is not on any treatment now.

What further investigations would you request?

How would you manage this patient's hyperglycaemia?

Background

This patient remains hyperglycaemic despite taking large amounts of insulin. His BMI is in the desirable range, but he clearly has an extreme insulin resistance state (IRS), arbitrarily defined on clinical grounds as the requirement of more than 200 units of insulin per day to attain glycaemia control and to prevent ketosis. While central obesity—the most common cause of insulin resistance—is characterized pathophysiologically by a decreased number of insulin receptors and post-receptor defects, two major variants of insulin receptor abnormalities have been described—type A and type B syndromes, depending on the aetiology. In the absence of other recognized familial insulin resistance syndromes (such as lipodystrophic state, Werner syndrome, Rabson-Mendenhall syndrome, Alström syndrome), poor patient compliance or any technical difficulties with insulin injections, both type A and type B insulin resistance syndrome should be considered when patients present with persistent hyperglycaemia despite taking large amounts of insulin.

Type A syndrome is defined by insulin resistance, acanthosis nigricans and hyper-androgenism without overt obesity or lipoatrophy. A variant known as the HAIR-AN syndrome (HyperAndrogenism, Insulin Resistance and Acanthosis Nigricans) affects female patients. Acanthosis nigricans is very common in both types of insulin resistance syndrome and is typically described as patchy, velvety brown hyperpigmentation plaques usually found in flexural areas, especially axillae and the nuchal region. The lesion may be due to the effect of high circulating levels of insulin on insulin-like growth factor (IGF-1) receptors in the skin. Patients with type A syndrome may also show features of acromegaly with acral enlargement but with normal growth hormone and IGF-1 levels—a form of pseudoacromegaly. The mechanism for the latter clinical presentation is thought to occur due to hyperinsulinaemia stimulating anabolic and growth effects via normally function-ing receptors in other tissues. The type B syndrome of severe insulin resistance is often acquired and is characterized by the presence of autoantibodies to the insulin receptor. The syndrome frequently results in symptomatic hyperglycaemia that is resistant to high doses of insulin, although ketosis is rare. It commonly occurs in conjunction with other autoimmune disorders. Symptoms related to immunological disorders (e.g. arthralgia, skin rash and hair loss) may also occur.

A thorough history and examination will reveal problems with compliance, complica-tions of insulin injection—which might affect insulin absorption (e.g. lipohypertro-phy)—or features of familial severe insulin resistance syndrome. Laboratory investigation should include a full lipid profile (IRS is characterized by elevated low-density lipoprotein [LDL]-cholesterol, high triglyceride levels and reduced high-density lipoprotein [HDL]-cholesterol), plasma glucose, glycosylated haemoglobin (HbA1c) and electrolytes. Novel biochemical markers of IRS are homocysteine, plasminogen activator inhibitor-1 and fib-rinogen levels, all of which are elevated in IRS. Increased fasting insulin level is an indirect measure of insulin resistance, while euglycaemic insulin clamp technique is the gold-stan-dard method to measure insulin resistance. In clinical practice, measurement of glucose response to intravenous infusion of insulin is useful to determine the appropriate insulin dose required by the patient. Electrocardiogram and assessment of microalbuminuria are useful determinants of patients' cardiovascular risk.

In female patients with type A syndrome, testosterone and free androgen index level may be raised, associated with low sex-hormone binding globulin levels. Whilst low titres of immunoglobulin G (IgG) anti-insulin antibodies are present in most patients receiv-ing insulin, rarely, a high titre may induce IRS by post-receptor failure. Thus, anti-insulin antibody titre levels should be checked, particularly in patients who gradually develop severe insulin resistance after taking long-term insulin, or if patients develop insulin resistance after converting from bovine to human insulin. Type B syndrome is often more severe and is characterized by the presence of a high titre of IgG anti-insulin receptor antibodies in the serum.

Treatment for patients with severe insulin resistance remains largely experimental.[1, 2] Patients are often prescribed high doses of insulin in combination with insulin sensitizers. In patients with intractable symptomatic hyperglycaemia, a trial of human recom-binant IGF-1 may be effective in selected cases. Immune-mediated insulin resistance may respond to immunosuppressive treatment such as steroids, cyclophosphamide and plasmapheresis.[3]

Recent Developments

1 A recent report[4] suggested that rituximab—a monoclonal antibody directed at the CD20 molecule on B lymphocytes—given as an intravenous infusion (375 mg/m² of body-surface area) once weekly for four weeks may induce remission of severe insulin resistance in a patient with type B syndrome. Mycophenolate was not effective in this case, but other case reports have shown remission of insulin resistance when patients were given a combination of mycophenolate and cyclophosphamide.

2 Human recombinant IGF-1 injection has been reported to be a potential therapy for individuals with severe insulin resistance.[5,6] In a study of eleven patients, glucose levels decreased in response to subcutaneous injections of human recombinant IGF-1 (0.1–0.3 mg/kg).[5] A long-term trial of IGF-1 (up to 16 months) showed that IGF-1 (0.1–0.4 mg/kg twice daily) was effective in lowering both fasting and post-prandial plasma glucose concentrations, with decreases in both fructosamine and

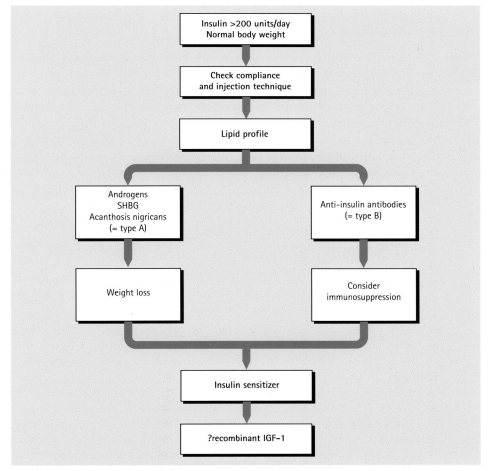

Fig. 6.1 Assessment and investigation for type A and type B insulin resistance syndrome. SHBG = sex-hormone binding globulin.

HbA1c values.[5] Improvement of acanthosis nigricans was observed in some patients. Recombinant IGF-1 (100 μg/kg twice daily) given subcutaneously to several patients with type A syndrome was associated with improvements in glycaemic control and insulin resistance.[6]

Conclusion

Severe IRS should be suspected in all patients with intractable hyperglycaemia despite taking large amounts of insulin (>200 units/day). A thorough history and clinical examination may reveal underlying phenotypes of severe IRS (Figure 6.1). A high serum titre of IgG anti-insulin antibody and/or anti-insulin-receptor antibody may suggest immune causes of IRS. Treatment with immunosuppressive agents (such as rituximab, prednisolone or cyclophosphamide) or human recombinant IGF-1 may be justified as a therapeutic trial in patients with intractable hyperglycaemia.

Further Reading

1 In't Veld PA, Bruining J. Genetic syndromes and diabetes mellitus. In: Pickup J, Williams G (eds). *Textbook of Diabetes*, 2nd edn. Oxford: Blackwell Science, 1997; 1–28.

2 Kahn CR, Flier JS, Bar RS, Archer JA, Gorden P, Martin MM, Roth J. The syndromes of insulin resistance and acanthosis nigricans. Insulin-receptor disorders in man. *N Engl J Med* 1976; **294**: 739–45.

3 Coll AP, Morganstein D, Jayne D, Soos MA, O'Rahilly S, Burke J. Successful treatment of Type B insulin resistance in a patient with otherwise quiescent systemic lupus erythematosus. *Diabet Med* 2005; **22**: 814–15.

4 Coll AP, Thomas S, Mufti GJ. Rituximab therapy for the type B syndrome of severe insulin resistance. *N Engl J Med* 2004; **350**: 310–11.

5 Kuzuya H, Matsuura N, Sakamoto M, Makino H, Sakamoto Y, Kadowaki T, Suzuki Y, Kobayashi M, Akazawa Y, Nomura M, *et al*. Trial of insulinlike growth factor I therapy for patients with extreme insulin resistance syndromes, *Diabetes* 1993; **42**: 696–705.

6 Morrow LA, O'Brien MB, Moller DE, Flier JS, Moses AC. Recombinant human insulin-like growth factor-I therapy improves glycemic control and insulin action in the type A syndrome of severe insulin resistance. *J Clin Endocrinol Metab* 1994; **79**: 205–10.

Acute Diabetes

7   Diabetic ketoacidosis

8   Hyperosmolar hyperglycaemic state

9   Recurrent hypoglycaemia

10   Diabetes and acute myocardial infarction

11   Diabetes and acute stroke

12   Diabetes and critical limb ischaemia

13   Perioperative management of diabetes

14   The hot foot

PROBLEM

7 Diabetic Ketoacidosis

Case History

You were called to see a 26-year-old Caucasian woman in the casualty department. Her partner informed you that she has had type 1 diabetes since the age of 12, which has previously been well controlled. Leading up to her presentation, she has had a two-day history of diarrhoea and vomiting. On your assessment, she was very drowsy, uncommunicative, hyperventilating and severely dehydrated. Arterial blood gas showed: pO_2 15.4 kPa; pCO_2 1.9 kPa; HCO_3 3.8 mmol/l; pH 6.92.

How would you manage her?

Is there a role for giving phosphate or bicarbonate?

Do analogue insulins have a role in the acute management?

Background

Diabetic ketoacidosis (DKA) is the most common hyperglycaemic emergency in patients with diabetes, and is now the leading cause of death in children with type 1 diabetes. The annual incidence rate for DKA, estimated from population-based studies, ranges from 4.6 to 8 episodes per 1000 patients with diabetes. Early diagnosis is important so that treatment can be initiated promptly with close monitoring of the patient's biochemical, haemodynamic and clinical status. Whilst the condition should ideally be managed by specialists, there remains limited evidence comparing clinical outcomes in the management of DKA between non-specialist physicians' care and diabetologists' care. In a study in a large teaching hospital in Scotland, patients with DKA treated by non-diabetologists showed a non-significant trend towards longer hospital stay. In the United States, a study showed that endocrinologists provided more cost-effective care than generalists when serving as a primary care providers for patients hospitalized with DKA. Thus, well-informed general physicians appear to manage DKA effectively although resources may be used more efficiently by diabetologists.

Insulin error (e.g. missed injection, abnormal injection sites) and intercurrent infection are the most common precipitating factors for developing DKA, accounting for more than two-thirds of cases. Other predisposing factors include autonomic neuropathy with delayed gastric emptying, alcohol binge, diarrhoea or vomiting illnesses and, rarely, drug use such as atypical antipsychotic use and cocaine abuse. The main features of DKA are hyperglycaemia (plasma glucose level >14 mmol/l), metabolic acidosis (serum bicarbonate <15 mmol/l), increased anion gap, heavy ketonuria (>2+) and/or ketonaemia (positive serum ketone level >1:4 dilution by the nitroprusside reaction and/or serum β-hydroxybutyrate >3.0 mmol/l). The sensitivity of urine ketone dip-test for ketonaemia in patients with DKA is 97%, and thus the absence of ketonuria makes the diagnosis of DKA unlikely. The mean difference between arterial and venous pH is negligible (approximately 0.03) and thus painful arterial sampling should be reserved for cases when respiratory failure is suspected. Diagnosis is often straightforward where there is a clear history of diabetes but can cause some difficulties when patients are unconscious or DKA is the first presentation of diabetes. Diagnostic clues are dehydration, drowsiness, acidotic hyperventilation, unexplained metabolic acidosis, hyperkalaemia and the smell of ketones on the patient's breath.

In the management of patients with DKA (Figure 7.1), early venous access is essential and standard measures of oxygen, regular assessment of pulse and blood pressure, as well as urinary catheterization for accurate measurement of urine output are important. Insertion of a central line is not routinely indicated except in severely ill patients, particularly in the elderly. A suitable fluid-replacement regimen for patients who are not shocked or oliguric is 500 ml/h of 0.9% saline for the first four hours, followed by 250 ml/h for the next four hours. This regimen has been shown to produce correction of acidosis and hyperglycaemia as rapidly as a regimen using twice these rates. Large fluid boluses may contribute to the increased risk of cerebral oedema. An alternative initial fluid regimen is to infuse 0.9% saline at 500–1000 ml/h for the first two hours followed by 0.45% saline at 250–500 ml/h until blood glucose level drops to <14.0 mmol/l. No formal studies comparing the outcome between these two regimens have been performed. Once plasma glucose has fallen to around 14 mmol/l (an arbitrary cut-off level), 5% dextrose infusion should then be added, to facilitate the clearance of ketone bodies and to buffer

Wirral Teaching Hospital
Self Service

Checkout summary

Name:
Date: 19/04/2023   02:15

Loaned today

Title: B12678
ID: B12678
Due back: 10/05/2023

Total item(s) loaned today: 1
Previous Amount Owed: 0.00   <INVALID>

Overdue: 0
Reservation(s) pending: 0
Reservation(s) to collect: 0
Total item(s) on loan 1
Thank you for using
Self Service

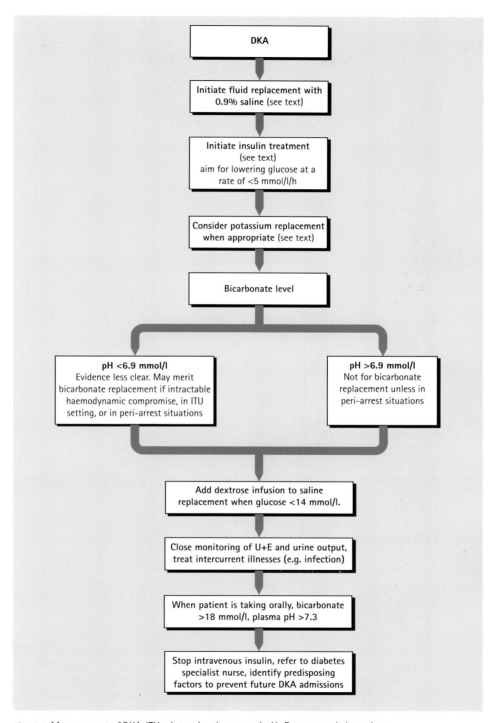

Fig. 7.1 Management of DKA. ITU = intensive therapy unit; U+E = urea and electrolytes.

against hypoglycaemia and a too-rapid fall in osmolarity. The combination of saline and dextrose could be given in the form of 5% or 10% dextrose with 0.45% saline or dextrose–saline solution (0.18% saline, 4% dextrose) until resolution of DKA.

Insulin replacement is normally given intravenously via a 'sliding scale' regimen. This involves an initial intravenous bolus of 0.1 unit/kg body weight, followed by a variable infusion rate determined by patients' hourly glucose levels. Glucose levels should not be reduced too quickly, and a rate of fall of <5 mmol/l/h is recommended. Alternatively, a regimen giving a continuous infusion rate of 0.1 unit/kg/h until plasma glucose is <14 mmol/l could be used, after which a 5% dextrose solution is added and the insulin infusion rate reduced to 0.05 units/kg/h. Failure to achieve a reduction in plasma glucose level with this regimen should prompt a search for mechanical failures (e.g. connections, infusion device) or unusual insulin resistance states where changes in the regimen's rate of insulin infusion will be required. The insulin infusion should be continued until ketosis and acidosis have cleared (serum bicarbonate >18 mmol/l and venous pH >7.30). The first subcutaneous insulin dose must be given at least one hour before the insulin infusion is stopped.

Insulin induces a shift of potassium into cells resulting in the risk of life-threatening hypokalaemia. Potassium levels are often normal or elevated at initial presentation and levels should be checked every two hours. A commonly used potassium regimen is:

- if serum K^+ >5.5 mmol/l, do not give K^+;

- if K^+ = 4–5.5 mmol/l, add 20 mmol of KCl to each litre of intravenous (IV) fluid;

- if K^+ = 3–4 mmol/l, add 40 mmol of KCl to each litre of IV fluid;

- if K^+ <3 mmol/l, 10–20 mmol of KCl hourly until serum K^+ >3 mmol/l.

Potassium replacement should not be started before insulin treatment and should be cautiously given in patients who are anuric or oliguric.

Prior to discharge from hospital, patients should be referred to a diabetes specialist nurse to help identify any practical or social problems associated with their insulin regimes, and provide education on sick rules and appropriate use of insulin during intercurrent illness.

Recent Developments

1 Recent controlled studies have shown that treatment of mild to moderate DKA with one- to two-hourly injections of subcutaneous short-acting insulin analogue represents a safe and effective alternative to the use of an intravenous, regular insulin protocol.[1,2]

2 Phosphate levels are often low in patients with DKA. Potential complications of severe hypophosphataemia include respiratory and skeletal muscle weakness, haemolytic anaemia and worsened cardiac systolic performance. Studies have not demonstrated clinical benefits from the routine use of phosphate replacement in DKA, but replacement should be given to patients with serum phosphate concentrations <1.0 mg/dl, or to patients with moderate hypophosphataemia and concomitant hypoxia, anaemia or cardiorespiratory compromise.

3   The role of bicarbonate infusion in patients with DKA and severe acidosis is also unclear.[3] Metabolic acidosis increases the risk of organ damage in the heart, liver and brain but, conversely, bicarbonate infusion is associated with significant adverse effects, such as worsening hypokalaemia and paradoxical central nervous system acidosis. The rise in blood pH after bicarbonate infusion may also adversely affect the haemoglobin–O_2 dissociation curve, thereby reducing tissue oxygenation and increasing lactate production and intracellular acidosis. Studies to date have failed to show evidence of earlier resolution of acidosis, or any improvement in short- or long-term outcomes, with bicarbonate treatment of DKA patients with blood pH between 6.9 and 7.1. No prospective, randomized studies concerning the use of bicarbonate in DKA with arterial pH values <6.9 have been reported. In the absence of such studies, the use of bicarbonate in patients with DKA should be restricted to the peri-arrest situation or to patients with life-threatening hyperkalaemia.

4   DKA may also occur in patients with type 2 diabetes or, more rarely, in patients with 'atypical diabetes'. The latter group are patients who presented with DKA but subsequently do not require insulin treatment; this has been reported in patients of African-American, African, Chinese and Japanese origin.

Conclusion

Development of local protocols and guidelines for management of DKA has greatly improved the outlook for patients when they safely reach hospital. Short-acting analogue insulins are a safe alternative to soluble insulin but probably do not offer any major advantage for use in this emergency. There is currently no justification for the routine use of bicarbonate or phosphate in the management of patients with DKA.[4]

Further Reading

1   Kitabchi AE, Umpierrez GE, Murphy MB, Barrett EJ, Kreisberg RA, Malone JI, Wall BM. Management of hyperglycemic crises in patients with diabetes. *Diabetes Care* 2001; **24**: 131–53.

2   Umpierrez GE, Cuervo R, Karabell A, Latif K, Freire AX, Kitabchi AE. Treatment of diabetic ketoacidosis with subcutaneous insulin aspart. *Diabetes Care* 2004; **27**: 1873–8.

3   Viallon A, Zeni F, Lafond P, Venet C, Tardy B, Page Y, Bertrand JC. Does bicarbonate therapy improve the management of severe diabetic ketoacidosis? *Crit Care Med* 1999; **27**: 2690–3.

4   Wallace TM, Matthews DR. Recent advances in the monitoring and management of diabetic ketoacidosis. *QJM* 2004; **97**: 773–80.

8 Hyperosmolar Hyperglycaemic State

Case History

A 67-year-old woman with no previous history of diabetes mellitus was admitted to the Acute Medical Admission Unit with a four-day history of progressive drowsiness and dehydration. An urgent blood test showed pre-renal uraemia (Na$^+$ 174 mmol/l; K$^+$ 4.0 mmol/l; urea 26.2 mmol/l; creatinine 168 μmol/l), severe hyperglycaemia (34.2 mmol/l) and arterial blood gas parameters of pO$_2$ 12.1 kPa, pCO$_2$ 5.2 kPa, HCO$_3^-$ 18.9 mmol/l and pH 7.32. Urinalysis showed 2+ protein, trace blood and nil else.

How would you manage this patient acutely?

What ongoing management is she likely to require?

Background

Although the incidence of hyperosmolar hyperglycaemic state (HHS) is less than that of DKA (approximately 1 per 1000 person-years for HHS compared with 5–8 per 1000 person-years for DKA), the estimated mortality rate in HHS is higher, (approximately 15% in HHS compared with <5% in DKA) and increases substantially with age and the presence of concomitant illnesses. Provided that standard, written therapeutic guidelines are followed, clinical outcomes of patients with HHS have not been shown to be altered by whether patients were managed by a generalist or a diabetologist.

HHS usually occurs in older patients, with or without pre-existing diabetes, and often takes days or weeks to develop fully. Progressive hyperglycaemia leads to increasing polyuria and de-hydration, and failure to compensate this by increasing fluid intake, especially in elderly patients, makes this group of patients particularly at risk. Abdominal pain with nausea and vomiting due to reduced mesenteric perfusion may perpetuate dehydration. Infection is a common precipitant, with urinary tract infection or pneumonia accounting for 30–50% of cases. Other common precipitants are myocardial infarction, stroke, acute pancreatitis, trauma, use of drugs which interfere with carbohydrate metabolism (e.g. steroids, thiazide diuretics or beta-blockers) or excessive use of diuretics. The diagnosis of HHS is based on increased serum osmolality, significant hyperglycaemia of >34 mmol/l and absence of severe ketoacidosis. Increasing serum osmolality has been shown to correlate significantly with reduced mental status in patients with HHS.

The definition of HHS is:

- Plasma pH >7.3

- Plasma bicarbonate >18 mmol/l

- Plasma osmolality >320 mOsm/kg*

- Only mild ketonaemia and ketonuria

*calculated as: [(2 × plasma Na$^+$) + plasma glucose]

Plasma urea is not included in the calculation of effective osmolality because it is freely permeable in and out of the intracellular compartment. Coma is often associated with serum osmolality of >400 mOsm/kg. Other common biochemical abnormalities at presentation are hypernatraemia and disproportionately raised urea levels. Initial laboratory tests should also include a complete blood count with differentials, bacterial cultures of blood, urine and other tissues, serum amylase, chest radiograph, electrocardiogram and serum creatinine kinase in patients with prolonged immobilization to exclude rhabdomyolisis. Differences in biochemical abnormalities associated with DKA and HHS are shown in Table 8.1 below.

Table 8.1   Comparison of blood biochemistry abnormalities in DKA and HHS

	Normal range	DKA	HHS
Glucose (mmol/l)	4.2–6.4	>14	>34
Arterial pH	7.35–7.45	<7.3	>7.3
Bicarbonate (mmol/l)	22–28	<15	>15
Effective serum osmolality (mOsm/kg)	275–295	<320	>320
Sodium (mmol/l)	136–145	134 (1.0)	149 (3.2)
Potassium (mmol/l)	3.5–5.0	4.5 (0.13)	3.9 (0.2)
Lactate (mmol/l)	0.56–2.2	2.4	3.9

Values for sodium and potassium in DKA and HHS are mean (standard deviation). *Source:* adapted from Chiasson *et al.* 2003.[1]

Patients with DKA tend to produce larger increases in some counter-regulatory hormones—catecholamines, growth hormones and cortisol—but not glucagon, inducing a greater degree of insulin resistance compared with patients with HHS.

The treatment goals for HHS are improving circulatory volume and tissue perfusion, reducing serum glucose and plasma osmolality and correcting electrolyte imbalances, as well as identifying and treating precipitating factors (Figure 8.1). The choice of initial replacement fluid in patients with HHS remains debated. Some authorities advocate the use of hypotonic fluid (e.g. 0.45% saline) from the outset, whereas others advocate the initial use of isotonic fluid (0.9% saline) in the first hour followed by the use of 0.45% or 0.9% saline, depending on corrected plasma sodium and the haemodynamic status of the patient. In the absence of clear evidence, it would be reasonable to firstly correct extracellular fluid depletion by infusing isotonic saline at a rate of 15–20 ml/kg/h (which is hypotonic to the patient's extracellular fluid and remains restricted to the extracellular fluid

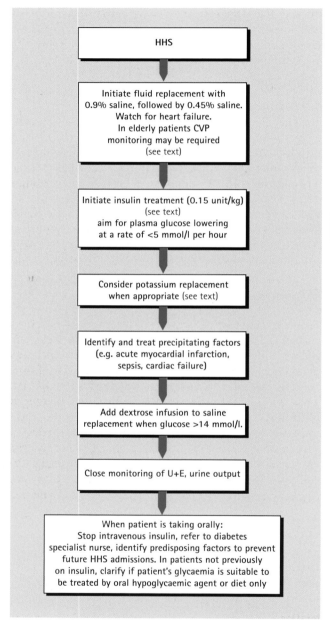

Fig. 8.1 Management of HHS.
CVP = central venous pressure;
U+E = urea and electrolytes.

compartment) in the first one to two hours until vital signs are stabilized, followed by the administration of hypotonic saline at a rate of 4–14 ml/kg/h with the aim of restoring deficits in both intracellular and extracellular compartments as well as ongoing fluid losses.[2] Dextrose should be added to replacement fluids when plasma glucose is around 14 mmol/l, with administration of 5% or even 10% dextrose depending on the patient's sodium level. Correction of the patient's dehydration and hyperglycaemic state may result in a transient false elevation of the observed plasma sodium, but when serum sodium is corrected for glucose levels—calculated as ([observed sodium] + 1.6 × [(plasma glucose −5.5)/5.5])—the level of serum sodium may, in fact, be stable or gradually improving. It is also important that changes in plasma osmolality do not exceed 3 mOsm/kg/h. In patients with renal or cardiac dysfunction, it is important to maintain close monitoring of fluid balance, occasionally by central venous pressure and/or pulmonary artery pressure monitoring, in order to avoid iatrogenic fluid overload.

Insulin treatment should be initiated while the patient is being rehydrated with an initial bolus of 0.15 unit/kg (or 10 units soluble insulin) followed by continuous intravenous insulin infusion at a rate of 0.1 unit/kg/h. Failure to reduce plasma glucose level by 3–4 mmol/l/h is often due to inadequate hydration. The appropriate level of hydration reduces the amount of counter-regulatory hormones such as cortisol, growth hormones, glucagon and catecholamines, produced in response to stress, making cells more responsive to insulin. If hydration status is acceptable, insulin rate should be increased hourly until a decrease in plasma glucose of 3–4 mmol/l/h is achieved. Patients are considered to have recovered from HHS if effective osmolality is <315 mOsm/kg and the patient is alert, at which time intravenous insulin treatment can be discontinued. Some patients with HHS may not require long-term subcutaneous insulin treatment, with some requiring only dietary treatment at follow-up.

Treatment with insulin and fluid typically results in a decline in plasma potassium levels, particularly in the first five hours of therapy. Potassium levels should therefore be monitored two-hourly in the first six hours and less frequently thereafter, with appropriate correction (see Chapter 7). High osmolality, dehydration, contracted vascular volume and increased blood viscosity associated with HHS increase the risk of thrombosis. Low-molecular-weight heparin should therefore be administered for prophylaxis in all patients with HHS. Physicians should also be aware of other potential treatment-related complications of HHS. Cerebral oedema can be prevented by correcting sodium and water deficits gradually and avoiding rapid decline in plasma glucose. A reduction in the partial pressure of oxygen caused by increased water in the lungs and reduced lung compliance may lead to adult respiratory distress syndrome. Finally, preventing, identifying and treating the underlying precipitant to HHS are paramount in order to reduce the incidence of HHS and to improve clinical outcomes of patients with this condition.

Recent Developments

1   While preliminary evidence supports the safety of subcutaneous insulin treatment in patients with mild to moderate DKA, the evidence for this mode of insulin replacement in patients with HHS is not available. Given the greater risks of drowsiness in patients with HHS, only the intravenous route of insulin replacement is recommended.

2   Hypophosphataemia is seen regularly in patients with HHS. The theoretical benefit of phosphate replacement includes the prevention of respiratory depression, skeletal muscle weakness and risks of cardiac dysfunction. Conversely, excessive phosphate replacement can lead to tetanus, hypocalcaemia and soft-tissue calcification. There are currently no studies on the use of phosphate therapy for HHS.

Conclusion

Patients who present with HHS are at high risk of death from their condition, often because of the presence of conditions other than diabetes (e.g. stroke, myocardial infarction or infection). The essential early management consists of rehydration, correcting hyperglycaemia, maintaining electrolyte balance as near normal as possible, anticoagulation and dealing with comorbidities.[3,4] The severe fluid and electrolyte abnormalities in HHS are a feature of the condition developing gradually. Once these are restored, renal function may return to normal and patients can often return to dietary or oral hypoglycaemic treatment for their diabetes.

Further Reading

1   Chiasson JL, Aris-Jilwan N, Belanger R, Bertrand S, Beauregard H, Ekoe JM, Fournier H, Havrankova J. Diagnosis and treatment of diabetic ketoacidosis and the hyperglycaemic hyperosmolar state. *CMAJ* 2003; **168**: 859–66.

2   Adrogue HJ, Madias NE. Hypernatremia. *N Engl J Med* 2000; **342**: 1493–9.

3   Kitabchi AE, Umpierrez GE, Murphy MB, Barrett EJ, Kreisberg RA, Malone JI, Wall BM. Management of hyperglycemic crises in patients with diabetes. *Diabetes Care* 2001; **24**: 131–53.

4   Marshall SM, Walker M, Alberti KGM. Diabetic ketoacidosis and hyperglycaemic non-ketotic coma. In: Alberti KGM, Zimmet P, DeFronzo RA (eds). *International Textbook of Diabetes Mellitus*. New York: John Wiley, 1997; 215–1229.

PROBLEM

9   Recurrent Hypoglycaemia

Case History

A 48-year-old man has had type 1 diabetes for 30 years and multiple sclerosis for ten years. He can walk around the house with help but is otherwise confined to a wheelchair. He attends with his wife complaining that he is having recurrent blackouts. His wife has checked his blood sugar twice during these episodes and found it to be below 2.0 mmol/l. He takes Mixtard 30/70 twice daily and his glycosylated haemoglobin (HbA1c) is 9.0%. His wife complains that his memory is deteriorating.

How should his hypoglycaemia be managed?

What is the differential diagnosis of his memory loss?

Does the presence of multiple sclerosis affect his diabetes management?

Background

While better glycaemic control decreases the risks from diabetes, particularly in relation to microvascular complications, hypoglycaemia, or the fear of hypoglycaemia, is the major barrier to obtaining tight blood sugar control in most patients. It is easy to understand why this is so: hypoglycaemia is thought to be the cause of death in 2–4% of patients with type 1 diabetes. Severe hypoglycaemia, requiring help from another individual, has an incidence of 50–150 episodes per 100 patient-years in type 1 diabetes; type 2 patients treated with insulin have an incidence of hypoglycaemia about one-tenth of this, presumably largely because of coexistent insulin resistance. Attempts to tighten glycaemic control with insulin or oral hypoglycaemic drugs almost invariably increase the risk of hypoglycaemia—65% of patients in the Diabetes Control and Complications Trial (DCCT, type 1 diabetes) had at least one episode of severe hypoglycaemia, while 2% of patients using oral hypoglycaemics and 11% using insulin in the United Kingdom Prospective Diabetes Study (UKPDS, type 2 diabetes) had at least one episode.[1] Episodes of symptomatic hypoglycaemia occur up to two times per week on average in patients with type 1 diabetes and tight glycaemic control.

Symptoms and signs of hypoglycaemia vary from person to person, as do the thresholds at which these develop, particularly if glycaemic control is poor or variable. Many episodes of hypoglycaemia are unrecognized, including those that occur during sleep. Patients with chronic hyperglycaemia may well experience hypoglycaemic symptoms at a higher threshold than those with tight control. The aim should be to achieve glycaemic control as tight as possible overall, while maintaining a blood glucose above 4.0 mmol/l. Triggers for hypoglycaemia include: excessive or mistimed insulin or insulin secretagogue; inadequate intake of carbohydrate—missed meals or dieting; decreased endogenous glucose production—alcohol intake or chronic liver disease; increased glucose utilization, as during exercise; increased sensitivity to insulin—after vigorous exercise, pituitary or adrenal failure; or decreased clearance of insulin in renal failure.

Patients who are taking insulin or high doses of potent insulin secretagogues have already lost the first line of defence against hypoglycaemia, which is to decrease the amount of insulin in the circulation (Table 9.1). The next immediate response to hypoglycaemia is to increase secretion of glucagon and adrenaline. Glucagon combats hypoglycaemia by stimulating both glycogenolysis and gluconeogenesis. Adrenaline and noradrenaline are responsible for some of the warning signs of hypoglycaemia (adrenergic) and help combat hypoglycaemia by mobilizing other metabolic substrates including free fatty acids, glycerol, amino acids and lactate. More medium- to long-term protection from hypoglycaemia comes from increased secretion of cortisol and growth hormone. In patients with type 1 diabetes, the glucagon response to hypoglycaemia is blunted or lost. Thus, the major protection from hypoglycaemia comes from increased catecholamine secretion. In patients with diabetes, the glycaemic threshold for adrenaline release is often shifted to a lower glucose value. The patient may not, therefore, experience symptoms until a lower blood glucose value is reached and they may not be so able to combat developing hypoglycaemia. This is particularly the case where there has been preceding repeated or severe hypoglycaemia. The concept of hypoglycaemia associated autonomic failure (HAAF) has been proposed.[2] Exercise, even of relatively modest intensity, has a similar effect on blunting autonomic responses.[3] This phenomenon can be reversed by two to three weeks of strict avoidance of hypoglycaemia.

Table 9.1	Responses to Low Blood Glucose		
Glucose (mmol/l)	**Response**		
4.0–6.0	Low physiologic blood glucose. In non-diabetic subjects insulin secretion is suppressed		
3.6–3.9	Start of counter-regulatory response. Increased secretion of glucagon and catecholamines		
3.1–3.5	Patient may begin to develop neurogenic symptoms:		
	Adrenergic	**Cholinergic**	
	Palpitations	Hunger	
	Anxiety	Sweating	
	Tremor	Paraesthesiae	
2.8–3.0	Neuroglycopaenic symptoms – behavioural change, cognitive dysfunction, focal neurological abnormalities, seizures, coma		

The above patient has both type 1 diabetes and multiple sclerosis. The pathogenesis of the latter is less well understood than that of type 1 diabetes but it is an inflammatory/immune condition, and the two diseases are associated.[4] Autonomic function is often impaired in patients with multiple sclerosis.[5] This is usually manifest as problems with bowel or bladder function or as abnormal cardiovascular reflexes, but may also lead to impaired hypoglycaemic warning signs. Repeated hypoglycaemia may lead to cognitive impairment. However, in this patient it is difficult to be clear that hypoglycaemia is leading to cognitive changes. Patients with multiple sclerosis, especially those with progressive forms of the disease, may also suffer cognitive impairment.[6]

The following might be useful in the management of the above patient (Figure 9.1).

● Review by a diabetes nurse specialist and a dietician to ensure that insulin is being given at the appropriate time and in the correct dose, and also that the patient knows how to deal with hypoglycaemic episodes.

● Psychological assessment should be considered to document the degree of cognitive impairment.

● Screen for contributory factors including psychological disturbance, renal impairment and adrenal failure.

● Review of his blood glucose diary to determine whether there is a pattern to hypoglycaemia and whether there are episodes that he is not detecting. If the patient is able, and willing, a full capillary blood glucose profile should be taken for several days—fasting, before and two hours after each meal, before bed and at least once during the night. If available, continuous subcutaneous blood glucose monitoring might be helpful.

● Even though his overall control is not good, cutting back on his insulin for a few weeks should decrease the risk of hypoglycaemic attacks and minimize wide variations in his blood glucose level.

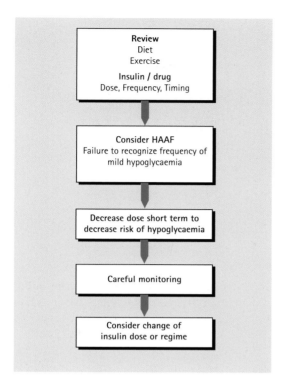

Fig. 9.1 Management of recurrent hypoglycaemia. HAAF = hypoglycaemia associated autonomic failure.

- Consider a change of insulin. His pre-mixed insulin means that most of his control is coming from long-acting isophane insulin. He may agree a change to a basal bolus regime, at least until his hypoglycaemic episodes have become less of a problem. Short-acting analogue insulin, titrated if possible to his two-hour post-prandial blood glucose, should minimize his exposure to insulin during the day. Long-acting analogues have a flatter profile than conventional long-acting insulins and, used as part of a basal bolus regime, may keep background exposure to insulin to a minimum.

Recent Developments

1. The effect of diabetes on cognitive function has been controversial. High-risk groups, including young children and the elderly, are at risk and may suffer mild to moderate impairment compared with their non-diabetic peers. Patients in the Diabetes Control and Complications Trial (DCCT) suffered an increased incidence of hypoglycaemia but they had no evidence of cognitive impairment. Chronic hyperglycaemia, as well as hypoglycaemia, is a risk factor for cognitive impairment in diabetes. A recent meta-analysis confirmed that patients with type 1 diabetes are at risk for mild to moderate cognitive impairment (Figure 9.2).[7]

2. There is a greater understanding of the mechanisms underlying hypoglycaemic awareness and the counter-regulatory response. Recent data[8] suggest that ATP-sensitive K^+ channels in the ventromedial hypothalamus play a critical role in sensing

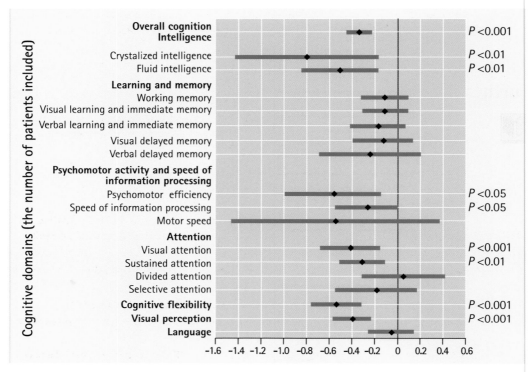

Fig. 9.2 Diabetes and Cognitive Performance. Effect sizes are shown with 95% confidence intervals comparing patients with type 1 diabetes and non–diabetic controls. *Source*: Brands *et al*. 2005.[7]

hypoglycaemia. Closing the channels blunted autonomic responses to low blood glucose. Work in this area may open the way to therapeutic advances that may allow us to maintain tight glucose control while minimizing hypoglycaemia.

3   One therapeutic advance that is attracting much attention is the use of incretin-like molecules to stimulate insulin release in response to food ingestion. Exenatide (synthetic exendin-4) is a 39 amino acid peptide with incretin activity. This molecule can improve glycaemic control in patients with type 2 diabetes and its use is not associated with blunting of the counter-regulatory response.[9]

Conclusion

Hypoglycaemia is a major problem for patients who have insulin-dependent diabetes and who wish to maintain reasonably tight glycaemic control. While the latter is important to minimize the risk of complications, the aim should be to keep blood glucose >4.0 mmol/l at all times. Particular caution should be exercised when patients experience repeated hypoglycaemia, where there is nocturnal hypoglycaemia, or where the patient has lost hypoglycaemic warning symptoms and signs. After screening for contributory causes, the aim should be to cut back on the insulin, understanding that overall control might temporarily be compromised, so as to avoid hypoglycaemia for two to three weeks. The appearance of hypoglycaemia should prompt a review of the dose and type of insulin, as well as the patient's diet. Before making any changes, ensure as far as possible that reported symptoms are due to hypoglycaemia.

Further Reading

1   Cryer PE, Davis SN, Shamoon H. Hypoglycemia in diabetes. *Diabetes Care* 2003; **26**: 1902–12.

2   Cryer PE. Hypoglycemia-associated autonomic failure in diabetes. *Am J Physiol Endocrinol Metab* 2001; **281**: E32–41.

3   Sandoval DA, Guy DLA, Richardson MA, Ertl AC, Davis SN. Effects of low and moderate antecedent exercise on counterregulatory responses to subsequent hypoglycemia in type 1 diabetes. *Diabetes* 2004; **53**: 1798–806.

4   Edwards LJ, Constantinescu CS. A prospective study of conditions associated with multiple sclerosis in a cohort of 658 consecutive outpatients attending a multiple sclerosis clinic. *Mult Scler* 2004; **10**: 575–81.

5   McDougall AJ, McLeod JG. Autonomic nervous system function in multiple sclerosis. *J Neurol Sci* 2003; **215**: 79–85.

6   Huijbregts SCJ, Kalkers NF, de Sonneville LMJ, de Groot V, Reuling IEW, Polman CH. Differences in cognitive impairment of relapsing remitting, secondary, and primary progressive MS. *Neurology* 2004; **63**: 335–9.

7   Brands AMA, Biessels GJ, de Haan EHF, Kappelle LJ, Kessels RPC. The effects of type 1 diabetes on cognitive performance. A meta-analysis. *Diabetes Care* 2005; **28**: 726–35.

8   Evans ML, McCrimmon RJ, Flanagan DE, Keshavarz T, Fan X, McNay EC, Jacob RJ, Sherwin RS. Hypothalamic ATP-sensitive K+ channels play a key role in sensing hypoglycemia and triggering counterregulatory epinephrine and glucagon responses. *Diabetes* 2004; **53**: 2542–51.

9   Degn KB, Brock B, Juhl CB, Djurhuus CB, Grubert J, Kim D, Han J, Taylor K, Fineman M, Schmitz O. Effect of intravenous infusion of exenatide (synthetic exendin-4) on glucose-dependent insulin secretion and counterregulation during hypoglycemia. *Diabetes* 2004; **53**: 2397–403.

10 Diabetes and Acute Myocardial Infarction

Case History

A 54-year-old man with metformin-treated type 2 diabetes is admitted with myocardial infarction. He was diagnosed with diabetes three years ago, and has no microvascular complications. He stopped smoking two years ago, and has been taking lisinopril 10 mg/day for hypertension.

How should glycaemia be managed on the coronary care unit?

Should he be discharged taking metformin?

Background

The risk of death and disability following myocardial infarction is higher in patients with diabetes or hyperglycaemia than in non-diabetic, euglycaemic patients.

There are a number of factors which complicate the diagnosis of myocardial infarction in diabetes.

● Silent myocardial infarction is more common in diabetes and can be missed without an adequate index of suspicion.

● There is uncertainty about appropriate management of glycaemia.

● The presence of retinopathy has previously been cited as a reason to avoid thrombolysis in the patient with diabetes.

● There is ongoing uncertainty about the most appropriate revascularization strategy in diabetes.

● There is probably a need for a more intensive approach to secondary prophylaxis given the increased risk for patients with diabetes.

Hyperglycaemia in response to myocardial infarction and an acute coronary syndrome is common—studies identify diabetes or 'stress hyperglycaemia' in up to 30% of admissions to coronary care units.[1] The focus in this scenario will be on management of hyperglycaemia in acute coronary syndromes.

The University Group Diabetes Program Study[2] raised doubts about the safety of sulphonylureas in cardiovascular disease in 1976, though the United Kingdom Prospective Diabetes Studies (UKPDS) 33 and 34[3,4] were reassuring that oral hypoglycaemics were not, in themselves, harmful. Indeed, UKPDS 34[4] suggested a 7% ten-year mortality reduction in newly diagnosed, overweight patients treated with metformin.

In 1995, the DIGAMI study[5] (Diabetes and Insulin-Glucose Infusion in Acute Myocardial Infarction) addressed whether intensive metabolic treatment with glucose insulin potassium (GIK) infusion followed by multidose insulin treatment in patients with diabetes or hyperglycaemia and acute myocardial infarction improved prognosis. Myocardial infarction was defined as at least two periods of chest pain >15 minutes in duration, elevation of creatine kinase (CK) or lactate dehydrogenase (LDH) two standard deviations above reference range or development of Q waves in two consecutive electrocardiogram leads. Intensive glucose management required GIK infusion in all patients with diabetes or admission blood glucose >11 mmol/l, aiming for a glucose level of 7–10 mmol/l, followed by four times daily insulin aiming for stable normoglycaemia. Of 1240 patients screened, 620 were subsequently randomized and the relative risk of death was 30% lower in the intensively managed group.

Recent Developments

1   DIGAMI-2[6] attempted to answer whether the reduction in mortality seen in DIGAMI was due to GIK, ongoing intensive glycaemic management with four-times daily insulin, both, or other factors such as structured follow-up or chance. Patients with diabetes or hyperglycaemia and myocardial infarction were randomized to GIK for 24 hours followed by long-term subcutaneous insulin, GIK for 24 hours followed by standard glucose control, or standard treatment. Myocardial infarction was defined as chest pain of >15 minutes duration in the previous 24 hours and Q waves / ST-T wave deviation. Unfortunately, this study achieved neither recruitment targets nor separation of glycaemia in the randomized groups. There was no evidence of harm or benefit in any of the groups. However, *post hoc* analysis of DIGAMI,[5] DIGAMI-2[6] and other studies, such as the Insulin in Intensive Care Study,[7] identifies that hyperglycaemia is closely associated with greater risk of death.

2   These trials mean that a strategy to manage hyperglycaemia on an acute cardiac unit is generally demanded, though there are insufficient data for this to be robustly evidence-based—particularly with the advent of more sensitive markers of cardiac damage such as troponins making even the diagnosis of myocardial infarction problematic. The suggested approach in patients with diabetes and acute coronary syndrome is therefore pragmatic and outlined in Figure 10.1. The selection of an insulin intervention threshold of HbA1c 8% is to target achievable long-term glycaemic control in patients where insulin therapy is most likely to succeed in reducing the long-term impact of microvascular complications. Data from Sweden[8] suggest that glucose tolerance remains abnormal in at least one-quarter of those with 'stress hyperglycaemia' and so glucose tolerance testing after recovery is also recommended in those not known previously to have diabetes.

Conclusion

The risk of death and disability in patients with diabetes or hyperglycaemia and an acute coronary syndrome is two or more times that of the non-diabetic, euglycaemic patients.

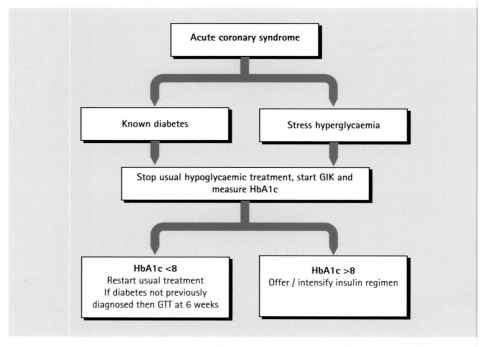

Fig. 10.1 Diabetes and myocardial infarction. GTT = glucose tolerance test; GIK = glucose insulin potassium.

Despite trials of intensive glycaemic management, there remains uncertainty about how best to manage these patients. A newer question of how to treat patients who have 'troponin-positive' ischaemic cardiac pain and diabetes or hyperglycaemia is unlikely to be subjected to randomized trial. A pragmatic approach to glycaemia is suggested that limits exposure to severe hyperglycaemia at the time of an acute coronary syndrome and identifies patients at highest risk of microvascular complications following discharge from hospital.

Further Reading

1 Savage MW, Mah PM, Weetman AP, Newell-Price J. Endocrine emergencies. *Postgrad Med J* 2004; **80**: 506–15.

2 Riveline JP, Danchin N, Ledru F, Varroud VM, Charpentier G. Sulfonylureas and cardiovascular effects: from experimental data to clinical use. Available data in humans and clinical applications. *Diabetes Metab* 2003; **29**: 207–22.

3 UKPDS Study Group. Intensive blood-glucose control with sulphonylureas or insulin compared with conventional treatment and risk of complications in patients with type 2 diabetes (UKPDS 33). *Lancet* 1998; **352**: 837–43.

4 UKPDS Study Group. Effect of intensive blood-glucose control with metformin on complications in overweight patients with type 2 diabetes (UKPDS 34). *Lancet* 1998; **352**: 854–65.

5 Malmberg K, Ryden L, Efendic S, Herlitz J, Nicol P, Waldenstrom A, Wedel H, Welin L. Randomized trial of insulin-glucose infusion followed by subcutaneous insulin treatment in diabetic patients with acute myocardial infarction (DIGAMI): effects on mortality at one year. *J Am Coll Cardiol* 1995; **26**: 57–65.

6 Malmberg K, Ryden L, Wedel H, Birkeland K, Bootsma A, Dickstein K, Efendic S, Fisher M, Hamsten A, Herlitz J, Hildebrandt P, MacLeod K, Laakso M, Torp-Pedersen C, Waldenstrom A. Intense metabolic control by means of insulin in patients with diabetes mellitus and acute myocardial infarction (DIGAMI 2): effects on mortality and morbidity. *Eur Heart J* 2005; **26**: 650–61.

7 Van den Berghe G, Wouters P, Weekers F, Verwaest C, Bruyninckx F, Schetz M, Vlasselaers D, Ferdinande P, Lauwers P, Bouillon R. Intensive insulin therapy in critically ill patients. *N Engl J Med* 2001; **345**: 1359–67.

8 Norhammar A, Tenerz A, Nilsson G, Hamsten A, Efendic S, Ryden L, Malmberg K. Glucose metabolism in patients with acute myocardial infarction and no previous diagnosis of diabetes mellitus: a prospective study. *Lancet* 2002; **359**: 2140–4.

PROBLEM

11 Diabetes and Acute Stroke

Case History

A 62-year-old man is admitted with a sudden episode of right hemiparesis consistent with an acute stroke. He is obese with a four-year history of type 2 diabetes and taking metformin and rosiglitazone. He does not smoke and drinks minimal amounts of alcohol. Clinically, he was in sinus rhythm and had no evidence of heart failure.

Consider his risk factors for stroke.

Consider short– and long–term outcome and acute management strategies.

Does he require insulin treatment during his acute stroke?

Background

The risk of stroke in patients with diabetes mellitus is two- to three-fold higher than in people without diabetes. Diabetes doubles the risk of stroke recurrence, while stroke outcomes are often worse among patients with diabetes, e.g. a higher hospital and long-term stroke mortality, more residual functional disability, higher risk of stroke-related dementia as well as longer hospital stay. At one year, mortality rate was two-fold higher in diabetes and after five years, only a fifth of patients with diabetes survive.[1] In the United Kingdom Prospective Diabetes Study (UKPDS), the odds ratio for case fatality in stroke was 1.37 per 1% increase in glycosylated haemoglobin (HbA1c).

Differences in the clinical presentation of stroke in patients with diabetes compared to those without diabetes have been reported. Diabetes confers a greater ischaemic to haemorrhagic stroke ratio compared with the general population, a higher incidence of lacunar infarcts (small infarcts, less than 15 mm in diameter, often resulting in pure motor strokes), and a higher frequency of infratentorial (i.e. cerebellar, midbrain and brainstem) infarcts. In the stroke population younger than 55 years old, diabetes increases the risk of stroke by more than ten-fold.

Hypertension, dyslipidaemia and atrial fibrillation are well-recognized risk factors for stroke. Components of the metabolic syndrome, both individually and collectively, such as insulin resistance, central obesity, impaired glucose tolerance, low high-density lipoprotein (HDL)-cholesterol and hyperinsulinaemia, have also been associated with an excess risk of stroke. Poor glycaemic control is an independent risk factor for fatal and non-fatal stroke, and plays an important role in the outcome from acute stroke. Preliminary evidence has also emerged on the relationship between post-prandial hyperglycaemia and stroke mortality, while stress hyperglycaemia is now recognized to be a predictor of poor stroke outcome. Similarly, degrees of albuminuria have been shown to be a predictor of stroke in patients with diabetes, although no clear association has been observed for stroke mortality. Diabetic autonomic neuropathy is also another risk factor for stroke, and diabetic retinopathy is associated with an increased risk of ischaemic stroke and lacunar infarcts.

Acute stroke should be treated aggressively in order to limit stroke volume and subsequent functional and neurological deficit. The mainstay of emergency treatment for stroke includes adequate control of hydration state, body temperature and blood glucose, early assessment for swallowing and the initiation of antiplatelet agents in patients with ischaemic stroke. A Cochrane meta-analysis involving 41 399 patients from nine randomized clinical trials, which includes many patients with diabetes, has shown that aspirin, 160–300 mg daily given by mouth, nasogastric tube or rectum, started within 48 hours of onset of a presumed ischaemic stroke, reduces the risk of death or dependency after six months without major risks of early haemorrhagic complications.[2] The standard maintenance dose of aspirin for secondary prevention, meanwhile, is usually 75–150 mg daily, although there is theoretical evidence that patients with diabetes may require slightly higher doses of aspirin to achieve similar antiplatelet effects. A meta-analysis of trials of anticoagulation for acute stroke, however, found no difference in stroke outcomes, even in patients with embolic stroke. Thrombolysis with alteplase[3] when administered within three hours of acute stroke reduces stroke volume, but this is only feasible within a specialized setting with immediate access to emergency neuroimaging performed by a neuroradiologist. The presence of diabetes on admission, however, is associated with poor neurological outcome despite early revascularization with recombinant tissue plasminogen activator (rTPA).

Early neurosurgical intervention is indicated in large posterior fossa stroke where evacuation of infarct or clot is clinically indicated, shunting for acute hydrocephalus and for patients with subarachnoid bleeds. The benefit of surgery in large hemispheric infarcts and moderate intracerebral bleeds is unclear and is being investigated. Neuroprotectant drugs have so far not been shown to be beneficial in ischaemic or haemorrhagic stroke, although several trials are still underway. A Cochrane meta-analysis, however, showed that early use of nimodipine in patients with subarachnoid haemorrhage is associated with a 30% relative risk reduction due to the prevention or reversal of cerebral vasospasm.

The presence of high blood pressure following an acute stroke is common and is in-dependently associated with an adverse prognosis due to promoting early recurrence and the development of fatal cerebral oedema in patients with ischaemic stroke and re-bleeding in those with haemorrhagic stroke. At present, the optimum management of blood pressure in the immediate post-stroke period is unclear. Acute blood pressure lowering could improve outcome by reducing the risks of acute stroke recurrence or secondary haemorrhagic complications while, conversely, may worsen outcome by reducing regional cerebral perfusion. It is suggested that in the absence of clear trial evidence, blood pressure should not be routinely lowered unless it is extreme (systolic blood pressure >220 mmHg) or associated with arterial dissection or cardiac ischaemia or failure, in which case cautious lowering (<15%) may be appropriate. Large studies are needed to address this important management issue.

Recent Developments

1   Benefits of intensive insulin treatment for ischaemic tissue protection have emerged. Insulin and glucose flux into ischaemic tissue is an important substrate for glycolysis and subsequent ATP synthesis, thereby attenuating ischaemia-induced decreases in ATP synthesis. This was supported by results from the Diabetes and Insulin-Glucose Infusion in Acute Myocardial Infarction (DIGAMI) study, where intensive insulin treatment improved survival at one year. Another study showed that intensive insulin therapy for patients admitted to a surgical intensive care unit (ICU) and treated to target glucose resulted in reduced in-hospital mortality, less neuropathy and shorter ICU stay. A 'proof of concept' pilot study was successfully implem-ented and forms the basis for a larger, ongoing Glucose Insulin in Stroke Trial (GIST) to assess the role of intravenous administration of glucose, potassium and insulin (GKI) for 24 hours on acute stroke.[4]

2   The Controlling Hypertension and Hypotension Immediately Post-Stroke (CHHIPS) pilot trial,[5] which is a UK-based multicentre, randomized, double-blind, placebo-controlled, titrated dose trial, is underway to assess whether hypertension and relative hypotension, manipulated therapeutically in the first 24 hours following acute stroke, affects short-term outcome measures.

3   Magnesium has been shown to be neuroprotective in experimental animal models of stroke. In a large randomized clinical trial, however, intravenous magnesium given within 12 hours of acute stroke did not significantly reduce mortality or disability, although it may be of benefit in lacunar strokes, a variant of stroke commonly seen in patients with diabetes.[6]

Conclusion

Patients with diabetes have considerably increased risk of cerebrovascular disease. However, general treatment recommendations as for non-diabetic patients apply

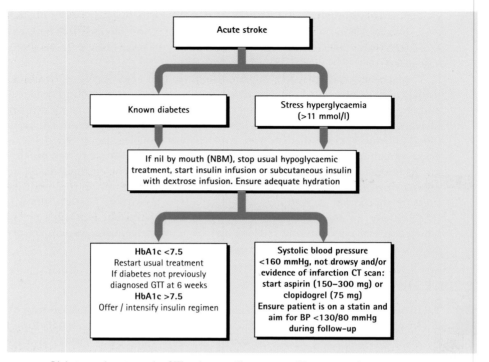

Fig. 11.1 Diabetes and acute stroke. GTT = glucose tolerance test; CT = computed tomography; BP = blood pressure.

(Figure 11.1). Supportive measures along with aspirin are now recommended in the acute phase, and aspirin is also considered beneficial for secondary prevention. Hypertension is the most important risk factor. Hyperlipidaemia and glycaemic control are also important.[7] At present, the role of intensive glycaemic control with insulin infusion in the acute phase followed by tight control with frequent insulin injections is not certain.

Further Reading

1 Megherbi S-E, Milan C, Minier D, Couvreur G, Osseby GV, Tilling K, Di Carlo A, Inzitari D, Wolfe CD, Moreau T, Giroud M. Association between diabetes and stroke subtype on survival and functional outcome 3 months after stroke. Data from the European BIOMED Stroke Project. *Stroke* 2003; **34**: 688–94.

2 Sandercock P, Gubitz G, Foley P, Counsell C. Antiplatelet therapy for acute ischaemic stroke. *Cochrane Database Syst Rev* 2003; **2**: CD000029.

3 Albert GW, Clark WM, Madden KP, Hamilton SA. Atlantis trial: results for patients treated within 3 hours of stroke onset. Alteplase Thrombolysis for Acute Noninterventional Therapy in Ischaemic Stroke. *Stroke* 2002; **33**: 493–5.

4 Scott JF, Robinson GM, French JM. Glucose potassium insulin infusions in the treatment of acute stroke patients with mild to moderate hyperglycaemia. The Glucose Insulin in Stroke Trial (GIST). *Stroke* 1999; **30**: 793–9.

5 Potter J, Robinson T, Ford G, James M, Jenkins, D, Mistri A, Bulpitt C, Drummond A, Jagger C, Knight J, Markus H, Beevers G, Dewey M, Lees K, Moore A, Paul S. CHHIPS (Controlling Hypertension and Hypotension Immediately Post-Stroke) pilot trial: rationale and design. *J Hypertens* 2005; **23**: 649–55.

6 Muir KW, Lees KR, Ford I, Davis S. Magnesium for acute stroke (Intravenous Magnesium Efficacy in Stroke trial): Randomised controlled trial. *Lancet* 2004; **363**: 439–45.

7 Mankovsky BN, Ziegler D. Stroke in patients with diabetes mellitus. *Diabetes Metab Res Rev* 2004; **20**: 268–87.

PROBLEM

12 Diabetes and Critical Limb Ischaemia

Case History

During a routine diabetes review, your patient tells you of the ongoing severe pains affecting his left foot. On examination, his left foot appeared very pale, was devoid of any pulses from his knee downwards and felt cold. His right foot was normal. He takes oral hypoglycaemics and his glycosylated haemoglobin (HbA1c) is reasonable at 7.3%

Describe how you would investigate the acute problem.

What are the likely outcomes of treatment?

What secondary prevention strategies are important?

Background

Peripheral arterial disease (PAD), defined as lower extremity arterial atherosclerosis, is common in people with diabetes.[1] It is estimated to affect up to 8% of the diabetic population at the time of diagnosis. Diabetes confers a 10- to 16-fold increase in the lifetime risk of lower limb amputation compared with non-diabetes. Diabetes tends to cause more diffuse and more distal (i.e. infrapopliteal and tibial) atherosclerotic disease, often associated with vascular calcification. Two-thirds of patients with symptomatic PAD improve spontaneously or remain stable with fixed exercise limitation, while the remaining third have progressively deteriorating symptoms. About 2% of patients with intermittent claudication will eventually require some sort of amputation. There is no easy way of identifying which patients will get worse, but a poor outcome is closely linked to smoking and suboptimal risk factor control (such as low high-density lipoprotein [HDL], high low-density lipoprotein [LDL], central obesity and hyperglycaemia). Patients are also at significant high risk of developing cardiovascular disease.[2] In one study, 20% of patients with intermittent claudication were shown to suffer a myocardial infarction over a 5-year period. Thus, the medical management of patients with PAD should not only be considered in the context of lower limb salvage but also in terms of cardiovascular risk protection.

PAD results in compromised blood supply to leg tissues, and to the vasa nervorum, resulting in ischaemic neuritis and continuous distal foot pain. Critical ischaemia occurs when lower limb circulation falls to a critical level at which the viability of distal tissues or the limb is at risk. This is defined by the European Consensus Document as 'persistently recurring rest pain requiring regular analgesia for more than two weeks, or ulceration or gangrene of the foot and toes in combination with an ankle systolic pressure less than 50 mmHg'. Patients with diabetes and severe PAD may, however, not experience rest or night pain due to coexisting peripheral neuropathy, and may present to healthcare professionals later in the course of disease. Not surprisingly, a much higher proportion of patients with diabetes will require surgical interventions.

Clinical signs

The limb is often cold and pale with hair-loss from the medial aspect of the leg. There is poor capillary refill and impaired venous filling of superficial veins. When critically ischaemic legs are elevated to an angle of 30 degrees, they will turn pale. Buerger's test will also be positive: elevate the leg and then in the dependent position the microvasculature becomes dilated with blood rushing into the foot to give the appearance of hyperaemia. Evidence of trophic changes such as ulceration on pressure points or gangrene at the extremities is common. The latter is associated with tissue pallor and mottling, progressing to purple and then the characteristic black appearance due to haemoglobin breakdown forming iron sulphide.

The ankle–brachial pressure index (ABPI) involves the measurement of ankle systolic blood pressure with an ordinary blood-pressure cuff around the calf and a hand-held Doppler over the dorsalis pedis or posterior tibial pulses; an ABPI value >0.9 is normal while an ABPI value of <0.8 indicates PAD. A cut-off of 0.8 for ABPI is often used in various epidemiological studies of diabetes and has been shown to be highly specific (99%) for PAD in the general population, while claudication and absence of pulses has a 95% specificity for PAD in the diabetic population. ABPI is usually <0.6 in patients with critical lower limb ischaemia. Patients with diabetes may have falsely high ABPI readings due to calcified vessels.

Treatment

The incidence and outcomes from critical limb ischaemia are significantly worse among patients with diabetes, e.g. higher amputation rates and less successful outcomes from revascularization procedures (angioplasty or bypass grafting).[3] Patients should be seen urgently by a vascular specialist for further investigations, e.g. duplex ultrasonography and/or angiography, and for urgent treatment (Figure 12.1). The preferred treatment option is angioplasty or surgical bypass grafting with either autologous saphenous vein or an artificial graft. Angioplasty is ideal if the stenotic lesions are short and proximal, with surgical bypass as the next solution if angioplasty fails. Critical ischaemia threatens the viability of the limb and therefore some attempt at improving blood flow surgically is justified. In cases of an acute embolus, where the vascular occlusion is sudden and com-

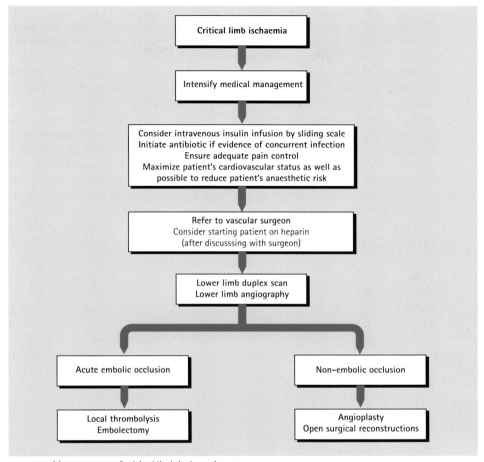

Fig. 12.1 Management of critical limb ischaemia.

plete, an embolectomy with a Fogarty catheter is the treatment of choice and can be done either with a local anaesthetic or with general anaesthesia. This is followed by anticoagulation. If the ischaemia is not severe and if the clot is more likely to be a thrombus, intra-arterial thrombolysis with recombinant tissue plasminogen activator (rTPA) may be the best method of treatment.[4]

Sympathectomy is no longer thought to have a role for providing symptomatic control in patients with critical limb ischaemia because sclerosed arteries in diabetic patients have very little capacity to dilate after a sympathectomy. Prostacyclin infusions, however, may prolong the survival of critically ischaemic legs.

Open surgical reconstructions for lower limb ischaemia are divided into supra- and infrainguinal reconstructions. Suprainguinal vascular reconstructions, e.g. aorta–bifemoral bypass with Dacron grafts, often achieve high patency rates in the presence of a patent superficial femoral artery, while femoral–popliteal bypass or bypass to the crural arteries are often performed for infrainguinal occlusive disease. The latter may be preferred for patients with diabetes since arterial occlusion in this group is often located more distally. Outcomes of percutaneous revascularization procedures, meanwhile, depend on various factors including the location and length of the lesion, stenosis and the presence of a collateral circulation. Patients with diabetes tend to have more severe arterial occlusive disease below the knee and reduced distal collateral supply, resulting in a less favourable outcome in patients with diabetes compared with those without diabetes. Iliac artery stenting in patients with diabetes achieves a 90% patency rate at one year, although some groups have shown lower patency rates. The one-year patency rates after femoral artery interventions range from 29% to 80%, with diabetes associated with a less favourable outcome due to poorer collateral circulation. Importantly, in those diabetic patients with good collaterals, the patency rates were comparable to those of non-diabetic patients. For infrainguinal ischaemia, the outcomes of surgical revascularization in diabetes are similar to those without diabetes in terms of limb salvage. Overall, however, it appears that in patients with severe claudication or critical limb ischaemia, surgery seems to be superior to percutaneous revascularization procedures in the femoral, popliteal and infrapopliteal vessels, but with higher risks of cardiovascular morbidity and mortality.[5]

Recent Developments

These are discussed in detail in Chapter 46 'Advances in management of peripheral vascular disease'.

Conclusion

The initial approach to the patient with critical limb ischaemia will depend on the severity of symptoms and the speed of onset. After thorough clinical assessment, and measurement of ABPI, consideration should be given to urgent angiography. Medical treatment of vascular risk factors is important in secondary prevention, but the major decisions to be made regarding acute treatment hinge upon whether embolectomy or reconstructive surgical treatment are indicated.

Further Reading

1   Beckman JA, Creager MA, Libby P. Diabetes and atherosclerosis: epidemiology, pathophysiology, and management. *JAMA* 2002; **287**: 2570–81.

2   Adler A, Stevens R, Neil A, Stratton I, Boulton A, Holman R. UKPDS 59: hyperglycaemia and other potentially modifiable risk factors for peripheral arterial disease in type 2 diabetes. *Diabetes Care* 2002; **25**: 894–9.

3   da Silva A, Desgranges P, Holdsworth J, Harris P, McCollum P, Jones SM, Beard J, Callam M. The management and outcome of critical limb ischaemia in diabetic patients: results of a national survey. Audit Committee of the Vascular Surgical Society of Great Britain and Ireland. *Diabet Med* 1996; **13**: 726–8.

4   Donnelly R, Yeung JC. Management of intermittent claudication: the importance of secondary prevention. *Eur J Vasc Endovasc Surg* 2002; **23**: 100–7.

5 Spittell PC. Peripheral vascular disease with suspected coronary artery disease. In: Gersh BJ, Yusuf S (eds). *Evidence Based Cardiology, Part IIIh: Specific Cardiovascular Disorders: Other conditions,* 2nd edn. London, BMJ Books, Blackwell Publishing Ltd, 2002; 87–102.

PROBLEM

13 Perioperative Management of Diabetes

Case History

An overweight 57-year-old woman who takes metformin and insulin to treat type 2 diabetes is to be admitted for elective hysterectomy. Blood pressure is well controlled and she is generally fit.

How should her diabetes be managed to minimize perioperative risk?

Background

Ten to twenty-five per cent of people in hospital will have diabetes – both diagnosed and undiagnosed.[1] Patients with diabetes are at higher risk of post-operative infection and transfer to intensive care settings. As many of these people will not be under the specific care of a diabetes specialist, clear guidance for patients and clinical staff is essential to reduce the risk of preventable errors in management. There is little research to support more than general recommendations about adjusting oral medications and using intravenous insulin in the perioperative period. Most guidance is therefore pragmatic, as is the approach outlined below.

Many factors will need to be considered to minimize the risk of surgery in this case. Some are generic to good surgical practice—such as the use of thromboprophylaxis—and others are more particular to a given patient and clinical setting, such as the degree of diabetes self-management that is desirable and possible. It is perhaps helpful to consider this problem in two stages—before and during elective admission.

Before admission

1 Risk factors for surgery associated with diabetes and being overweight, for example atheromatous vascular disease, renal dysfunction and thromboembolic risk, should be identified and a plan made.

2 The presence of diabetes, current treatment regime and complications of diabetes should be recorded in the clinical notes.

3   There should be specific assessment of diabetes self-management skills so that the supervision of management of glycaemia while in hospital is appropriate. For example, if the patient administers their own insulin at home, clinical staff may be able to allow the patient to administer subcutaneous insulin doses while in hospital. Similarly, if the patient does home blood glucose monitoring, staff may allow the patient to monitor blood glucose levels where possible during admission.

4   A plan for diabetes self-management arrangements while in hospital should be recorded in the clinical notes.

5   There should be clear information about managing hypoglycaemic therapy in the lead-up to surgery. For example, the British National Formulary[2] recommends that metformin is suspended two days prior to general surgery because of the risk of lactic acidosis. Local guidance should be in place to organize timing of admission and starvation in the hours prior to surgery. Consequent insulin adjustment will be necessary—perhaps halving usual doses with breakfast for an afternoon operation and altering the timing/necessity of intravenous insulin. The plan for adjustment of usual hypoglycaemic therapy prior to admission should be recorded in the clinical notes and clearly communicated with the patient.

6   When pre-operative bloods are drawn, a glycosylated haemoglobin (HbA1c) should be taken if none is available from the previous 2–3 months. This helps identify patients with poor glycaemic control where hyperglycaemia is likely to be more problematic during admission and in planning discharge and follow-up.

During admission

1   Assuming that starvation and pre-admission management of glycaemia has been satisfactory, the next step is ensuring glycaemia is controlled during general anaesthesia. This may require a titrated continuous intravenous insulin and dextrose infusion—see recommendations in Figure 13.1.

2   Clear parameters for the use of a titrated continuous intravenous insulin infusion should be recorded in the clinical notes.

3   Hyperglycaemia alone is generally not a reason to cancel surgery. The financial and emotional costs of late cancellation can be high. If the patient is otherwise well, the use of a titrated continuous intravenous insulin infusion will be sufficient to achieve adequate glycaemic control. The suggested practice is to start an intravenous insulin infusion if fingerprick glucose is outside specific glucose parameters (5–15 mmol/l) or if a patient will not or is not able to eat and drink postoperatively within one or two hours. Evidence from intensive care settings suggests that tighter glycaemic control may be preferable if admission to a critical care bed is needed.[4]

4   Hypoglycaemia (fingerprick glucose <4 mmol/l) will require correction with intravenous glucose if the operation is not to be delayed or cancelled—see recommendations in Figure 13.2.

5   Once normal eating and drinking is re-established postoperatively, usual hypoglycaemic therapy can be instituted. The pre-operative HbA1c and monitoring of pre-meal and pre-bed fingerprick glucose levels will identify patients with poor glycaemic

control prior to discharge. Early referral to the diabetes team then ensures early adaptation of current management and early follow-up after discharge.

6   Clear recommendations about monitoring glycaemia postoperatively should be recorded in the clinical notes. Clear follow-up arrangements should also be recorded in the clinical notes.

Management of hypoglycaemic therapy

1.   **Omit all oral hypoglycaemic agents on day of operation and sulphonylureas (gliclazide, glibenclamide, glimepiride etc.) from the evening before**

  1.1   **Morning list**

   1.1.1   Omit morning insulin

   1.1.2   Follow usual pre-operative fasting guidance for a morning list

   1.1.3   Check and record fingerprick glucose hourly from 06:00 am or time of admission
   - **If less than 5 mmol/l** start IV insulin, dextrose and potassium regimen. **Only in this case**, the first bag of fluid prescribed should be 500 ml 10% dextrose with 10 mmol KCl at 85 ml/h
   - **If greater than 15 mmol/l** start IV insulin, dextrose and potassium regimen

   1.1.4   If patient able to eat on return to the ward, give usual oral hypoglycaemic agents and *half usual morning insulin doses*

   1.1.5   If patient cannot eat or drink, IV insulin, dextrose and potassium regimen should be started/continued

  1.2   **Afternoon list**

   1.2.1   Light breakfast, finished before 08:00 am with half usual morning insulin doses

   1.2.2   Follow usual pre-operative fasting guidance for an afternoon list

   1.2.3   Check fingerprick glucose hourly from 08:00 am or time of admission and record on insulin card
   - **If less than 5 mmol/l** start IV insulin, dextrose and potassium regimen. **Only in this case**, the first bag of fluid prescribed should be 500 ml 10% dextrose with 10 mmol KCl at 85 ml/h
   - **If greater than 15 mmol/l** start IV insulin, dextrose and potassium regimen

   1.2.4   If patient able to eat on return to the ward, give usual oral hypoglycaemic agents and *usual insulin doses*

   1.2.5   If patient cannot eat or drink, IV insulin, dextrose and potassium regimen should be started/continued

2.   **Where IV insulin, dextrose and potassium regimen has been used, stop these and restart usual treatment when the patient is eating and drinking normally**

Fig. 13.1 Management of hypoglycaemic therapy. *Source:* Nottingham Diabetes Guidelines.[3]

Continuous Intravenous Insulin Regimen

1. Where IV insulin is used, aim to maintain glucose between 8 and 11 mmol/l to maintain adequate metabolic control and reduce the risk of hypoglycaemia, particularly under anaesthesia.

2. Suggested regimen in boxes to right

    2.1 Insulin and dextrose should both be delivered via dedicated infusion devices through a non-return device;

    2.2 A dedicated cannula should be used for this purpose only;

    2.3 Renew infusion equipment (syringes, tubing etc.) every 24 hours and cannula every 48 hours.

3. Stopping the regimen

    3.1 Stop when the patient is eating and drinking normally and nausea/vomiting are controlled.

    3.2 As the patient has type 2 diabetes, the insulin can be stopped at any time and the usual therapy started at the time it is usually given.

4. Institute fingerprick glucose monitoring before meals and before bed.

Insulin Infusion

Add 50 units of soluble insulin to 49.5 ml of 0.9% saline to give a 1 unit/ml solution.

Scale 2 most commonly used.

Aim to maintain glucose between 8 and 11 mmol/l.

Test stick glucose	Scale 1 Units/h	Scale 2 Units/h	Scale 3 Units/h
<3.9	0.5	0.5	0.5
4–6.9	0.5	1	2
7–9.9	1	2	3
10–14.9	2	3	4
15–19.9	3	4	5
>20	4	5	6

Scale 1: Daily insulin requirements   <30 units
Scale 2: Daily insulin requirements   30–60 units
Scale 3: Daily insulin requirements   >60 units

- Insulin requirements may increase with intercurrent illness.
- Use scale 2 unless BMI over 35 kg/m² where scale 3 is advised.

Glucose Monitoring

1. Initially, monitor fingerprick glucose hourly.

2. When insulin infusion stable for 2 hours and patient conscious and no clinical changes, then monitor 2 hourly.

Dextrose Infusion

1. 1000 ml 5% dextrose with 40 mmol/l KCl.

2. Start and continue infusion at 85 ml/h (1000 ml in 12 hours) until insulin infusion ceases.

3. Prescribe additional fluid requirements separately.

Fig. 13.2 Continuous Intravenous Insulin Regimen. BMI = body mass index. *Source*: Nottingham Diabetes Guidelines.[3]

Conclusion

Most perioperative diabetes management is managed by non-specialists. This requires guidance and support from diabetes teams to reduce the risk of preventable errors in management of glycaemia. Errors in management can delay procedures, delay discharge or expose the patient to unnecessary perioperative risk. The key to a successful outcome is clear communication between patient and clinicians and, perhaps more critically, between clinicians themselves.

Further Reading

1 American Diabetes Association. Standards of Medical Care in Diabetes. *Diabetes Care* 2005; **28**: S4–36.

2 British National Formulary 2005; **6**: 1.2.2.

3 Nottingham Diabetes Guidelines. www.nottinghamdiabetes.nhs.uk/gppages.html

4 Van den Berghe G, Wouters P, Weekers F, Verwaest C, Bruyninckx F, Schetz M, Vlasselaers D, Ferdinande P, Lauwers P, Bouillon R. Intensive insulin therapy in critically ill patients. *N Engl J Med* 2001; **345**: 1359–67.

PROBLEM

14 The Hot Foot

Case History

You are called to see a 38-year-old warehouseman with long-standing type 1 diabetes. He has a painful, hot, red foot. There is a small plantar ulcer which has been present for some weeks. He has missed a number of recent clinic appointments, and his control is poor (glycosylated haemoglobin, HbA1c = 9.6%).

How should he be managed?

Does he need to come into hospital?

Will he benefit from intensive insulin therapy?

Background

A 'hot' foot in a patient with diabetes is an emergency as the integrity of the limb may be threatened. Rapid and structured treatment (Figure 14.1) allows timely attendance by physician, surgeon, podiatrist, orthotist and educator, acutely and for longer-term care.

As the foot is hot, red and ulcerated, the likeliest diagnosis is infection. Alternate diagnoses should be considered where the diagnosis is less clear:

● Radiolucent foreign body

● Fracture

● Acute (Charcot) neuroarthropathy

● Deep vein thrombosis

Diabetic peripheral sensory neuropathy may mask a history of trauma sufficient for foreign body penetration. A radiolucent foreign body—such as a splinter or glass—may be invisible on plain X-ray. If a radiolucent foreign body is suspected, ultrasound examination with a high-frequency transducer should be requested.

Fracture, particularly of a metatarsal bone or fibula, can be overlooked on plain X-ray. Metatarsal fracture or minor tarsal fracture/dislocation in an insensate foot may herald acute (Charcot) neuroarthropathy. A high index of suspicion is needed to ensure appropriate early immobilization. Chapter 44 deals with the acute neuroarthropathic (Charcot) foot in more detail.

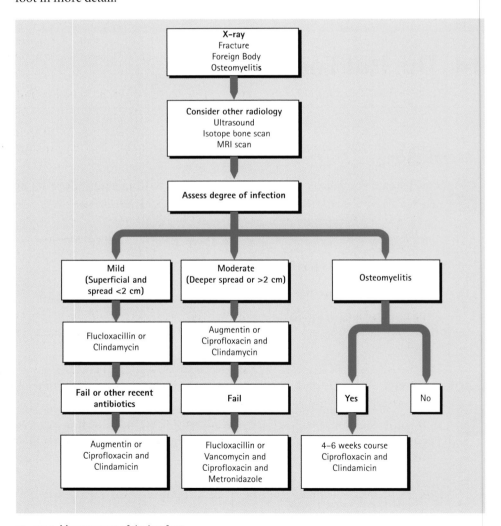

Fig. 14.1 Management of the hot foot.

It is difficult to provide definitive treatment guidance for diabetic foot ulceration with infection. However, a clinical assessment of the severity and likely organisms should provide sufficient information to select appropriate blind antibiotic therapy.

Severity of infection

● Mild—limited and superficial with no spread beyond 2 cm from the ulcer

● Moderate—superficial spread beyond 2 cm or to deeper structures

● Severe—infection with systemic upset

Inpatient care is generally desirable to treat more severe infection.

Microbiology

● Infections are commonly polymicrobial[1] – gram-positive cocci can be associated with gram-negative bacilli and/or anaerobes in a quarter of cases. Anaerobes are more commonly associated with a foul-smelling ulcer.[2]

● Ulcer-base curettage and culture provides a better guide to the infecting (rather than colonizing) organism when compared with superficial swabs or needle aspiration.[2]

● Exposed bone is always associated with osteomyelitis. An ability to probe to bone, and larger (>2 cm by 2 cm) or deeper (>3 mm) ulcers are more likely to be associated with osteomyelitis.

● A plain X-ray at baseline (repeated after 2–4 weeks if normal), magnetic resonance imaging (MRI) scanning or empiric treatment of osteomyelitis are all reasonable approaches in suspected osteomyelitis.[3] MRI scanning has a sensitivity of approximately 90% and specificity of nearly 100% for osteomyelitis.

Appropriate choice of antibiotic[3]

Mild infection (mainly outpatient therapy):

1   Flucloxacillin or clindamycin (penicillin-allergic patients) will target gram-positive organisms and are reasonable choices where there has been no recent antibiotic exposure.

2   Where these antibiotics fail, or there has been other recent antibiotic exposure, the addition of ciprofloxacin or a change to amoxicillin/clavulinic acid will broaden cover to include gram-negative organisms.

3   If methicillin-resistant *Staphylococcus aureus* (MRSA) is suspected and clindamycin has been ineffective, discussion with a microbiologist about local bacterial resistance would be appropriate.

Moderate/severe infection (inpatient or outpatient therapy):

1   Mixed infection should be treated with either amoxicillin/clavulanic acid or ciprofloxacin and clindamycin.

2   Where this is ineffective or oral therapy is inappropriate, the suggested practice is to use high-dose flucloxacillin (or vancomycin), ciprofloxacin and metronidazole until culture results are available to direct therapy.

Osteomyelitis (inpatient or outpatient therapy):

1   Where avoidance of amputation is a goal of therapy, a four- to six-week course of antibiotics may delay amputation or provide cure depending on the extent of bone involvement. Treatment frequently comprises initial intravenous therapy, followed by a prolonged course of oral antibiotics once response to therapy and sensitivities are known.

2   Where blind outpatient therapy of osteomyelitis is appropriate, the suggested practice is to use a combination of oral ciprofloxacin and clindamycin and adjust this once response to therapy and sensitivities are known.

3   The risk of failure is substantial and surgery may be necessary.

The aetiology of ulceration is also usually mixed, with coexisting neuropathic and vascular disease. Each aetiology requires a focused approach to support resolution of the acute infection and healing of the ulcerated site.

● Approximately half of all people with diabetes will develop some degree of peripheral neuropathy. Coexisting motor neuropathy with abnormalities of joint flexibility caused by glycation of collagen causes clawing of toes and reduced flexibility of small joints. Muscular imbalance causes abnormal weight transfer during walking, with consequent ulceration and inhibition of healing—frequently at the first metatarsal head. A bespoke temporary walking cast with a cut-out over the ulcer can promote healing, pending transfer into bespoke footwear with a large toebox and pressure-relieving insoles.

● Critical ischaemia is unlikely in this case because the foot is warm. However, a bedside assessment of vascular supply—using Doppler ultrasound if necessary—may identify less severe degrees of peripheral vascular disease. Incompressible, calcified blood vessels—particularly associated with renal failure—can make clinical and Doppler assessment of peripheral vessels difficult to interpret. Treatment of infection with antibiotics would usually precede vascular intervention unless there is apparent critical ischaemia or slow resolution of infection.

● Autonomic neuropathy with impaired sympathetic activity and abnormal arteriovenous shunting causes functional impairment of vascular supply[4] with inappropriate diversion of blood flow, impaired control of infection and slow healing. Decreased sweat and sebaceous secretion causes dryness of the skin which is then prone to cracking and secondary infection. The use of a daily moisturizing routine may improve the suppleness of the skin.

Recent Developments

1   Multiresistant strains of bacteria, particularly MRSA, are of increasing concern. Resistance to vancomycin as well as isolated resistance to the oxazolidinone, linezolid,

to the streptogramins, quinupristin and dalfopristin, and to the cyclic lipopeptide, daptomycin, has been identified. Spread by cross-contamination has the potential to establish resistant clones, causing endemic, untreatable infections. Rigorous attention to infection control and rapid MRSA testing are increasingly on the agenda of health-care providers and are needed to facilitate patient isolation and reduce cross-infection rates in healthcare institutions.

2 Granulocyte colony–stimulating factor (G-CSF) induces neutrophil release from the bone marrow, improves neutrophil function and enhances host response to infection. A recent meta-analysis of five trials (167 patients) of G-CSF as adjunctive therapy for diabetic foot infections without critical ischaemia showed a reduction in likelihood of any surgical intervention (relative risk [RR] 0.38; 95% CI 0.20–0.69) and amputation (RR 0.41; CI 0.17–0.95).[5] Clinical improvement in infection and overall healing were not affected. The authors suggest that adjunctive G-CSF may be considered in limb-threatening infection, but identify long-term outcomes and overall cost effectiveness as important areas for study before definitive conclusions can de drawn.

Conclusion

In this case, infection seems the likeliest diagnosis, though a high index of suspicion for alternate diagnoses is needed. An assessment of general clinical status—including a careful examination of the contralateral limb—will guide a decision about admission for treatment. Usual bloods should be drawn to support this assessment, as well as evaluation of inflammatory markers (to track response to treatment) and blood cultures. A clinical assessment of the vascular supply and likelihood of osteomyelitis should be made, as should an attempt to gain material for culture by curettage of the base of the ulcer. X-ray in two planes should be requested and further imaging studies with MRI may be appropriate.

Blind antibiotic therapy should be instituted, then adjusted once the initial response to therapy, antibiotic sensitivities and the likelihood of osteomyelitis are clearer. Poor glycaemic control is associated with poorer leucocyte response to infection and glycaemic control should be intensified.

Longer-term measures to support ulcer healing with pressure-relieving footwear should be instituted with immediate advice to temporarily cease work and reduce weight-bearing to an absolute minimum.

Further Reading

1 Lipsky BA, Pecoraro RE, Larson SA, Hanley ME, Ahroni JH. Outpatient management of uncomplicated lower-extremity infections in diabetic patients. *Arch Int Med* 1990; **150**: 790–7.

2 Sapico FL, Witte JL, Canawati HN, Montgomerie JZ, Bessman AN. The infected foot of the diabetic patient: quantitative microbiology and analysis of clinical features. *Rev Infect Dis* 1984; **6**: S171–6.

3 Lipsky BA, Berendt AR, Deery HG, Embil JM, Joseph WS, Karchmer AW, LeFrock JL, Lew DP, Mader JT, Norden C, Tan JS. Diagnosis and treatment of diabetic foot infections. *Clin Infect Dis* 2004; **39**: 885–910.

4   Cacciatori V, Dellera A, Bellavere F, Bongiovanni LG, Teatini F, Gemma ML, Muggeo M. Comparative assessment of peripheral sympathetic function by postural vasoconstriction arteriolar reflex and sympathetic skin response in NIDDM patients. *Am J Med* 1997; **102**: 365–70.

5   Cruciani M, Lipsky BA, Mengoli C, de Lalla F. Are granulocyte colony–stimulating factors beneficial in treating diabetic foot infections? A meta-analysis. *Diabetes Care* 2005; **28**: 454–60.

Managing Diabetes

15   Insulin pumps

16   Type 1 diabetes and exercise

17   Adolescent diabetes

18   Low-carbohydrate diets

19   Treatments that stimulate insulin production

20   Treatments that improve insulin resistance

21   Diabetes and enteral feeding

22   Obesity and diabetes

23   Diabetes in the elderly

PROBLEM

15 Insulin Pumps

Case History

A 25-year-old teacher with type 1 diabetes has unpredictable hypoglycaemia which she finds embarrassing in front of her class. She has been running her sugars high to avoid this and is worried about the consequences. She has read about insulin pump therapy and wishes to try this.

Is she a candidate for treatment with an insulin pump?

What are the potential benefits?

Are there any pitfalls?

Background

Insulin pump therapy uses a portable, programmable infusion pump to deliver a continuous subcutaneous infusion of insulin (CSII) to the patient. The infused insulin is generally a rapid-acting insulin analogue to minimize lag in insulin delivery to the bloodstream caused by di- and hexamerization of soluble insulin in subcutaneous tissues. A basal infusion rate is set to mimic physiological background insulin production and carbohydrate intake is matched to insulin boluses to mimic physiological prandial insulin release—as far as possible. This requires significant patient motivation so that the basal rate does not cause fasting hypo- or hyperglycaemia and prandial insulin boluses correspond appropriately to carbohydrate intake.

Uptake of CSII has increased significantly following the publication of the DCCT (Diabetes Control and Complications Trial)[1] in which 42% of patients in the tight control group were on CSII for the last full year of study. Increased uptake of CSII has been supported by technological developments that have reduced the size of insulin pumps and improved the systems to alert the user to equipment failure. Equipment failure was responsible for ketoacidosis and death in some of the earliest trials of insulin pump therapy.

In many European industrialized nations and the United States, approximately 10% of patients with type 1 diabetes now use CSII to manage their diabetes. An economic analysis carried out by the National Institute for Health and Clinical Excellence in the United Kingdom identified the annual cost of CSII compared to multiple daily injections (MDI) as approximately £1400. This took into account the initial cost of the pump—designed for a three-year lifecycle before servicing/replacement, the cost of consumables and subtracted savings from reducing complications through improved glycaemic control. As these savings are reliant on reducing complications through improved glycaemic control, the guidance concluded that CSII should be reserved for patients with a high level of self-care who cannot maintain a glycosylated haemoglobin (HbA1c) <7.5% (<6.5% with microalbuminuria) without disabling hypoglycaemia, despite MDI with insulin analogues. It also concluded that a meaningful estimate of the cost of a quality-adjusted life-year for a patient with type 1 diabetes using CSII rather than MDI was impossible to calculate. This was because of the difficulties in quantifying the economic cost of unpredictable hypoglycaemia and because MDI with newer insulin analogues had not been compared to CSII with newer insulin pumps.

CSII is effective in treating diabetes, but works best following structured education and with the support of an experienced diabetes care team (Figure 15.1). CSII is most effective in treating type 1 diabetes in a relatively narrow range of indications:

● where the dawn phenomenon makes nocturnal and morning blood sugar difficult to control;

● where there is significant day-to-day variability of glycaemia;

● where insulin requirements are relatively low.

Reduction in HbA1c with CSII is, on average, 0.5%, though observational studies suggest that this is in conjunction with a reduction in severe hypoglycaemic events,[2] body weight stability and modest improvement in quality of life measures.

Recent Developments

1   A recent pooled analysis of randomized trials of CSII versus MDI regimens with prandial rapid-acting insulin analogues[3] showed that CSII was associated with a lowering of HbA1c of approximately 0.3%. However, high patient motivation within a trial setting and an inability to blind studies of CSII makes interpretation of data difficult.

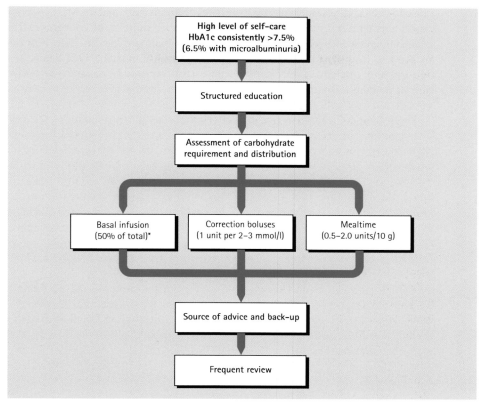

Fig. 15.1 Approach to insulin pump therapy. *the background insulin dose usually varies during the 24-hour period.

2   The role of CSII in children is not yet clear. There are undoubtedly patients in whom CSII reduces hospital admission and improves metabolic control by ensuring a constant supply of insulin. However, randomized trials of CSII and MDI have shown little difference in HbA1c or quality of life.[4]

Conclusion

 It is important to assess the patient's motivation for pump use and understanding of diabetes, and assess whether there are psychological barriers to effective insulin pump use. For example, there may be a misunderstanding that an insulin pump is a closed-loop system that requires little or no user input. Also, body self-image is frequently affected in insulin pump users because diabetes becomes externally visible, and well-being becomes dependent upon technology rather than an injection that the patient knows has been given.

Insulin pump therapy may also require significant educational input. The suggested usual practice is to ensure that carbohydrate counting and pre-prandial and bedtime blood glucose monitoring are incorporated as part of usual diabetes self-management prior to a final decision about a trial of CSII. This ensures that an MDI regimen is optimized through dose adjustment of appropriate prandial and background insulins—including trials of both short- and long-acting analogue insulin. This may sufficiently reduce the impact of the unexpected hypoglycaemic attacks. CSII, then, remains an option but is unlikely to provide better glycaemic control. If, despite a high level of self-care of diabetes, disabling hypoglycaemia persists, then a trial of CSII is probably warranted.

There is no definitive way to calculate starting rates of insulin administration for CSII. The suggested practice is to subtract 10–20% of the total daily dose of insulin used for MDI and to give half of this as background insulin, evenly delivered over 24 hours. The remainder is given as prandial insulin. Fine-tuning requires experience in insulin pump use. For example, checking the afternoon basal insulin rate requires measurement of blood glucose before, two hours after and four hours after deliberate omission of the lunchtime meal to ensure that the basal insulin rate does not cause fasting hypo- or hyperglycaemia. This process needs to be repeated for the basal rate overnight, at breakfast and at the evening meal. Prandial insulin is then adjusted by defining and adjusting a ratio of carbohydrate to insulin. The glycaemic index of the meal can be accounted for by varying the duration of administration of the mealtime bolus.

With long-term commitment, CSII may mitigate some of the problems that this 25-year-old teacher is having with inter-prandial hypoglycaemia. However, efforts to optimize an MDI regime with dietetic support, education and trial of insulin analogue therapy would be reasonable; not least because such intervention is likely to provide a secure foundation for an effective trial of CSII.

Further Reading

1 The Diabetes Control and Complications Trial Research Group. The effect of intensive treatment of diabetes on the development and progression of long-term complications in insulin-dependent diabetes mellitus. *N Engl J Med* 1993; **329**: 977–86.

2 Bode B, Steed R, Davidson P. Reduction in severe hypoglycemia with long-term continuous subcutaneous insulin infusion in type I diabetes. *Diabetes Care* 1996; **19**: 324–7.

3 Retnakaran R, Hochman J, DeVries JH, Hanaire BH, Heine RJ, Melki V, Zinman B. Continuous subcutaneous insulin infusion versus multiple daily injections: the impact of baseline A1c. *Diabetes Care* 2004; **27**: 2590–6.

4 Fox LA, Buckloh LM, Smith SD, Wysocki T, Mauras N. A randomized controlled trial of insulin pump therapy in young children with type 1 diabetes. *Diabetes Care* 2005; **28**: 1277–81.

16 Type 1 Diabetes and Exercise

Case History

A 28-year-old office worker with type 1 diabetes is training for a 10 km fun run. She can run for 3–4 km without problems but is finding it difficult to extend her training runs without becoming hypoglycaemic. Her general level of glycaemic control is satisfactory and she has no diabetic complications or other health problems.

How would you manage her insulin therapy?

What dietary advice would you give?

Background

The body selects fuel for muscles depending on the duration and intensity of exercise. Maintaining fuel supply for endurance running requires significant physiological adaptability. Initially, muscle activity is dependent upon muscle glucose, muscle glycogen and glucose from the peripheral circulation which enters muscle cells via the glucose transporter, GLUT4, which is an insulin-dependent mechanism. As exercise continues, insulin levels drop, while glucagon, adrenaline, noradrenaline, cortisol and growth hormone levels rise. This shift stimulates hepatic glycogenolysis and mobilization of triglycerides from fat. This allows muscle fuel supply to be maintained by sources not based on exhaustible muscle glycogen—glycerol is a substrate for hepatic gluconeogenesis, free fatty acids are used directly by exercising muscles and glucose derives from hepatic glycogenolysis. Training for endurance running also enhances efficiency in fuel use by increasing mitochondrial activity, the proportion of slow twitch muscle fibres and muscle capillary density.

Type 1 diabetes may interfere with exercise in a number of ways:

- very fine adjustment of circulating insulin levels is difficult with subcutaneous insulin administration;

- inadequate insulin may inhibit initial uptake of glucose by muscle and cause exercise-induced hyperglycaemia and performance to suffer;

- excessive insulin may cause early hypoglycaemia or inhibition of lipolysis and hepatic glycogenolysis;

- physiological counter-regulatory hormone release during exercise may interfere with the recognition of hypoglycaemia;

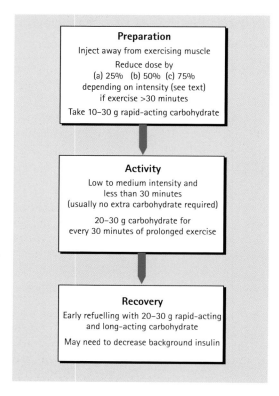

Preparation
Inject away from exercising muscle
Reduce dose by
(a) 25% (b) 50% (c) 75%
depending on intensity (see text)
if exercise >30 minutes
Take 10–30 g rapid-acting carbohydrate

Activity
Low to medium intensity and
less than 30 minutes
(usually no extra carbohydrate required)

20–30 g carbohydrate for
every 30 minutes of prolonged exercise

Recovery
Early refuelling with 20–30 g rapid-acting
and long-acting carbohydrate

May need to decrease background insulin

Fig. 16.1 Management of insulin and carbohydrate intake for exercise in a patient with type 1 diabetes.

● patients with longer duration of diabetes or antecedent hypoglycaemia may have blunted release of counter-regulatory hormones. This may also make hypoglycaemia difficult to detect[1,2] and inhibit energy supply from triglycerides.

The suggested approach is to divide exercise into preparation, activity and recovery to ensure that each phase is appropriately managed (Figure 16.1). Appropriate adjustment of insulin and carbohydrate intake for exercise will allow normal athletic performance in a patient with type 1 diabetes. However, a significant amount of trial and error is usually necessary.

Preparation

Insulin may be absorbed more rapidly from subcutaneous fat overlying exercising muscle, so use of an alternative insulin administration site is suggested—for example the abdomen, prior to jogging. Prandial insulin prior to exercise should also be reduced, particularly if the exercise duration is over 30 minutes or so. To some extent this mimics normal physiological lowering of insulin levels, and may reduce the risk of hypoglycaemia and allow a switch from carbohydrate to fatty acid as fuel. It is difficult to be prescriptive about prandial insulin reduction and experimentation is necessary.

It is usual to reduce the insulin dose in proportion to perceived exercise intensity:

● by 25% if conversation is easy while exercising (walking—<65% of maximal oxygen uptake [VO_2max]);

- by 50% if it is difficult to complete a sentence (jogging—~75% VO₂max);

- by 75% if talking is impossible (fast running, football—>80% VO₂max).

However, if blood sugar is high (>15 mmol/l) prior to exercise, this suggests that there is insufficient insulin to allow glucose entry into muscle and a small dose (1 or 2 units) of quick-acting insulin may be needed.

Conversely, low blood sugar (<5 mmol/l) prior to exercise increases the risk of hypoglycaemia, and 10–30 grams of rapid-acting carbohydrate should be taken in advance of exercise. Also, if it has not been possible to reduce insulin prior to exercise, rapid-acting carbohydrate usually needs to be taken.

Activity

Where exercise duration is less than 30 minutes, extra carbohydrate does not usually need to be taken during exercise. However, 20–30 grams of rapidly absorbed carbohydrate is usually needed every 30 minutes during prolonged exercise. This is usually taken either as a sports drink or as solid, rapidly digested carbohydrate. A sports drink has the benefit of supporting hydration.

Recovery

After exercise, the body replenishes depleted glycogen stores. This may cause a tendency toward hypoglycaemia for 4–8 hours or more, depending on the intensity and duration of exercise. Early refuelling is usually advised, with 10–30 grams of fast-acting carbohydrate after exercise, and longer-acting carbohydrate taken at the same time. The background insulin dose following exercise may also need to be cut by 30% or so to prevent late hypoglycaemia. This will usually be the insulin taken before bed. Long-acting insulin analogues can be difficult to adjust in this situation because of their long half-life.

Recent Developments

1   Nuclear magnetic resonance (NMR) spectroscopy is a technique described relatively recently for non-invasive study of the metabolism of glucose. Glucose is labelled with ¹³C—a stable isotope of carbon. ¹³C-enriched glucose is infused at a fixed rate and insulin is co-administered to 'clamp' glycaemia and the stability of ¹³C enrichment. Once at steady state, ¹³C glucose has a characteristic NMR signal and glucose disposal to muscle and liver can be followed.[3] This minimally invasive technique has significantly reduced or eliminated the need for liver and muscle biopsy during physiological study. One recent study has shown that carbohydrate during exercise is derived more from gluconeogenesis than from glycogenolysis in patients with type 1 diabetes compared to people without diabetes.[4] This observation and other ongoing studies should provide further insights into exercise physiology and so aid adaptation of insulin regimens for exercise in patients with diabetes.

Conclusion

The patient should be supported in her cardiovascular training because of the general benefits of increased physical activity. Early hypoglycaemia during activity suggests inadequate preparation for exercise. The advice given will depend significantly on her insulin regimen.

1 If she is on a basal bolus regimen, preparation for exercise is advised, as outlined above.

2 If she uses insulin pump therapy, preparation for exercise is again advised, as outlined above. The background insulin should be reduced approximately two hours prior to exercise, and may need to remain reduced for many hours after exercise.

3 If she is on a twice daily mixed regimen and does not wish to change to a basal bolus regimen, reduction in insulin dose prior to exercise may be difficult. The time–action profile of mixed insulins means that insulin reduction prior to exercise is likely to cause significant hyperglycaemia. It may be simpler to leave the insulin regimen stable, but take fast-acting carbohydrate prior to exercise.

Finally, as her exercise programme improves insulin sensitivity, she may need to reduce both background and mealtime insulin doses to prevent hypoglycaemia.

Further Reading

1   Sandoval DA, Guy DLA, Richardson MA, Ertl AC, Davis SN. Effects of low and moderate antecedent exercise on counterregulatory responses to subsequent hypoglycemia in type 1 diabetes. *Diabetes* 2004; **53**: 1798–806.

2   Ertl AC, Davis SN. Evidence for a vicious cycle of exercise and hypoglycemia in type 1 diabetes mellitus. *Diabetes Metab Res Rev* 2004; **20**: 124–30.

3   Bloch G, Velho G. Metabolic investigations in humans by in vivo nuclear magnetic resonance. Recommendations of ALFEDIAM (French Language Association for the Study of Diabetes and Metabolic Diseases). *Diabetes Metab* 1997; **23**: 343–50.

4   Petersen KF, Price TB, Bergeron R. Regulation of net hepatic glycogenolysis and gluconeogenesis during exercise: impact of type 1 diabetes. *J Clin Endocrinol Metab* 2004; **89**: 4656–64.

17 Adolescent Diabetes

Case History

A 16-year-old student has very poor glycaemic control with glycosylated haemoglobin (HbA1c) 12.2%. At his first visit to the adult diabetes service he says that he does very few blood tests. He wishes to improve his control as he appreciates the potential for problems in the future.

What approach would you take?

How would you manage his insulin therapy?

Background

Type 1 diabetes in adolescence can pose challenges to healthcare systems for which there are no easy answers. Adolescence is a time when patients take more responsibility for diabetes self-management. Boundary-testing and risk-taking behaviour mean that poor glycaemic control in type 1 diabetes is not unusual in adolescence and transition to adult services.[1] Influencing diabetes self-management at this stage may have long-standing effects on beliefs and attitudes toward diabetes in adulthood. Diabetes education in childhood is often directed toward parents or guardians. The greater independence that comes with adolescence often means that self-care strategies are inadequately applied and insufficient to maintain good glycaemic control. Though adolescence confers some protection against incident complications of diabetes, these will develop as adult physiology becomes established.

It is not unusual for adolescents with poor glycaemic control to have suffered repeated admissions to hospital—often with ketoacidosis—despite repeated efforts by healthcare staff to support lower-risk behaviour. The term 'brittle diabetes' has been coined to identify 'the patient whose life is constantly disrupted by episodes of hyper- or hypoglycaemia, whatever their cause'.[2] Referral to adult/transitional services often means that the patient is re-evaluated by a new clinical team. Adequate handover of previous psychological interventions and social circumstances is important as these are likely to be more useful in developing a successful treatment strategy than more 'mechanistic' medical information about insulin doses and sugar levels.

A consultation—particularly in adolescence—is more likely to be effective if it is structured toward an agreed common agenda than if it is disease- and complication-focused (Figure 17.1). The American Medical Association has developed guidance on a strategy to integrate preventive care into routine consultation with adolescents.[3] Though not specifically targeted to diabetes, it is a useful model.

1   Gather information

2   Further assess

3   Identify and prioritize problems together

4   Develop solutions together

5   Follow up

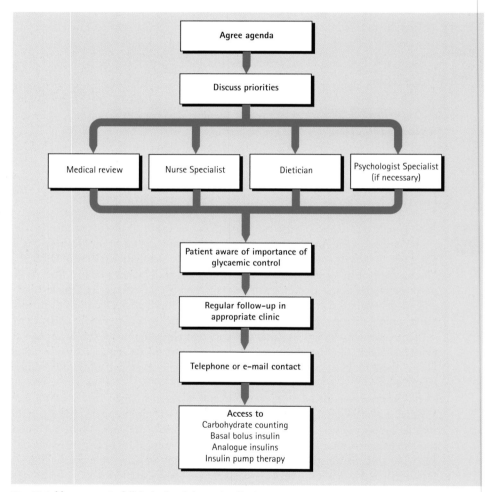

Fig. 17.1 Management of diabetes in adolescent patients.

Recent Developments

1   The National Health Service in the United Kingdom recently commissioned a review of educational and psychological interventions for adolescents with diabetes.[4] This was to determine if there were interventions which were effective in improving biological or psychosocial outcomes. Sixty-two studies were included, which examined

interventions such as learning social and coping skills, individual and family therapy, learning problem-solving skills and diabetes-related education in both individual and group settings. Many had small to medium beneficial effects and the review noted that such interventions are already generally regarded as integral to clinical services. However, the review also commented that it was not clear whether stratification of interventions should be by stage of diabetes, age of patient or specific problem, and whether individual or group intervention was more effective.

Conclusion

Ideally, the first contact with adult services should be as part of a managed transition from paediatric services, rather than during an intercurrent metabolic crisis. Joint clinics and consultations are probably most effective in achieving this. Comprehensive psychological, medical and educational input may all be needed and it is important that these are appropriately prioritized as part of a jointly agreed management plan. For example, dysfunctional home or school relationships, depression, illicit drug or alcohol use, lipohypertrophy and poor knowledge or skills in diabetes management may individually or jointly contribute to poor overall control.

Adolescence and the transition to adult diabetes services is frequently marked by intermittent outpatient attendance. Though this can be frustrating for healthcare providers, an overly punitive attitude is counter-productive, further reducing attendance and opportunities to support lower-risk behaviours.

The HbA1c of 12.2% suggests significant under-dosing of insulin. If long-standing, this has potentially life-threatening consequences—if accompanied by episodes of metabolic decompensation—and also increases long-term risks of microvascular complications. It is likely that the patient is aware of these risks. The most serious potential consequence of poor glycaemic control is death from ketoacidosis. It is important to ensure that the patient has access to clear information about self-management of hyperglycaemia/illness and knows when and how to seek help. The family, school and other significant individuals or institutions should have access to a personalized diabetes management plan and supplies so that a metabolic crisis can be swiftly and appropriately treated if the patient is unable to do this.

For a female patient it is important to discuss pregnancy, as the poor glycaemic control described in this case history puts a foetus at unnecessary risk of malformation, and increases risk of pre-eclampsia and pre-term delivery.

It is unlikely that the insulin regimen alone is the cause of poor glycaemic control. However, transition to adult services is an opportunity to provide structured diabetes education to ensure appropriate access to carbohydrate counting, basal bolus regimens, analogue insulin and insulin pump therapy.

Further Reading

1 Wills CJ, Scott A, Swift PGF, Davies MJ, Mackie ADR, Mansell P. Retrospective review of care and outcomes in young adults with type 1 diabetes. *BMJ* 2003; **327**: 260–1.

2 Tattersall R. Brittle diabetes. *Clin Endocrinol Metab* 1977; **6**: 403–19.

3 Levenberg PB, Elster AB. Guidelines for Adolescent Preventive Services: Clinical Evaluation and Management Handbook. Chicago: American Medical Association, 1995.

4 Hampson SE, Skinner TC, Hart J, Storey L, Gage H, Foxcroft D, Kimber A, Shaw K, Walker J. Effects of educational and psychosocial interventions for adolescents with diabetes mellitus: a systematic review. *Health Technol Assess* 2001; **5**: 1–79.

PROBLEM

18 Low-Carbohydrate Diets

Case History

A 55-year-old business man is referred to you because his diabetic control is deteriorating. He is overweight (body mass index 32 kg/m²) and is currently treated with metformin 500 mg and gliclazide 80 mg—both twice daily. He has tried a number of diets without success and would like to know whether he might benefit from a low-carbohydrate diet.

Is this dietary approach sensible in view of his diabetes?

How should his oral hypoglycaemic drugs be managed?

What benefits can he expect from the diet?

Are there any ill effects he should be warned about?

Background

The notion that a low-carbohydrate diet may be beneficial has been around for well over a century. The diets have become very popular and the popular literature in this area has, until recently, advanced considerably more rapidly than the scientific literature. The book describing the Atkins diet has sold over ten million copies, and around a million people in the United Kingdom are currently using the diets at any one time. The macronutrient content of low-carbohydrate, high-protein diets is very different to that of the traditional diabetic diet (55% carbohydrate, 15% protein and 30% fat). The reluctance of the health professions to recommend and support patients in using these diets is, therefore, understandable.

The literature on low-carbohydrate diets in relation to diabetes was recently reviewed.[1] Under normal circumstances, carbohydrate is the preferred metabolic fuel, and is oxidized in the body in preference to other fuels. When carbohydrate is consumed in excess, it is turned into fat and stored. The body has very limited capacity to store either carbohydrate or protein, but an enormous capacity to store fat. There has been considerable debate over the years about the optimal macronutrient content for a healthy diet. The current recommendations for a diet relatively high in carbohydrate arose from observations that a diet high in carbohydrate, including substantial amounts of complex carbohydrate, had a favourable effect on glucose tolerance and lipid profile. Consumption of carbohydrate in excess of caloric needs gives rise to fat deposition, not only from the excess carbohydrate that is consumed, but also from other metabolic fuels. Low-carbohydrate diets tend to be relatively high in protein. High-protein diets are not recommended in the long-term for patients with diabetes since they tend to increase progression of renal disease. However, there is evidence from short-term metabolic studies that high-protein intake improves carbohydrate tolerance.

Severe carbohydrate restriction induces ketosis. This is an important adaptation to starvation. Ketone bodies are critical energy substrates for the brain and heart in times of calorie restriction. They allow vital organs to adapt to very low glucose concentrations by inducing expression of glucose transporter (GLUT4) and key enzymes in intermediary metabolism. It is not clear at present how strict carbohydrate restriction has to be for a low-carbohydrate diet to be effective. However, from published trials, it does appear that diets that at least have a period of severe restriction are more effective than those that advocate only modest carbohydrate restriction. What is clear from the published trials is that the diets are only effective if they are hypocaloric. Patients who are prone to, or have, type 2 diabetes experience wider fluctuations in their blood glucose than those without diabetes. This may be an important mechanism driving hunger: high blood glucose in a patient who is hyperinsulinaemic leads to a relative reactive hypoglycaemia, and the normal response to this is to eat. Decreased glucose fluctuations, adaptation to a relatively low glucose state, and satiety induced by the high-protein content of the diets may all contribute to their effectiveness. There is now sufficient literature on this subject to allow the conclusion that the diets are safe for short- to medium-term use, and that they are effective for periods up to six months. Care has to be taken that the diets are calorie restricted, and there are no grounds for recommending unrestricted consumption of fat to compensate for the reduction in carbohydrate. Like all diets, they will be most effective if they are used in conjunction with a programme of regular exercise (Figure 18.1).

A recent short-term study by Boden et al.[2] confirmed that a low-carbohydrate diet decreased weight and improved insulin sensitivity in severely obese subjects (Figure 18.2). Even though subjects were allowed unrestricted fat and protein, the restricted nature of the diet led to a voluntary decrease in energy intake. A recent randomized trial by Aude and colleagues[3] demonstrates that a calorie-controlled diet with only modest carbohydrate restriction is more effective than a standard low-calorie, low-fat diet. Gannon and Nuttall[4] studied the effects of a low-carbohydrate diet in a short-term study involving patients with type 2 diabetes. Dramatic improvements in glucose control were demonstrated. Fears that low-carbohydrate diets may worsen lipid profile are not borne out by recent studies. Indeed, a number of studies now clearly demonstrate improvements in features of the metabolic syndrome. We do not know about the long-term effects of low-carbohydrate diets, but we know enough to support patients in the use of these diets for periods up to six months.

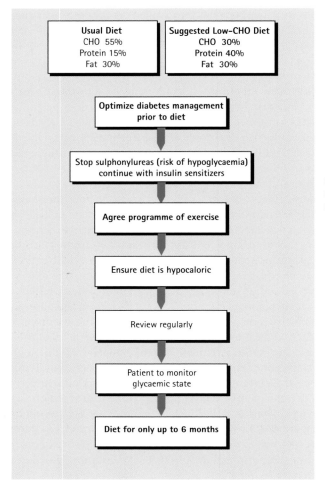

Fig. 18.1 Managing low-carbohydrate diet in patients with diabetes. CHO = carbohydrate.

Recent Developments

1   Low-carbohydrate diets are not recommended for routine management of patients with diabetes.[5] This is because carbohydrates are important sources of energy and carbohydrate-containing foods also contain other important nutrients. The concept of glycaemic load has emerged. This is a notional product of the amount of carbohydrate consumed and the availability of the carbohydrate. High glycaemic load predisposes to obesity and glucose intolerance. Low glycaemic index (GI) diets, in which the carbohydrate is slowly broken down and released, are currently very popular. A recent randomized, controlled trial of a low GI diet[6] confirmed the potential of such diets to improve glycaemic control in patients with type 2 diabetes.

2   There is now considerable evidence that consumption of foods rich in whole-grain also improves carbohydrate tolerance. Extensive population-based studies have confirmed that whole-grain consumption improves insulin sensitivity[7] and decreases the

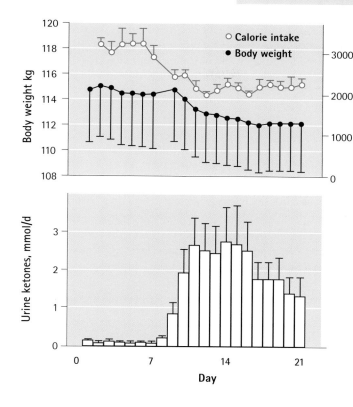

Fig. 18.2 A comparison of the effect of usual diet (days 1 to 7) with low-carbohydrate diet (days 8 to 21) in patients with type 2 diabetes. As subjects develop ketonuria on the low-carbohydrate diet (bottom panel), both calorie intake and body weight decrease (top panel).
Source: Boden et al. 2005.[2]

risk of developing type 2 diabetes.[8] It is not known whether these benefits are attributable to the complex carbohydrate components of whole-grain food or to micronutrients contained in such foods.

Conclusion

 The patient is overweight and has poor diabetic control. Standard dietary approaches often do not work in such patients. Calorie restriction by whatever means will lead to weight loss and thus improvement in metabolic parameters. We are not in a position to recommend low-carbohydrate diets at present. However, many patients choose these diets and we need to offer sensible advice to them. There is no evidence that, when used for periods up to six months, there is any harmful effect from the use of a low-carbohydrate diet.

There is no evidence base from which to draw recommendations on use of oral hypoglycaemic drugs during this type of diet. The diet needs to be regarded as a short-term intervention rather than a long-term lifestyle change. It is certainly suggested that the patient stop taking gliclazide for the duration of his diet. The drug may limit his weight loss and could cause hypoglycaemia. His insulin sensitivity should improve as he loses weight and there would be an argument for seeing if he can manage without metformin as well. With limited carbohydrate intake, his glycaemic control is likely to improve. However, as with any situation where treatment is altered, he should monitor his blood glucose carefully and report any changes. The demonstration of improved glucose control, weight loss and reduction in therapy, in association with a diet that is not too restricted and does not leave the patient feeling permanently hungry, can be quite empowering for the patient who is sufficiently motivated and knowledgeable to adhere to a low-carbohydrate diet.

Further Reading

1 Kennedy R, Chokkalingam K, Farshchi H. Nutrition in patients with type 2 diabetes: are low-carbohydrate diets effective, safe or desirable? *Diabet Med* 2005; **22**: 821–32.

2 Boden G, Sargrad K, Homko C, Mozzoli M, Stein TP. Effect of a low-carbohydrate diet on appetite, blood glucose levels, and insulin resistance in obese patients with type 2 diabetes. *Ann Intern Med* 2005; **142**: 403–11.

3 Aude YW, Agatston AS, Lopez-Jimenez F, Lieberman EH, Almon M, Hansen M, Rojas G, Lamas GA, Hennekens CHl. The National Cholesterol Education Program Diet vs a diet lower in carbohydrates and higher in protein and monounsaturated fat: a randomized trial. *Arch Intern Med* 2004; **164**: 2141–6.

4 Gannon MC, Nuttall FQ. Effect of a high-protein, low-carbohydrate diet on blood glucose control in people with type 2 diabetes. *Diabetes* 2004; **53**: 2375–82.

5 Sheard NF, Clark NG, Brand-Miller JC, Franz MJ, Pi-Sunyer FX, Mayer-Davis E, Kulkarni K, Geil P. Dietary carbohydrate (amount and type) in the prevention and management of diabetes: a statement by the American Diabetes Association. *Diabetes Care* 2004; **27**: 2266–71.

6 Rizkalla SW, Taghrid L, Laromiguiere M, Huet D, Boillot J, Rigoir A, Elgrably F, Slama G. Improved plasma glucose control, whole-body glucose utilization, and lipid profile on a low-glycemic index diet in type 2 diabetic men: a randomized controlled trial. *Diabetes Care* 2004; **27**: 1866–72.

7 Liese AD, Roach AK, Sparks KC, Marquart L, D'Agostino RB, Mayer DEJ. Whole-grain intake and insulin sensitivity: the Insulin Resistance Atherosclerosis Study. *Am J Clin Nutr* 2003; **78**: 965–71.

8 Montonen J, Knekt P, Järvinen R, Aromaa A, Reunanen A. Whole-grain and fiber intake and the incidence of type 2 diabetes. *Am J Clin Nutr* 2003; **77**: 622–9.

19 Treatments that Stimulate Insulin Production

Case History

A 62-year-old man with mild essential hypertension, but generally fit, was diagnosed with type 2 diabetes six months ago. He has altered his diet as suggested by his general practitioner and dietician, but his blood glucose remains high at 12–15 mmol/l, and is particularly high later in the day. He is not overweight and he has no family history of note.

What is the best treatment for his diabetes?

He would like to know if he is likely to require insulin therapy in the future.

What are the chances of the first line of treatment chosen keeping his diabetes under control?

Background

In the United States in 1990, there were around 23 million prescriptions issued for oral hypoglycaemic drugs. These were almost entirely for sulphonylureas. A decade later, the number of prescriptions had risen to over 90 million. While the variety of drugs had increased, sulphonylureas were still the most commonly prescribed drugs for type 2 diabetes, and are the initial treatment of choice for patients who are not overweight (Figure 19.1). The drugs bind to a complex of the sulphonylurea receptor (SUR) and an ATP-sensitive potassium channel (kir6.2) on the surface of the pancreatic beta cell. Binding of the drug leads to closure of the potassium channels, as a result of which potassium efflux is inhibited, the cell becomes depolarized, and calcium channels in the endoplasmic reticulum open. Contraction of microtubules in response to this leads to exocytosis of insulin.[1] The available sulphonylurea drugs include gliclazide, glibenclamide and glimepiride. All have similar potency in decreasing glycosylated haemoglobin (HbA1c) by between 1.0% and 1.5% in the short to medium term. The older sulphonylureas, tolbutamide (short-acting) and chlorpopamide (long-acting), are now rarely used. This group of drugs is generally well tolerated, sometimes causing mild gastrointestinal upset and occasionally causing allergic reactions. The most common side effects are weight gain and hypoglycaemia. One can expect a patient starting sulphonylureas to gain 2–5 kg in the first few months. Hypoglycaemia is generally mild but may affect up to 2% of treated patients per year. Glimepiride and modified-release gliclazide are convenient preparations as they can be taken once daily.

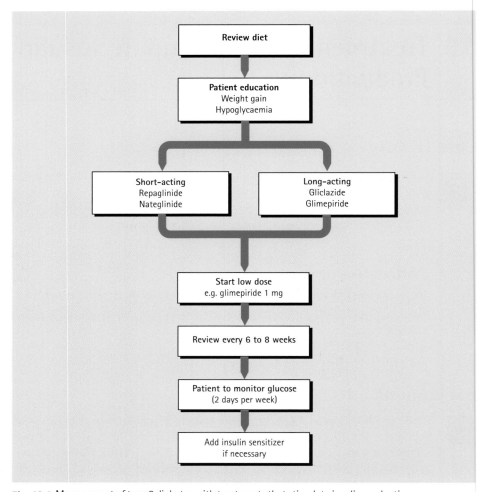

Fig. 19.1 Management of type 2 diabetes with treatments that stimulate insulin production.

Repaglinide, a benzoic acid derivative, and nateglinide, a phenylalanine derivative, bind to sites on the SUR distinct to those to which sulphonylureas bind. However, these agents have a more rapid onset of action and a shorter half-life. These agents specifically target the post-prandial increase in blood glucose. Repaglinide has potency, in terms of decreasing HbA1c, similar to that of the sulphonylureas, while nateglinide is a little less potent. Because of their shorter duration of action they are less likely to cause either hypoglycaemia or weight gain. Their major disadvantage is that they have to be taken three times per day with meals. Use is flexible in that the drug may be omitted if the patient chooses to skip a meal.

Improved glycaemic control with insulin secretagogue treatment is often not sustained. Treatment failure is probably determined largely by factors within the beta cell leading to decreased insulin production with time, and with prolonged exposure to high glucose concentration. Secondary treatment failure occurs in about 5–7% of sulphony-

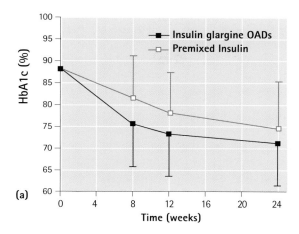

(a)

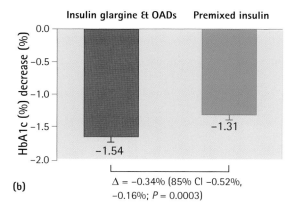

(b)

$\Delta = -0.34\%$ (85% CI −0.52%, −0.16%; $P = 0.0003$)

Fig. 19.2 Addition of basal insulin to oral hypoglycaemic drugs. Data shown are from a 24-week study comparing the effects of twice daily premixed insulin and the combination of basal insulin plus oral antidiabetic drugs (oral antidiabetic agents, OADs). In this study, the combination of insulin and drug achieved superior glycaemic control. Many patients prefer a staged introduction to insulin therapy and as few injections as possible. *Source:* Janka *et al.* 2005.[3]

lurea-treated patients per year. A number of factors may contribute to failure, including deteriorating compliance with diet and exercise, the aging process, weight gain and progressive insulin resistance. Recent data,[2] examining polymorphisms in insulin receptor substrate-1, confirm that both peripheral factors (i.e. outside the beta cell) and genetic factors may be important determinants of treatment failure. For patients who require insulin, a stepwise treatment approach is preferred. Janka *et al.*[3] recently compared two groups of patients with poor control on oral hypoglycaemic drugs: one group changed to twice daily mixed insulin, while the other group continued with metformin plus glimepiride but additionally took a single daily dose of insulin glargine. The latter group achieved better glycaemic control, with less hypoglycaemia, and a greater proportion of them reached the target HbA1c of 7.0% (Figure 19.2).

Recent Developments

1 The 37 amino acid hormone amylin is co-secreted with insulin and, like insulin, is deficient in patients with diabetes. Administration of pramlintide, a synthetic analogue of amylin, has been shown to improve glycaemic control, both in type 1 and

type 2 diabetes.[4,5] The drug both decreases post-prandial excursions in glucagon and delays gastric emptying. By the combination of these two mechanisms, delivery of both exogenous glucose and endogenously produced glucose into the circulation is decreased. Glucose delivery is better matched to the available insulin. Use of the drug leads to decreased peak of glucose after eating, less pre-prandial hypoglycaemia and decreased oxidative stress associated with food intake.

2   Glucagon-like peptide-1 (GLP-1) is an incretin hormone that when secreted physio-logically in response to food intake or administered exogenously both enhances insulin secretion and decreases secretion of glucagon. The hormone also has trophic effects on the pancreatic beta cell, a slowing effect on gastric emptying thus delaying glucose absorption, and a central effect in promoting satiety.[6] Analogues of GLP-1 including exenatide and liraglutide are now in an advanced stage of clinical trials. An alternative approach is inhibition of the enzyme dipeptidyl peptidase IV (DPP-IV), which is responsible for inactivating GLP-1.[7] One major advantage of the DPP-IV inhibitors is that they can be administered orally.

Conclusion

As a lean individual who has almost certainly developed type 2 diabetes, the patient would be most suitably treated with a sulphonylurea drug. The dose of this can be gradually titrated upwards, according to response, in the two months after commencing treatment. The patient should be taught to understand what the treatment goals are and that the drug may not keep his diabetes under control indefinitely. He is relatively young and, with a sulphonylurea failure rate of around 5% per year, he may well require additional treat-ment in time. If treatment with sulphonylurea fails, the next step would generally be to consider treatment with an insulin sensitizer (metformin or a glitazone). Progressive pan-creatic failure with age and duration of diabetes, particularly if glycaemic control is poor, occurs in many patients with type 2 diabetes, but is by no means inevitable. A single daily bolus of long-acting insulin along with oral hypoglycaemic drugs may improve control for many years before the patient eventually becomes fully insulin dependent.

Further Reading

1   Cheng AYY, Fantus IG. Oral antihyperglycemic therapy for type 2 diabetes mellitus. *CMAJ* 2005; **172**: 213–26.

2   Sesti G, Marini MA, Cardellini M, Sciacqua A, Frontoni S, Andreozzi F, Irace C, Lauro D, Gnasso A, Federici M, Perticone F, Lauro R. The Arg972 variant in insulin receptor substrate-1 is associated with an increased risk of secondary failure to sulfonylurea in patients with type 2 diabetes. *Diabetes Care* 2004; **27**: 1394–8.

3   Janka HU, Plewe G, Riddle MC, Kliebe FC, Schweitzer MA, Yki-Järvinen H. Comparison of basal insulin added to oral agents versus twice-daily premixed insulin as initial insulin therapy for type 2 diabetes. *Diabetes Care* 2005; **28**: 254–9.

4   Ceriello A, Piconi L, Quagliaro L, Wang Y, Schnabel CA, Ruggles JA, Gloster MA, Maggs DG, Weyer C. Effects of pramlintide on postprandial glucose excursions and measures of oxidative stress in patients with type 1 diabetes. *Diabetes Care* 2005; **28**: 632–7.

5   Heptulla RA, Rodriguez LM, Bomgaars L, Haymond MW. The role of amylin and glucagon in the dampening of glycemic excursions in children with type 1 diabetes. *Diabetes* 2005; **54**: 1100–7.

6   Holst JJ, Orskov C. The incretin approach for diabetes treatment: modulation of islet hormone release by GLP-1 agonism. *Diabetes* 2004; **53**: S197–204.

7   Ahren B, Gomis R, Standl E, Mills D, Schweizer A. Twelve- and 52-week efficacy of the dipeptidyl peptidase IV inhibitor LAF237 in metformin-treated patients with type 2 diabetes. *Diabetes Care* 2004; **27**: 2874–80.

PROBLEM

20 Treatments that Improve Insulin Resistance

Case History

A 55-year-old woman with hypertension and high cholesterol was diagnosed with diabetes six months ago. She has a body mass index of 29 kg/m² and has not lost significant weight since diagnosis. Her glycosylated haemoglobin (HbA1c) is 8.5%. She is a non-smoker.

Would you start her on drug therapy at this stage?

If so, which would be your first drug of choice?

How long would you wait to either start the first drug or step up her therapy?

What would be the next drug of choice?

Background

Metformin is generally the first drug of choice for the overweight patient with type 2 diabetes. It is the only biguanide drug in general usage. It is inexpensive and safe. The drug acts peripherally by increasing insulin sensitivity, increasing peripheral glucose uptake and decreasing hepatic glucose output. Because the drug can cause severe lactic acidosis, it is relatively contraindicated in patients with renal, cardiac or hepatic failure. The drug can cause nausea, diarrhoea or other gastrointestinal side effects in up to 30% of patients. Sometimes these symptoms improve with time, and the vast majority of patients started on the drug are able to tolerate it. Because of its side effects, it is best administered with food. If only given once a day, the drug is best administered in the evening as it will decrease hepatic over-production of glucose overnight. In the United Kingdom Prospective Diabetes Study (UKPDS), 753 overweight, newly diagnosed type 2 diabetic patients with persisting fasting hyperglycaemia in spite of dietary treatment were randomized in a trial.[1] The patients received diet therapy alone or with metformin. Those allocated metformin achieved a lower HbA1c (7.4% vs 8.0%), and experienced a 32% risk reduction for any diabetes-related endpoint, 42% reduction in diabetes-related death and 36% reduction for all-cause mortality. When compared to patients intensively treated with sulphonylureas or insulin, metformin-treated patients had fewer diabetes-related endpoints, fewer deaths from all causes and fewer strokes. Metformin remains the only hypoglycaemic drug that has been shown to decrease mortality in patients with type 2 diabetes. Recent data from the UKPDS group suggest that insulin resistance *per se* is not a potent cardiovascular risk factor, and the mechanisms through which metformin exerts its protective effect have yet to be elucidated. Apart from its ability to improve glycaemic control and protect against complications, the major advantages of metformin are that it does not provoke weight gain or cause hypoglycaemia.

Thiazolidinediones[2] are agonists at peroxisome proliferator-activated receptors-γ (PPAR-γ), which are predominantly present in adipocytes, pancreatic beta cells, vascular endothelial cells and macrophages. The drugs decrease fasting and post-prandial levels of both glucose and free fatty acids. Generally, use of the drugs decreases HbA1c by 1.0% to 1.5%. This is slightly less than the hypoglycaemic effect seen with maximum doses of glibenclamide, glimepiride or metformin. It was initially hoped that the thiazolidine-diones might improve multiple features of the metabolic syndrome. However, no consistent effects on blood pressure have been documented. Various effects on lipid profile have been reported, with decreased plasma triglycerides being shown more often with pioglitazone than rosiglitazone. PPAR-γ is an essential transcription factor in the differentiation of adipocytes. PPAR-γ agonists increase the number of small adipocytes in subcutaneous tissue. Enhanced lipogenesis through this mechanism, with consequent lowering of free fatty acid levels, may be one of the mechanisms through which the drugs improve insulin sensitivity. The drugs also have beneficial effects on adipocyte hormones, including increasing circulating levels of the protective hormone adiponectin.

Increased subcutaneous adipose tissue is largely responsible for the 2–3 kg weight gain commonly experienced by patients starting a thiazolidinedione. It is possible that this weight gain may partially offset some of the benefits of the drug's action on insulin resistance. In addition, the drugs also increase plasma renin activity leading to salt and water retention with oedema in some patients. Mild decreases in haemoglobin and haematocrit are also apparent in many patients. A liver test should be checked every six weeks or so after starting treatment and the drugs should probably be withdrawn if transaminase levels reach greater than three times normal. Thiazolidinediones are best regarded as second-line insulin-sensitizing drugs, for use in patients who are intolerant of metformin, and in those in whom first-line treatment with metformin or sulphonylurea fails. Thiazolidinediones can be given safely alone, in combination with either metformin or sulphonylurea, or as part of triple therapy with metformin plus sulphonylurea. They are not licensed for use with insulin because of risk of heart failure, although they may help in cases of severe insulin resistance. There are no long-term studies to demonstrate their benefit in preventing the progression of diabetic complications.

In patients whose first-line treatment with sulphonylurea fails, glitazones or metformin probably have similar effects in lowering HbA1c. The glitazones are probably preferable where insulin resistance is severe or where beta cell function is relatively normal. A recent meta-analysis[3] of 23 randomized controlled trials confirms that pioglitazone is slightly superior to rosiglitazone in decreasing triglycerides and increasing high-density lipo-protein (HDL)-cholesterol levels. There has been considerable focus recently on post-prandial excursions of glucose and lipids as independent risk factors for cardiovascular disease. The glitazones may be slightly better than either metformin or sulphonylurea in blunting post-prandial increases in glucose.[4]

Recent Developments

1 A new class of drugs that combines PPAR-α and PPAR-γ agonism is being developed. Ragaglitazar and ertiprotafib are drugs with such properties.[5] These drugs have similar hypoglycaemic potency to the existing glitazones but they have more potent actions in improving diabetic dyslipidaemia (Figure 20.1). PPAR-α is the molecular target for the fibrate group of drugs.

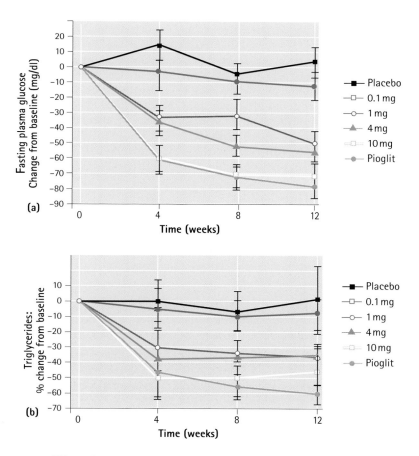

Fig. 20.1 Effects of a combined PPAR-α and PPAR-γ agonist. Data shown are following treatment with the drug ragaglitazar over a 12-week period in patients with hypertriglyceridaemia and type 2 diabetes. The drug improved both glycaemic control (a) and lipid profile (b). At higher doses, ragaglitazar was more potent than pioglitazone (Pioglit). *Source:* Saad *et al.* 2004.[5]

2   The role of pro-inflammatory cytokines and adipokines in the pathogenesis of the metabolic syndrome is well documented. A novel compound that inhibits the inhibitor of kappa B kinase-β (IKKβ) upregulates adiponectin and decreases insulin resistance.[6]

3   A completely new class of drugs are small-molecule insulino-mimetic drugs. A variety of vanadium compounds have the ability to activate components of the insulin signalling pathway,[7] and other molecules act directly at the insulin receptor to produce insulin-like effects.[8] These agents are in the preliminary stages of development at present.

Conclusion

This woman has multiple features of the metabolic syndrome and is at high risk of both micro- and macrovascular complications. Tight glycaemic control will help preserve her residual beta cell function and thus simplify her hypoglycaemic therapy in the medium to long term. The initial drug of first choice would be metformin. There are theoretical grounds in some patients (see above) for starting with a glitazone drug if the predominant abnormality is insulin resistance or if the major abnormality of glucose is in the post-prandial state. There is no ready access to measures of these abnormalities in routine clinical practice. The dose of metformin may be gradually adjusted, according to her response, over a period of about three months. If she remained hyperglycaemic, add-in therapy with either sulphonylurea or glitazone should be considered. For most patients, sulphonylurea seems a logical choice since the patient would then be taking an insulin sensitizer and a secretagogue. However, there is strong evidence that metformin and glitazone together are beneficial, particularly in patients with insulin resistance as the major abnormality.

Further Reading

1   UK Prospective Diabetes Study (UKPDS) Group. Effect of intensive blood-glucose control with metformin on complications in overweight patients with type 2 diabetes (UKPDS 34). *Lancet* 1998; **352**: 854–65.

2   Yki JH. Thiazolidinediones. *N Engl J Med* 2004; **351**: 1106–18.

3   Chiquette E, Ramirez G, Defronzo R. A meta-analysis comparing the effect of thiazolidinediones on cardiovascular risk factors. *Arch Intern Med* 2004; **164**: 2097–2104.

4   Ceriello A, Johns D, Widel M, Eckland DJ, Gilmore KJ, Tan MH. Comparison of effect of pioglitazone with metformin or sulfonylurea (monotherapy and combination therapy) on post load glycemia and composite insulin sensitivity index during an oral glucose tolerance test in patients with type 2 diabetes. *Diabetes Care* 2005; **28**: 266–72.

5   Saad MF, Greco S, Osei K, Lewin AJ, Edwards C, Nunez M, Reinhardt RR. Ragaglitazar improves glycemic control and lipid profile in type 2 diabetic subjects: a 12-week, double-blind, placebo-controlled dose-ranging study with an open pioglitazone arm. *Diabetes Care* 2004; **27**: 1324–9.

6   Kamon J, Yamauchi T, Muto S, Takekawa S, Ito Y, Hada Y, Ogawa W, Itai A, Kasuga M, Tobe K, Kadowaki T. A novel IKKbeta inhibitor stimulates adiponectin levels and ameliorates obesity-linked insulin resistance. *Biochem Biophys Res Commun* 2004; **323**: 242–8.

7 Srivastava AK, Mehdi MZ. Insulino-mimetic and anti-diabetic effects of vanadium compounds. *Diabet Med* 2005; **22**: 2–13.

8 Strowski MZ, Li Z, Szalkowski D, Shen X, Guan XM, Juttner S, Moller DE, Zhang BB. Small-molecule insulin mimetic reduces hyperglycemia and obesity in a nongenetic mouse model of type 2 diabetes. *Endocrinology* 2004; **145**: 5259–68.

PROBLEM

21 Diabetes and Enteral Feeding

Case History

A 64-year-old woman who had a stroke eight weeks ago is referred to you because her diabetes control is erratic. She made a good functional recovery from her stroke but had persistent difficulty swallowing afterwards. Her calorie intake was judged to be insufficient and, after consultation with the patient and her family, she underwent insertion of a percutaneous endoscopic gastrostomy (PEG) tube. She has had diagnosed diabetes for eight years and was taking Mixtard insulin, 26 units in the morning and 20 units in the evening. She will be able to be discharged once her nutrition and diabetes management is sorted out.

How would you advise approaching her nutritional management?

What would be the best approach to her insulin therapy?

Is there any place for oral hypoglycaemic drugs?

Should insulin–requiring diabetes be considered a relative contraindication to PEG feeding?

Background

Around 5% of the general population in the United Kingdom has a body mass index below 20 kg/m^2 and is, therefore, by definition underweight. Ten per cent of patients with chronic diseases are undernourished, and the figure rises to 20% when we consider those hospitalized for medical or surgical reasons. Undernutrition leads to impaired wound healing, decreased muscle strength and thus slower functional recovery, impaired immunity leading to infection, decreased psychological health, and longer hospital stays. With recognition of these factors, along with availability of feeding methods and formulations to meet individual patients' needs, interest in the nutrition of the acutely and chronically unwell patient has increased.

Enteral tube feeding (ETF)—nasogastric, nasojejunal, or through gastrostomy—is the preferred mode of feeding when nutritional support is required and the gastrointestinal tract is functionally intact. It should be considered in any patient who has a good prognosis but is unlikely to be able to sustain their projected calorie intake for more than 5–7 days.[1] The decision to feed may be deferred if the patient is taking in more than 50% of their projected requirement. In general, feeds contain 1 kcal/ml, and use of 30 ml/kg body weight is recommended as a baseline requirement. More concentrated feeds (1.5 kcal/ml) are available. These may be appropriate for patients whose gastrointestinal losses are increased through diarrhoea or malabsorption, or whose calorie intake is increased because of wounds, burns, surgery or other hypercatabolic states. It follows that a 70 kg patient may require over 2 litres of feed per day, and this may give rise to problems because of the tonicity and volume of the feed. The available regimens and formulation types are summarized in Table 21.1.

Table 21.1	Formulations and regimens for enteral feeding	
Formulation	Regimen
Polymeric	Bolus
Oligomeric	Overnight
Elemental	Intermittent
	Continuous

Polymeric or oligomeric (partially hydrolysed) feeds are preferable for patients with diabetes as they are less likely to cause large excursions in blood glucose. The carbohydrate content of feeds is generally high (45–90%). High-carbohydrate feeds tend to decrease high-density lipoprotein (HDL)-cholesterol and increase triglycerides. Formulations with added fibre may decrease diarrhoea associated with feeding, but it is not clear whether they are of benefit metabolically. Disease-specific formulations have proved to be of benefit in a number of areas. Diabetic formulations contain carbohydrate as starch and as fructose. While these do decrease excursions in blood glucose, it is not clear whether they are of long-term benefit in metabolic terms. It is important that the patient receives adequate calories and that this is covered by an appropriate amount of insulin in a suitable regimen.

For the very ill patient, continuous feeding, with insulin administered intravenously in titrated doses using a pump, is probably the treatment of choice.[2] For recuperating, ambulant or out-of-hospital patients, intermittent or bolus feeding is preferred. By estimating energy requirements and tailoring oral hypoglycaemic or insulin therapy to the chosen regimen, it is possible to maintain good glycaemic control in patients with diabetes who are fed via a PEG tube.[3] For insulin-requiring patients, the approach chosen will depend on the target level of control and the ability of the patient and their carers to cooperate. If PEG feed is administered continuously over a substantial part of the day, this may be best covered by an injection of isophane insulin given 15–30 minutes before the onset of feeding. Patients fed with a bolus regimen are best covered by injections of soluble or short-acting analogue insulin (depending on the length of the infusion) given before, or at the start of, each feed. In addition, patients who are truly insulin-dependent may require background insulin, the dose of which should be adjusted according to fasting glucose.

Complications of PEG feeding include diarrhoea, bloating, reflux, constipation, skin infection and tube blockage or displacement. Patients should be monitored closely for metabolic abnormalities, particularly in the early days after starting feeding. These include hypo- or hypernatraemia, depending upon whether other fluid is being administered. Ten per cent to 30% of patients (irrespective of whether they have diabetes or not) become hyperglycaemic. Severely malnourished patients may develop refeeding syndrome where initiation of feeding is associated with loss of intracellular, and therefore whole body, potassium, calcium, magnesium and phosphate. Many of these problems can be avoided by starting feeding gradually.

Recent Developments

1 The recently published FOOD (feed or ordinary diet) trials[4] add considerably to the body of knowledge on the approach to nutritional support following stroke. Routine oral dietary supplementation appeared not to influence outcome. Early, as opposed to late, ETF decreased mortality by 5.8%. Early PEG feeding was associated with increased adverse events. It seems clear, therefore, that nasogastric feeding should be considered early in dysphagic stroke patients whose prognosis is thought to be reasonable. PEG feeding should be reserved for a later stage if nasogastric feeding is not tolerated or PEG is the preferred option of the patient and carers for the longer term.

2 In a randomized trial[5] a traditional high-carbohydrate, low-fat feed was compared with a low-carbohydrate, high-monounsaturated fat feed in hospitalized patients with type 2 diabetes. The low-carbohydrate feed showed significant benefits in terms of glycaemic and lipid parameters. It is clear that further studies are required to determine the optimal feed composition for patients with diabetes who require enteral feeding.

Conclusion

Early ETF via nasogastric tube is indicated in stroke patients. Those who make a good recovery and require long-term feeding may benefit from PEG feeding, if that is the wish of the patient and their carers, and if they are able to cope with it (Figure 21.1). Ideally, the diabetes management should be planned directly with the nutrition team. An assessment of the calorie needs should be made and periodic nutritional assessment should be undertaken. If the patient lacks endogenous insulin and is not administered suitable doses of exogenous insulin, they are unlikely to benefit from enteral feeding. Attempts should be made to match the profile of the insulin regimen to that of their food intake and to provide sufficient background insulin to control fasting glucose. Oral hypoglycaemic drugs are not contraindicated, and are indeed preferred when the patient is not markedly hyperglycaemic, where tight control is not sought, and where the patient, or their carers, would have difficulty coping with regular injections and monitoring. There is not a substantial body of published evidence in this area. However, there is every reason to believe that

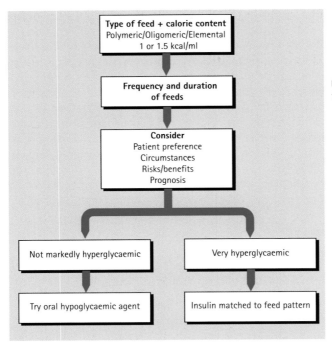

Fig. 21.1 Diabetes and enteral feeding.

stroke patients who require long-term nutritional support will benefit from tight glycaemic control as much as other patient groups do.

Further Reading

1   Stroud M, Duncan H, Nightingale J. Guidelines for enteral feeding in adult hospital patients. *Gut* 2003; **52**: vii1–vii12.

2   Rhoney DH, Parker D, Formea CM, Yap C, Coplin WM. Tolerability of bolus versus continuous gastric feeding in brain-injured patients. *Neurol Res* 2002; **24**: 613–20.

3   Kerr D, Hamilton P, Cavan DA. Preventing glycaemic excursions in diabetic patients requiring percutaneous endoscopic gastrostomy (PEG) feeding after a stroke. *Diabet Med* 2002; **19**: 1006–8.

4   Dennis MS, Lewis SC, Warlow C. Effect of timing and method of enteral tube feeding for dysphagic stroke patients (FOOD): a multicentre randomised controlled trial. *Lancet* 2005; **365**: 764–72.

5   León-Sanz M, García-Luna PP, Sanz-París A, Gómez-Candela C, Casimiro C, Chamorro J, Pereira-Cunill JL, Martin-Palmero A, Trallero R, Martinez J, Ordonez FJ, Garcia-Peris P, Camarero E, Gomez-Enterria P, Cabrerizo L, Perez-de-la-Cruz A, Sanchez C, Garcia-de-Lorenzo A, Rodriguez N, Usan L. Glycemic and lipid control in hospitalized type 2 diabetic patients: evaluation of 2 enteral nutrition formulas (low carbohydrate–high monounsaturated fat vs high carbohydrate). *J Parenter Enteral Nutr* 2005; **29**: 21–9.

22 Obesity and Diabetes

Case History

A 48-year-old man who has been obese all his adult life is referred because his diabetic control is deteriorating (glycosylated haemoglobin, HbA1c, 9.6%). Diabetes was diagnosed three years ago. He takes metformin, 1 g three times daily, and is also taking three different antihypertensive drugs and a statin. His current body mass index (BMI) is 36 kg/m².

What are the options for his further management?

Should pharmacological management of his obesity be considered?

If so, which drug, and what should be done with his current drugs?

Is he a candidate for surgical management of his obesity?

Background

The metabolic syndrome now affects approximately one in four adults in the United States. The increased frequency of this cluster of risk factors in recent years is partly due to the increased proportion of elderly individuals in the population, but is principally attributable to the increased prevalence of obesity. In most developed countries, around one in five of the population is classed as obese (BMI >30 kg/m²) and half are classed as overweight or obese (BMI >25 kg/m²). There is a close association between being overweight and the risk of developing diabetes. Even modestly overweight individuals (BMI 27–28 kg/m²) have double the risk of diabetes of their ideal-weight counterparts; at a BMI of 40 kg/m², this risk is increased 40-fold. On the other hand, even modest weight loss in those who are overweight can dramatically improve glucose tolerance—10% weight loss may decrease fasting blood glucose by up to 50%.

The first stage in managing a patient who is overweight and has comorbidities is always to examine lifestyle factors (Figure 22.1). The range of options that are now known to be effective for both diet and exercise has increased in recent years. The patient's drug treatment should also be reviewed since many of the drugs (including insulin) used for diabetes lead to weight gain as do other drugs—for example beta-blockers used in the management of hypertension. The two drugs widely available for weight loss and weight maintenance are orlistat and sibutramine. Other drugs are in advanced stages of development, and experience with surgical techniques to bring about weight loss is increasing, as is the evidence base relating to this modality.

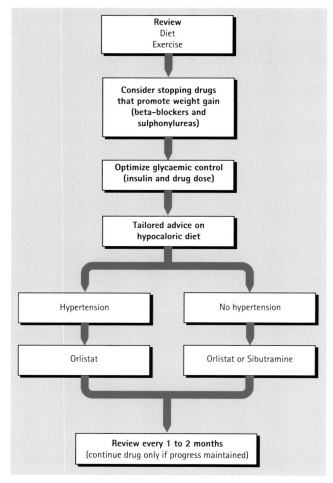

Fig. 22.1 Management of obesity and diabetes.

Orlistat is a safe drug that is now licensed in the United Kingdom for long-term management of obesity. The drug is an inhibitor of the lipase enzyme in the gut, and decreases dietary fat absorption by up to 30%. Gastrointestinal side effects are frequent, particularly if adherence to a low-fat diet is not strict. In a recent meta-analysis of published studies, mean weight loss over 12 months treatment with orlistat was 2.89 kg.[1] The most extensive single study with this drug is the XENDOS study (XENical in the prevention of Diabetes in Obese Subjects),[2] in which a large cohort of patients at high risk of diabetes were followed over four years. The modest weight loss observed was accompanied by a decreased incidence of new diabetes (6.2% in the treated group compared with 9.0% in the placebo arm). This study adds to a number of other important recent trials showing that lifestyle or pharmacological interventions to promote weight loss are effective in preventing, or delaying the onset of, type 2 diabetes.

Sibutramine is a drug that promotes early satiety, thus reducing food intake and promoting weight loss. It is related to the selective serotonin reuptake inhibitor (SSRI) group of antidepressants and acts centrally by inhibiting the reuptake of serotonin and noradrenaline. Because of its mechanism of action, the drug tends to increase pulse rate and blood pressure (mainly diastolic). Sibutramine can be used in hypertensive patients if their blood pressure is well controlled with other drugs. It should only be used with extreme caution and close monitoring in patients with ischaemic heart disease. Meta-analysis of trials confirms that sibutramine is slightly more effective than orlistat, promoting a mean weight reduction of 4.45 kg over twelve months. The drug is not recommended for longer-term use because of its effects on pulse rate and blood pressure. When used in conjunction with metformin in patients with type 2 diabetes, the drug promotes weight loss, improves glucose tolerance, and has a favourable effect on lipid profile.

Recent Developments

1 Endogenous and exogenous cannabinoids have been shown, in a large number of studies, to stimulate appetite. This effect is mediated through the CB1 receptor in the brain, and is involved in mediating the central effects of appetite-modulating peptides such as leptin. Pharmacological CB1 receptor blockade decreases appetite, and increases adiponectin expression and peripheral thermogenesis through effects at receptors on adipocytes and skeletal muscle, respectively. The recently published RIO (Rimonabant In Obesity)-Europe trial[5] was a multicentre, randomized controlled trial of the CB1 antagonist rimonabant in over 1500 subjects who were either overweight or obese and had a high prevalence of dyslipidaemia or hypertension. In association with a hypocaloric diet, subjects taking 20 mg of rimonabant once daily lost a mean of 6.6 kg over a year. Weight loss was accompanied by improved insulin sensitivity and decreased waist circumference.

2 The range of drugs available for patients who are overweight and have type 2 diabetes is increasing. These include agents related to glucagon-like peptide-1, or which prolong the action of endogenous incretins (see Chapter 19). The antiepileptic drug topiramate has been shown in a number of studies to facilitate weight loss and has potential as a therapeutic agent in this area when other measures fail.

3 There is now considerable evidence demonstrating the effectiveness of bariatric surgical procedures, and the number of operations being performed is increasing dramatically. A meta-analysis published recently[7] confirms that diabetes resolves in around 77% of cases. There is also improvement in hypertension, dyslipidaemia and obstructive sleep apnoea. Important long-term data are beginning to emerge from the Swedish Obese Subjects Study[8] demonstrating improved activity and risk factor profile up to ten years after bariatric procedures. The effectiveness of surgical procedures to help those at high risk lose weight is now beyond dispute. However, it must be remembered that there is an appreciable complication rate from these procedures and that patients need dietetic, medical and other health professional input both before and long after surgery.

Conclusion

The patient's risk factor profile will improve if he manages to lose significant weight. Ten per cent total body weight loss is a suitable early target. Many patients find this hard to achieve with standard medical and dietetic input. Safe and effective drug treatments have been a major development in this area, but need to be used in conjunction with lifestyle management. This patient may benefit from drug treatment. His hypertension is problematic. Sibutramine could be used for up to twelve months with careful monitoring of his blood pressure, but he requires three antihypertensive drugs, suggesting that his blood pressure has been difficult to control previously. Orlistat might be the preferred option initially. If he manages to achieve weight loss with this drug, and his blood pressure control is not problematic, sibutramine might be considered at a later date.

He should remain on his antihypertensives, although the need for three drugs should be reviewed if he loses weight. Metformin and orlistat together might give rise to gastrointestinal side effects. However, metformin will help to keep blood glucose under control and may have the additional benefit of preserving his residual beta cell function. Bariatric surgery would be an option for this patient if medical treatment of his obesity failed. The most appropriate surgical approach would almost certainly be laparoscopic gastric banding. The decision to proceed to surgery is generally a matter of patient preference in the main. The diabetes team should try to ensure that he is medically fit for such a procedure, psychologically able to cope with it, and fully informed of the risks as well as the potential benefits.

Further Reading

1   Li Z, Maglione M, Tu W, Mojica W, Arterburn D, Shugarman LR, Hilton L, Suttorp M, Solomon V, Shekelle PG, Morton SC. Meta-analysis: pharmacologic treatment of obesity. *Ann Intern Med* 2005; **142**: 532–46.

2   Torgerson JS, Hauptman J, Boldrin MN, Sjöström L. XENical in the prevention of diabetes in obese subjects (XENDOS) study: a randomized study of orlistat as an adjunct to lifestyle changes for the prevention of type 2 diabetes in obese patients. *Diabetes Care* 2004; **27**: 155–61.

3   Arterburn DE, Crane PK, Veenstra DL. The efficacy and safety of sibutramine for weight loss: a systematic review. *Arch Intern Med* 2004; **164**: 994–1003.

4   McNulty SJ, Ur E, Williams G. A randomized trial of sibutramine in the management of obese type 2 diabetic patients treated with metformin. *Diabetes Care* 2003; **26**: 125–31.

5   Van Gaal LF, Rissanen AM, Scheen AJ, Ziegler O, Rössner S. Effects of the cannabinoid-1 receptor blocker rimonabant on weight reduction and cardiovascular risk factors in overweight patients: 1-year experience from the RIO-Europe study. *Lancet* 2005; **365**: 1389–97.

6   Wilkes JJ, Nelson E, Osborne M, Demarest KT, Olefsky JM. Topiramate is an insulin-sensitizing compound in vivo with direct effects on adipocytes in female ZDF rats. *Am J Physiol Endocrinol Metab* 2005; **288**: E617–24.

7   Buchwald H, Avidor Y, Braunwald E, Jensen MD, Pories W, Fahrbach K, Schoelles K. Bariatric surgery: a systematic review and meta-analysis. *JAMA* 2004; **292**: 1724–37.

8   Sjöström L, Lindroos AK, Peltonen M, Torgerson J, Bouchard C, Carlsson B, Dahlgren S, Larsson B, Narbro K, Sjöström CD, Sullivan M, Wedel H. Lifestyle, diabetes, and cardiovascular risk factors 10 years after bariatric surgery. *N Engl J Med* 2004; **351**: 2683–93.

23 Diabetes in the Elderly

Case History

An 85-year-old woman who lives alone is referred because of deteriorating glycaemic control. She takes gliclazide 160 mg twice daily and metformin 850 mg three times daily. Glycosylated haemoglobin (HbA1c) is 10.4% and she has hyperglycaemic symptoms. She rarely goes out and has latterly become quite forgetful.

Does she require insulin?

What are reasonable targets for her therapy?

Background

Type 2 diabetes is common in the elderly, and becoming more common. Data from the National Health and Nutrition Evaluation Study (NHANES III) suggest that, by the age of 75, up to 20% of the population will have developed diabetes with only half being diagnosed.[1] The very elderly appear to be relatively protected from developing diabetes. There are a number of reasons for increased insulin resistance with age: alteration of body composition with increased fat and decreased muscle (sarcopoenic obesity); decreased physical activity; hormone changes that contribute to altered body composition and insulin resistance, including decreased growth hormone and insulin-like growth factor-1, decreased adrenal androgens and decreased testosterone in men; and increased production of cytokines including tumour necrosis factor-α and interleukin-6. Pancreatic beta cell function also declines with age, particularly in relation to the response to glucose.

Type 1 diabetes can develop at any age, and many people with long-standing type 2 diabetes become insulin dependent. Age should not, in itself, be a barrier to considering insulin therapy. Alterations in the innate immune system occur in individuals prone to type 2 diabetes. Autoantibodies are more common in the elderly, and up to 10% of elderly patients with diabetes have circulating autoantibodies directed against beta-cell antigens including glutamic acid decarboxylase and the protein tyrosine phosphatase IA-2.[2] Patients with this latent onset form of autoimmune diabetes may require insulin at an earlier stage than patients with type 2 diabetes.

Symptoms of diabetes are similar to those in younger people, but may be masked because of general frailty or the presence of other chronic diseases. The thirst mechanism becomes blunted with age and the renal threshold for glucose increases. The classic symptoms of thirst and polyuria may thus be less apparent in the elderly. There are some associations with diabetes that are generally only seen in the elderly: diabetic amyotrophy (usually in men); malignant otitis externa; renal papillary necrosis; painful, limited movement of the shoulders; and a form of cachexia associated with diabetic neuropathy.

Diabetes is the sixth most common cause of death in the elderly. In general, the presence of diabetes in an elderly person diminishes life expectancy by four years. Death is commonly due to macrovascular complications. The condition is also linked to decreased quality of life, functional impairment and decreased cognitive function. Thus, as in the young, effective treatment of diabetes generally improves health and well-being. Risk of complications is related to duration of diabetes and the degree of glycaemic control. Note that other causes of visual or renal impairment are also much more common in the elderly. The target for glycaemic control depends on functional status, perceived prognosis and life expectancy, symptoms from diabetes and residential circumstances. There is a lack of evidence from randomized trials conducted specifically in the elderly population. Guide therapeutic targets are suggested in Table 23.1. Prevention of macrovascular disease requires attention to multiple risk factors including dyslipidaemia and hypertension. For many patients, it may be of more benefit to focus on these risk factors rather than on trying to achieve very tight glycaemic control.

A realistic approach to managing diabetes in the elderly is required. Many patients will not achieve target levels of control. The number of elderly patients taking medication, and the number of medications they are taking, is increasing. As the treatment regime becomes more complex, patient compliance becomes more of an issue. Around a third of elderly patients on oral hypoglycaemics use their drugs inconsistently. This should be considered before making the treatment regime more complex in a patient with deteriorating control.

Lifestyle factors should be reviewed before intensifying therapy. As with drugs, there is a limited evidence base relating to diet. Moderate, but not severe, calorie restriction is appropriate for obese subjects. Advice on reducing intake of refined carbohydrate and saturated fat should be reinforced. Many nutritional factors may influence glycaemic control in the elderly patient with diabetes. These include relative deficiencies of magnesium and zinc. Exercise is important, where this is possible, and even modest increases in walking activity or armchair exercises may help to improve glucose control.

Sulphonylureas are the most widely used hypoglycaemic drugs, and are the first-line choice for those who are not very overweight. Potent and long-acting agents such as chlorpropamide and glibenclamide should be avoided. Once daily preparations such as glimepiride (1–6 mg/day) or the recently introduced gliclazide MR (30–120 mg/day) are preferred.[3] Metformin is the treatment of first choice for the obese patient. Age *per se* is not a risk factor for lactic acidosis but impairment of renal, hepatic and cardiac function

Table 23.1 Therapeutic targets for the elderly			
	Fasting Glucose (mmol/l)	2 Hour Glucose	HbA1c (%) (mmol/l)
Tight Control	<7.0	<11.0	7.1
Less Tight Control	<10.0	<14.0	8.5

Tight control is appropriate for a patient who is reasonably self-sufficient, able to deal with hypoglycaemia and intercurrent illness, and has a reasonable life expectancy. Less tight control is acceptable for patients who would not easily manage more intensive therapy and whose quality of life or life expectancy is limited.

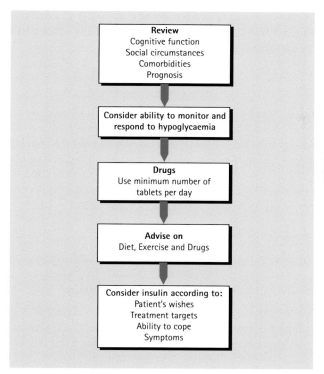

Fig. 23.1 Management of diabetes in the elderly.

is more common in the elderly. The α-glucosidase inhibitors, miglitol and acarbose, can reduce HbA1c modestly (0.5–0.8%). Although their use may be associated with gastrointestinal side effects, they are very safe drugs. There is evidence supporting the use of the thiazolidinedione drugs, rosiglitazone and pioglitazone. The kinetics of these drugs are no different to those in younger subjects but there is increased tendency to anaemia and oedema in older patients. Blood count and liver tests should be monitored at regular intervals. Finally, the post-prandial glucose regulators, repaglinide and nateglinide, may be useful and may cause fewer problems with weight gain or hypoglycaemia compared with the sulphonylureas.[4] Their major problem is that they have to be taken three times a day.

The use of insulin amongst elderly patients with diabetes is increasing. Diet, exercise and drug treatments should be reviewed prior to starting insulin (Figure 23.1). The patient's prognosis, cognitive function, social circumstances, vision and willingness to comply should be taken into account prior to starting insulin and in setting realistic treatment goals. The possibility of depression or other mood disturbance should be considered. All patients need to be educated about hypoglycaemia. Relatives, friends, carers or staff of residential facilities should be involved in the education process wherever possible. Possible regimens include: a single dose of isophane at night; twice daily isophane; twice daily premixed insulin; basal bolus with short-acting insulin at each meal; and background long-acting insulin. Analogue insulins, both short-acting (lispro, aspart) and long-acting (glargine, detemir) are suitable for use in the elderly. Concurrent use of metformin helps to minimize the insulin dose and reduces weight gain. Night-time isophane can often be combined with day-time sulphonylurea or post-prandial glucose regulator. A follow-up plan should be generated at the outset, and patients or their carers should have contact details in case problems should arise.

Recent Developments

1   Understanding of the nutritional factors that lead to obesity and insulin resistance is increasing rapidly. Nutritional management of the metabolic syndrome is likely to improve as this knowledge base develops and patients are increasingly diagnosed at an earlier stage. The role of vitamins and trace elements is increasingly recognized. Volpi and colleagues[5] recently demonstrated an anabolic effect of essential amino acid supplementation in the elderly. The potential to favourably influence body composition and insulin sensitivity without resort to pharmacological agents is becoming a real possibility.

2   Management of obesity is improving generally, and there is an evolving core of knowledge specifically relating to the elderly.[6] Diet, exercise, drugs and surgery are as effective as in younger patient groups. Primary management of obesity can reduce a number of risk factors concurrently and can simplify drug regimes.

3   The range of available treatments is increasing. A recent limited trial with glucagon-like peptide-1 (GLP-1)[7] has shown that this peptide, delivered subcutaneously, can contribute to improved glycaemic control in the elderly without the risk of undesirable weight gain.

Conclusion

Age is no barrier to insulin therapy. Indeed, increasing numbers of elderly patients are requiring insulin. Before starting insulin, careful consideration should be given to the risks, as well as the potential benefits, and to the ability of the patient to cope with the treatment. Realistic treatment goals are required, as is a follow-up plan. Attention to diet and exercise, along with imaginative combinations of oral hypoglycaemic agents may obviate the need for insulin in some cases. Combination of insulin with metformin or other oral hypoglycaemic drugs may reduce both the dose of insulin and the number of injections.

Further Reading

1   Meneilly GS, Tessier D. Diabetes in elderly adults. *J Gerontol A Biol Sci Med Sci* 2001; **56**: M5–13.

2   Pietropaolo M, Barinas-Mitchell E, Pietropaolo SL, Kuller LH, Trucco M. Evidence of islet cell autoimmunity in elderly patients with type 2 diabetes. *Diabetes* 2000; **49**: 32–8.

3   Drouin P, Standl E. Gliclazide modified release: results of a 2-year study in patients with type 2 diabetes. *Diabetes Obes Metab* 2004; **6**: 414–21.

4   Fonseca VA, Kelley DE, Cefalu W, Baron MA, Purkayastha D, Nestler JE, Hsia S, Gerich JE. Hypoglycemic potential of nateglinide versus glyburide in patients with type 2 diabetes mellitus. *Metabolism* 2004; **53**: 1331–5.

5 Volpi E, Kobayashi H, Sheffield MM, Mittendorfer B, Wolfe RR. Essential amino acids are primarily responsible for the amino acid stimulation of muscle protein anabolism in healthy elderly adults. *Am J Clin Nutr* 2003; **78**: 250–8.

6 Kennedy RL, Chokkalingham K, Srinivasan R. Obesity in the elderly: who should we be treating, and why, and how? *Curr Opin Clin Nutr Metab Care* 2004; **7**: 3–9.

7 Meneilly GS, Greig N, Tildesley H, Habener JF, Egan JM, Elahi D. Effects of 3 months of continuous subcutaneous administration of glucagon-like peptide 1 in elderly patients with type 2 diabetes. *Diabetes Care* 2003; **26**: 2835–41.

Reproductive Complications

24   Polycystic Ovarian Syndrome

25   Gestational diabetes

26   Type 1 diabetes and pregnancy

27   Erectile dysfunction

28   Pre-eclampsia

PROBLEM

24 Polycystic Ovarian Syndrome

Case History

A 34-year-old social worker is referred from the fertility clinic. She has recently married and wants to start a family. She has been trying to conceive for two years. Her periods are irregular, and she has a body mass index (BMI) of 34 kg/m² and mild hirsutism. A diagnosis of polycystic ovarian syndrome (PCOS) has been made previously. She takes metformin 500 mg three times daily, and has had diabetes for three years. Glycosylated haemoglobin (HbA1c) is 8.2%.

What are the considerations in her further treatment?

What options are there for fertility treatment?

How should her diabetes be managed?

Will metformin help her to conceive?

Should she continue metformin during pregnancy?

Is there increased risk associated with the pregnancy?

Background

Management is difficult and is best undertaken in a combined medical/gynaecology clinic. At least 75% of cases of anovulatory infertility are due to PCOS, and the condition may affect at least 7% of the young female population. The syndrome is associated with morphological changes in the ovary (increased stroma and multiple 2–9 mm cysts), defective gonadotrophin (follicle-stimulating hormone [FSH]) action leading to impaired follicular development, increased luteinizing hormone (LH), hyperinsulin-aemia and high androgen levels.

The primary aim of treatment should be to achieve weight loss (Figure 24.1), which will improve glycaemia control, increase the chances of conceiving and decrease the risks associated with pregnancy. Additionally, many local protocols exclude fertility treatment when the patient's BMI is greater than 30 kg/m^2. Loss of 10% body weight will allow 50% of women with PCOS to regain spontaneous ovulation within six months. Though patients with PCOS are generally overweight, 40% of relatively lean patients are insulin resistant and may also benefit from modest weight loss.

Poor diabetic control increases the risk of fetal abnormalities, miscarriage and macrosomia. As with all diabetic patients, she should aim for near-normal glycaemia in advance of conceiving. There is probably no role for oral hypoglycaemics other than metformin as these would be stopped if she conceived. Strenuous attempts to improve glycaemic control should be made with diet and exercise. This is best monitored with self-monitored blood glucose profiles as there is an intrinsic lag with HbA1c improvements. Mealtime, short-acting insulin may be needed at an early stage, with metformin used to treat fasting hyperglycaemia. The obvious disadvantage of insulin therapy is the potential for weight gain or impaired ability to lose weight.

The potential benefits of metformin treatment in PCOS have attracted a great deal of interest in recent years.[1,2] At 1.5–2.5 grams per day, the drug decreases insulin and androgen levels, and restores ovulation in a high proportion of patients. However, inducing spontaneous ovulation does not seem to normalize the rate of pregnancy. The drug does improve success rate when used alongside clomiphene (see below). The spontaneous abortion rate is increased in women with PCOS, and may affect as many as 40% of pregnancies. This complication is decreased by metformin, perhaps through a decrease in plasminogen activator inhibitor-1. In women without pre-existing diabetes who become pregnant, metformin treatment decreases the risk of gestational diabetes. It may also improve the outcome of *in vitro* fertilization (IVF) treatment, particularly in non-obese women. Studies using metformin have generally been too short to document an improvement in hirsutism or acne, although there is slight evidence in favour of benefit.

If lifestyle intervention and metformin treatment do not lead to successful pregnancy, clomiphene citrate is generally used as second-line treatment. This drug blocks the central oestrogen feedback mechanism and helps restore normal gonadotrophin secretion. A dose of 50–250 mg daily for five days, starting on day 2–5 after spontaneous bleeding, restores ovulation in 80% of cases, half of which become pregnant within six months. Obese and hyperinsulinaemic patients are less likely to respond. Clomiphene may usefully be combined with dexamethasone to reduce androgen levels or with metformin to improve insulin sensitivity. There is current interest in the use of aromatase inhibitors to reduce oestrogenic feedback and thus restore normal, pulsatile gonadotrophin secretion. If these measures fail, most gynaecologists would then treat with exogenous gonadotrophin, starting with 50 IU per day of recombinant FSH repeated every 5–7 days, or given continuously in low dose. Human chorionic gonadotrophin can be given to induce ovulation once suitable follicle development has taken place. Success of gonadotrophin treatment may be increased by the concurrent use of gonadotrophin-releasing hormone

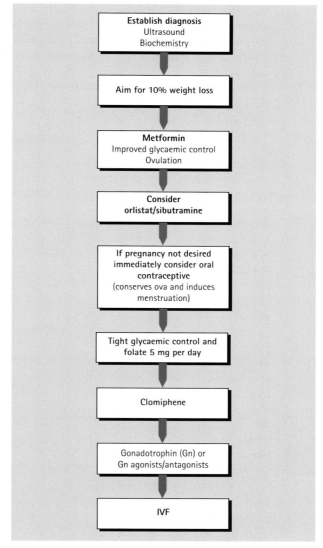

Fig. 24.1 Management of diabetes and PCOS.

agonists or antagonists. For patients who do not achieve pregnancy with drug treatment, laparoscopic ovarian drilling, in which diathermy or laser is used to induce 4–10 lesions 4–10 mm deep in the ovary, may be a useful option. Finally, for some patients the only option is IVF with embryo transfer.

Recent Developments

1 Metformin treatment appears to be safe during pregnancy.[3] Benefits with continuing treatment may include decreased risk of spontaneous abortion, lower likelihood of gestational diabetes in those without pre-existing diabetes, and decreased insulin requirement in those who do need treatment for diabetes during pregnancy.

2   States of insulin resistance, including PCOS, are associated with a number of risk factors for cardiovascular disease. This forms the basis for the current approach to treatment, but can provoke anxiety in generally healthy young women. It is not clear whether PCOS *per se* is actually associated with a marked increase in cardiovascular complications, and the risk profiles of PCOS patients may not differ substantially from age- and body weight-matched controls.[4]

3   Other drugs that improve insulin sensitivity may have a role in management of PCOS, although experience of using these drugs around the time of pregnancy is very limited at present. Both pioglitazone[5] and rosiglitazone[6] have recently been shown to have beneficial effects in insulin-resistant women with PCOS.

Conclusion

Attention to diet and exercise with the aim of improving glycaemic control and restoring normal ovulatory function should be the primary goals in this case. However, this lady has been trying to conceive for two years and she is already in her mid-30s. The chances of her requiring treatment to help her conceive are, therefore, very high. The choice of fertility treatment should take into account her age and metabolic state as well as her, and her partner's, preference. Her glycaemic control is a matter for concern and she will probably require insulin treatment to achieve near-normal glycaemic control. She will require careful weight management, particularly if fertility treatment is contemplated. Anticipating that she may become pregnant, folic acid at a dose of 5 mg per day should be used from an early stage. Metformin does not appear to pose a risk in pregnancy and continued treatment during pregnancy may confer some benefits.

Further Reading

1   Stadtmauer LA, Wong BC, Oehninger S. Should patients with polycystic ovary syndrome be treated with metformin? Benefits of insulin sensitizing drugs in polycystic ovary syndrome—beyond ovulation induction. *Hum Reprod* 2002; **17**: 3016–26.

2   Lam PM, Cheung LP, Haines C. Revisit of metformin treatment in polycystic ovarian syndrome. *Gynecol Endocrinol* 2004; **19**: 33–9.

3   Glueck CJ, Bornovali S, Pranikoff J, Goldenberg N, Dharashivkar S, Wang P. Metformin, pre-eclampsia, and pregnancy outcomes in women with polycystic ovary syndrome. *Diabet Med* 2004; **21**: 829–36.

4   Bickerton AST, Clark N, Meeking D, Shaw KM, Crook M, Lumb P, Turner C, Cummings MH. Cardiovascular risk in women with polycystic ovarian syndrome (PCOS). *J Clin Pathol* 2005; **58**: 151–4.

5   Guido M, Romualdi D, Suriano R, Giuliani M, Costantini B, Apa R, Lanzone A. Effect of pioglitazone treatment on the adrenal androgen response to corticotrophin in obese patients with polycystic ovary syndrome. *Hum Reprod* 2004; **19**: 534–9.

6   Sepilian V, Nagamani M. Effects of rosiglitazone in obese women with polycystic ovary syndrome and severe insulin resistance. *J Clin Endocrinol Metab* 2005; **90**: 60–5.

25 Gestational Diabetes

Case History

At 27 weeks' gestation, glycosuria is detected in an overweight 31-year-old woman with no prior history of diabetes. The midwife checked a random fingerprick glucose level at 8.2 mmol/l. The woman's pregnancy has been otherwise uncomplicated.

What will you advise the primary care physician when he telephones?

Is she likely to require insulin therapy?

Background

In normal pregnancy, placental production of diabetogenic hormones, such as growth hormone, corticotrophin-releasing hormone, placental lactogen and progesterone, induces maternal insulin resistance and compensatory hyperinsulinaemia. In some women, pancreatic insulin production cannot compensate for this insulin resistance and carbohydrate intolerance develops. Gestational diabetes mellitus (GDM) is defined as carbohydrate intolerance that begins or is first diagnosed in pregnancy. Type 1 diabetes, type 2 diabetes and monogenic diabetes can also present in pregnancy and care must be taken to differentiate these from true GDM, which should resolve after delivery.

GDM is associated with significantly increased feto-maternal morbidity, with increased rates of pre-eclampsia, polyhydramnios and macrosomia. Feto-maternal injuries during birth and subsequent development of diabetes in the mother are also increased. Though the associations are clear, there is significant disagreement about screening and treatment strategies. This is largely because, until very recently, there have been no data linking screening for GDM to improved feto-maternal outcome. Because GDM is frequently associated with other adverse features, such as maternal obesity, it has not been clear whether intervening to treat modest hyperglycaemia is beneficial. Indeed, excessive lowering of maternal glycaemia has been hypothesized to cause fetal growth retardation. Birth injury consequent upon macrosomia is also rarely permanent. It has been estimated that 450 caesarean sections would need to be performed to prevent one permanent neurological disability from shoulder dystocia.

There are a number of screening strategies.

1   Some centres advocate a stringent practice of universal screening for GDM.

2   The American Diabetes Association[1] currently recommends using an assessment of clinical risk factors at the first antenatal visit to support selective screening for GDM as

shown in Table 25.1. One-step or two-step screening/diagnostic strategies are then supported:

- The one-step approach may be more cost effective in women from ethnic groups at higher risk of GDM. A 100 gram 3-hour, or 75 gram 2-hour, oral glucose tolerance test (oGTT) is performed with samples obtained at baseline and then hourly. GDM is diagnosed if two or more glucose values are abnormal (thresholds are 5.3, 10.0, 8.6 and 7.8 mmol/l at 0, +1, +2 and +3 hours, respectively);

- The two-step strategy uses an initial 50 gram oral glucose challenge test (threshold of 7.8 mmol/l at +1 hour) to identify women at risk of GDM, who are then offered an oGTT as above.

3 Another approach is to use risk factors to selectively screen women at high risk for gestational diabetes using a 75 gram oGTT at 28 weeks' gestation. GDM is diagnosed if fasting glucose is ⩾7.0 mmol/l or 2-hour glucose is ⩾7.8 mmol/l.

A recent review concluded that a lack of high-quality evidence meant that it was impossible to determine the effect that any of these strategies might have on neonatal and maternal outcomes.[2]

Once GDM is diagnosed, there are three aspects to treatment: dietary modification, self-monitoring of blood glucose levels and insulin administration. Dietary modification stresses selection of a varied diet containing complex rather than simple carbohydrates. Some limitation of carbohydrate and fat intake is also usual—particularly carbohydrate at breakfast when insulin resistance is greatest. Emphasis is placed on weight maintenance rather than weight reduction.

Current technologies mean that self-monitoring of blood glucose is relatively simple. The suggested practice is to advise pre- and post-prandial monitoring, with a pre-prandial target of 4–6 mmol/l and a 2-hour post-prandial target of 6–8 mmol/l. Post-prandial monitoring is recommended because one study reported that a 1-hour

Table 25.1 American Diabetes Association screening protocol for GDM		
Risk of GDM	Risk factors	Action
High risk	Any of: Marked obesity Personal history of GDM Glycosuria Strong family history of diabetes	Screen at first visit. If normal, rescreen between 24 and 28 weeks' gestation
Average risk	Neither high nor low risk	Screen between 24 and 28 weeks' gestation
Low risk	Any of: Age <25 years Weight normal before pregnancy Member of an ethnic group with a low prevalence of GDM No known diabetes in first-degree relatives No history of abnormal glucose tolerance No history of poor obstetric outcome	No screening necessary

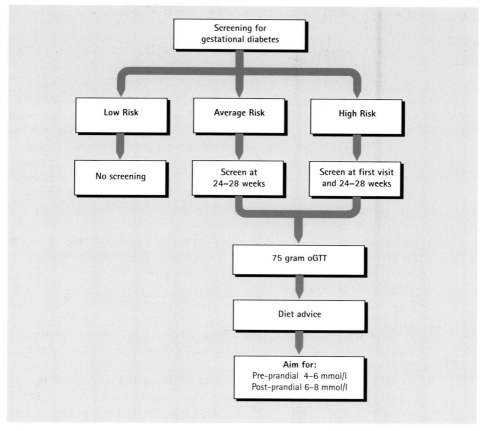

Fig. 25.1 Screening for gestational diabetes.

post-prandial target of <7.8 mmol/l compared with a pre-prandial target of 3.3–5.9 mmol/l was associated with a macrosomia rate of 12% versus 42% and a caesarean section rate of 12% versus 36%, respectively.[3] Similar pregnancy outcomes have been identified if insulin is initiated, if either of maternal glycaemic targets of 6.7 mmol/l pre-prandially and 11.1 mmol/l post-prandially are breached, or if fetal abdominal circumference is greater than the 75th percentile for gestational age.[4]

The suggested practice is to initiate twice daily pre-prandial insulin that contains a pre-mixed rapid-acting insulin analogue and intermediate-acting insulin. If glycaemic targets cannot be achieved with twice daily insulin, extra rapid-acting insulin or a basal bolus regimen is used. Oral hypoglycaemic agents are not routinely used, though small studies support the use of glibenclamide—which crosses the placenta minimally—in gestational diabetes.

Once the placenta is delivered, carbohydrate intolerance improves. However, as the lifetime risk of developing diabetes is 50% or greater following gestational diabetes, it is usual to perform a 75 gram oGTT six weeks after delivery to determine glucose tolerance and then carry out further assessment every two to three years thereafter if this is normal.

Recent Developments

1 The Australian Carbohydrate Intolerance Study in Pregnant Women (ACHOIS) trial[5] has demonstrated a clear association between selective screening/intervention for gestational diabetes and improved pregnancy outcome. Women between 24 and 34 weeks' gestation with a fasting glucose <7.8 mmol/l and blood glucose of 7.8 and 11.0 mmol/l before and two hours after a 75 gram oral glucose challenge, respectively, were randomized to either obstetric care with no further intervention in glycaemia, or active management of glycaemia to maintain pre-prandial glucose <5.5 mmol/l and 2-hour post-prandial glucose <7.0 mmol/l—an approach consistent with routine screening and treatment of gestational diabetes. Amongst 1000 women randomized, the composite primary outcome of perinatal death, shoulder dystocia, bone fracture and nerve palsy was 1% in the intervention group and 4% in the other group. There were no perinatal deaths in the intervention group and five deaths in the other group. Macrosomia rates were also lower in the intervention group, but the caesarean section rate of approximately 30% was similar in both groups. Though intervention is clearly of benefit in some pregnancies, optimal screening and intervention thresholds are not yet clear. Two further studies are currently underway which should help answer these questions.[6,7]

Conclusion

The woman in this case is at high risk of having gestational diabetes as she is overweight and the random glucose level is elevated. Although glycosuria may be the consequence of a low renal threshold for glucose, and there is no information given about the timing of the glucose sample, it would be reasonable to assess her carbohydrate tolerance further.

Attendance is advised at a joint antenatal diabetes/obstetric clinic within a week, in a fasted state, to have a 75 gram oGTT performed as well as an assessment of fetal well-being and growth. A fasting glucose ≥7.0 mmol/l or 2-hour glucose ≥7.8 mmol/l would be diagnostic of gestational diabetes. A strong family history of diabetes, a personal or family history of autoimmune disease, ketonuria or a lean body habitus may indicate pre-existing type 2, monogenic or type 1 diabetes. She should receive dietetic education and test fingerprick plasma glucose pre-prandially, two hours post-prandially and before bed on a daily basis. The suggested approach to initiation of insulin is based upon the criteria of Schaefer-Graf et al.[4] as described above. Fortnightly obstetric/diabetes review should be organized, with delivery planned for the 38th week of gestation unless other problems supervene. Six weeks after delivery, she should have a 75 gram oGTT performed to define glucose tolerance. If this is normal, further assessment should take place on a two to three yearly basis.

Further Reading

1 American Diabetes Association. Gestational diabetes mellitus. *Diabetes Care* 2004; **27** (Suppl 1): S88–90.

2 Brody SC, Harris R, Lohr K. Screening for gestational diabetes: a summary of the evidence for the U.S. Preventive Services Task Force. *Obstet Gynecol* 2003; **101**: 380–92.

3 de Veciana M, Major CA, Morgan MA, Astrat T, Toohey JS, Lien JM, Evans AT. Postprandial versus preprandial blood glucose monitoring in women with gestational diabetes mellitus requiring insulin therapy. *N Engl J Med* 1995; **333**: 1237–41.

4 Schaefer-Graf UM, Kjos SL, Fauzan OH, Buhling KJ, Siebert G, Buhrer C, Ladendorf B, Dudenhausen JW, Vetter K. A randomized trial evaluating a predominately fetal growth-based strategy to guide management of gestational diabetes in caucasian women. *Diabetes Care* 2004; **27**: 297–302.

5 Crowther CA, Hiller JE, Moss JR, McPhee AJ, Jeffries WS, Robinson JS. Effect of treatment of gestational diabetes mellitus on pregnancy outcomes. *N Engl J Med* 2005; **352**: 2477–86.

6 HAPO Study Cooperative Research Group. The Hyperglycemia and Adverse Pregnancy Outcome (HAPO) Study. *Int J Gynaecol Obstet* 2002; **78**: 69–77.

7 Landon MB, Thom E, Spong CY, Gabbe SG, Leindecker S, Johnson F, Lain K, Miodovnik M, Carpenter M. A planned randomized clinical trial of treatment for mild gestational diabetes mellitus. *J Matern Fetal Neonatal Med* 2002; **11**: 226–31.

PROBLEM

26 Type 1 Diabetes and Pregnancy

Case History

A 32-year-old solicitor with type 1 diabetes and glycosylated haemoglobin (HbA1c) of 8.2% states that she is trying for a baby. She has had type 1 diabetes for 16 years and has mild background retinopathy. She takes lisinopril 10 mg per day as she has previously been noted to have microalbuminuria. She has never been pregnant before. She takes Mixtard insulin 32 units in the morning and 28 units in the evening.

How would you advise her?

Would you advise a change of insulin?

When would you stop her lisinopril?

Background

The St Vincent declaration of 1989 'to achieve pregnancy outcome in the diabetic woman that approximates that of the non-diabetic woman' has not yet been met. Recent reports from Northern European centres show that up to 20% of all pregnancies in women with type 1 diabetes are complicated by pre-eclampsia and 50% by macrosomia. Approximately 30% of deliveries are before 37 weeks' gestation and at least 4% of babies have severe congenital malformations—double the background population. However, where pregnancy is planned and the HbA1c in the first trimester is <7%, this excess risk is reduced by two-thirds—but it remains above the level of the background population. In the case described, a delay in conception would allow a fuller assessment of maternal health, specific interventions to prepare for pregnancy and an expectation of a reduction in potential complications.

Issues generic to all pregnancies include usual pre-pregnancy assessments of general health, nutrition and vaccination status. Attention should be paid to the outcome of previous attempts at conception and whether these are likely to influence a further potential pregnancy or delivery. Smoking should be discouraged and teratogenic medications should be stopped or modified if possible.

In a woman with type 1 diabetes planning pregnancy, the commonest drug that requires intervention is an angiotensin-converting enzyme (ACE) inhibitor—usually prescribed for microalbuminuria. ACE inhibitors significantly disrupt normal fetal development in the second and third trimesters and have been associated with oligohydramnios, fetal and neonatal renal failure, bony malformations, limb contractures, pulmonary hypoplasia, prolonged hypotension and neonatal death. However, in pregnancies where ACE inhibitors are stopped in the first trimester there is no clear evidence of adverse outcome. Some clinicians continue an ACE inhibitor until pregnancy is established to maximize maternal renoprotection.

Neural tube defects (NTD—anencephaly, spina bifida, encephalocele) are more common in women with diabetes. Folic acid supplementation reduces the incidence of NTD by 70% or more in women at high risk of these defects[1] and is recommended for all women with diabetes. A dose of 5 mg daily is used in the United Kingdom (UK) for women with diabetes, which is a higher dose than that recommended to the general population. There is no evidence of harm from these higher doses of folic acid.

Intensification of glycaemic control is advisable, aiming for a HbA1c <7% in line with the Diabetes Control and Complications Trial (DCCT) findings. With support and significant effort, many women who are usually unable to maintain good glycaemic control can achieve excellent control in preparation for and during pregnancy. Most centres recommend a seven-point glucose profile—testing fingerprick glucose before and 1.5 to 2 hours after meals and before bed. The suggested practice is to aim for a pre-prandial glucose value between 4 and 6 mmol/l and post-prandial values between 6 and 8 mmol/l. Intermittent testing during the night, at 2 or 3 am, is also usually recommended to identify nocturnal hypoglycaemia that may otherwise go unrecognized. There is an acknowledged increased risk of hypoglycaemia with intensive glucose control and studies are relatively consistent in reporting that 40% of women will suffer at least one episode of (severe) hypoglycaemia requiring external assistance during pregnancy—a particular risk during the first trimester.[2] Warnings of hypoglycaemia may become reduced during pregnancy. One episode of hypoglycaemia may reduce the warning symptoms of subsequent hypoglycaemia, so meticulous testing is also necessary to try and avoid the development of hypoglycaemia unawareness.

Pregnancy is also associated with the development or worsening of diabetic retinopathy. It is not clear whether pregnancy itself worsens retinopathy and how much a rapid improvement in glycaemic control may contribute—a situation analogous to the worsening of retinopathy seen initially in the intensively treated cohort of the DCCT. The same risk factors for retinopathy outside pregnancy can identify patients at high risk of retinopathy progressing during pregnancy—long duration of diabetes, higher grade of retinopathy, poor glycaemic control, hypertension and proteinuria. Laser photocoagulation can and should be offered if there is sight-threatening disease.

Feto-maternal surveillance during pregnancy is frequent and will involve the diabetologist, obstetrician, diabetes specialist nurse, dietician and midwife.

- Up to 20 weeks' gestation, standard obstetric surveillance is offered, including screening for Down's syndrome and a detailed anatomical scan. Visits to intensify glycaemic control are as frequent as necessary.

- From 20 weeks' to 28 weeks' gestation, four-weekly ultrasound examination is offered, and two-weekly examination from 28 weeks to delivery. This is to assess growth (macrosomia or intrauterine growth restriction), amniotic fluid volume and fetal health through Doppler and biophysical studies.

- Unless there are particular indications, the aim is to continue the pregnancy to term (37 weeks' gestation)—with delivery ideally at, or around, 38 weeks' gestation. This balances the risks of macrosomia-related complications at delivery with the potential risk of late intrauterine fetal death. Late intrauterine fetal death still occurs in approximately 1 in 40 pregnancies, though modern obstetric and diabetes care mean that the incidence is much lower than in the 1950s where this rate was 1 in 3.

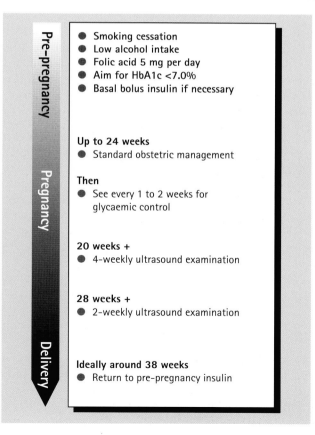

Fig. 26.1 Management of type 1 diabetes in pregnancy.

- There is no unequivocal evidence that routine caesarean section in women with diabetes is necessary. There is also no unequivocal evidence that routine removal of the newborn to a neonatal intensive care bed is necessary.

Recent Developments

1   The safety of both short- and long-acting insulin analogues during pregnancy has been the subject of significant debate. It is unlikely that formal prospective, randomized controlled trials will be done. The data that exist are mainly from retrospective or observational studies. Available data suggest that the rapid-acting insulin analogue, lispro, can be safely used in pregnancy and may even offer advantages in providing better glycaemic control.[3] Indeed, experimental data suggest that insulin lispro at usual therapeutic concentrations does not cross the placenta.[4]

2   There are concerns over the long-acting insulin analogues, glargine and detemir—partly because of a lack of clinical experience in pregnancy. Insulin glargine has a higher insulin-like growth factor (IGF)-1 receptor affinity than human insulin. One study has identified a mitogenic effect on an osteosarcoma cell line.[5] Human ovarian, breast and bone tumour growth and progression of diabetic retinopathy have also all been linked to IGF-1 stimulation. Detemir is not demonstrably safe in pregnancy, though many women have now completed pregnancies while using detemir as the background insulin. A large audit of these pregnancies is underway in the UK. Insulin detemir has a lower IGF-1 receptor affinity but has not been available long enough for study in pregnancy.

Conclusion

Smoking and alcohol consumption should be discouraged and daily folic acid supplementation should be encouraged—5 mg daily is recommended in the UK. Drugs that are potentially toxic to a fetus should be stopped. Glycaemic control should be intensified, with measurement of blood glucose before and 1.5 to 2 hours after meals, before bed and intermittently in the very early morning, aiming for a pre-conception HbA1c <7%. The types of insulin used should be discussed and optimized—perhaps avoiding long-acting analogues, but using short-acting analogues if appropriate to minimize prandial glycaemic excursion. There should be a careful examination for complications of diabetes—particularly retinopathy and nephropathy (including an assessment of albumin excretion rate).

It should be made clear that there will be an expectation of frequent feto-maternal monitoring and a hospital birth involving a joint obstetric/diabetes team. The risks of pre-eclampsia, pre-term delivery, Caesarean section, congenital malformation and perinatal morbidity should all be explained. Finally, it is probably reasonable to state that the majority of pregnancies have a happy outcome—once mother and baby have left hospital.

Further Reading

1   MRC Vitamin Research Group. Prevention of neural tube defects: results of the Medical Research Council Vitamin Study. *Lancet* 1991; **338**: 131–7.

2 Evers IM, de Valk HW, Visser GHA. Risk of complications of pregnancy in women with type 1 diabetes: nationwide prospective study in the Netherlands. *BMJ* 2004; **328**: 915.

3 Loukovaara S, Immonen I, Teramo KA, Kaaja R. Progression of retinopathy during pregnancy in type 1 diabetic women treated with insulin lispro. *Diabetes Care* 2003; **26**: 1193–8.

4 Boskovic R, Feig DS, Derewlany L, Knie B, Portnoi G, Koren G. Transfer of insulin lispro across the human placenta: in vitro perfusion studies. *Diabetes Care* 2003; **26**: 1390–4.

5 Kurtzhals P, Schaffer L, Sorensen A, Kristensen C, Jonassen I, Schmid C, Trub T. Correlations of receptor binding and metabolic and mitogenic potencies of insulin analogs designed for clinical use. *Diabetes* 2000; **49**: 999–1005.

PROBLEM

27 Erectile Dysfunction

Case History

A divorced 58-year-old publican with hypertension, dyslipidaemia and type 2 diabetes attends for annual review of diabetes. He is unable to get an erection satisfactory for intercourse and wishes to discuss treatments for erectile dysfunction.

What investigations should be requested?

What treatment can you offer?

Background

Erectile dysfunction is defined as 'an inability to acquire or maintain an erection satisfactory for sexual intercourse'. It is estimated to affect half of all men with diabetes in their 50s, with an increasing prevalence each decade. As effective and acceptable treatments are now available, it is usual practice to ask specifically about erectile dysfunction at review of diabetes. An unambiguous enquiry is often needed because of reticence of the patient about such a discussion. A clear description of the problem is needed to clarify exactly what happens during attempted intercourse, so that appropriate investigation and treatment is planned. For example, performance anxiety or premature ejaculation may respond to non-pharmacological therapies. Depression or alcohol-induced erectile dysfunction may respond to pharmacological therapy directed toward erectile dysfunction, but it may be more appropriate to treat the underlying problem.

Normal erectile function requires integration of libido, sexual stimuli, relevant hormones and control of vascular inflow/outflow by local and central neurological activity. One or more sexual stimuli induce a local increase in parasympathetic tone and decrease in sympathetic tone. Nitric oxide release then generates cyclic-GMP which relaxes local vasculature, increases blood flow into the corpus cavernosum and decreases blood flow out as trabecular muscle rapidly relaxes. Phosphodiesterase (PDE) type 5 breaks down cyclic-GMP in the penis. When breakdown exceeds generation, the process reverses and detumescence occurs. Disturbance of this complex system can result in erectile dysfunction:

- diabetes, hypertension and dyslipidaemia can induce neurovascular damage;

- hyperprolactinaemia, hypothyroidism or a low testosterone may all induce erectile dysfunction through effects on mood and testosterone-sensitive nitric oxide production in the penis. Ten per cent of men with erectile dysfunction who undergo hormonal testing have abnormal laboratory results. Hyperprolactinaemia and hypothyroidism are relatively clear-cut diagnoses. A borderline testosterone can be difficult to interpret and treat—particularly in men who are overweight or have heavy alcohol consumption;

- spironolactone and cimetidine have oestrogenic properties and may interfere with hormonal control of erection;

- some antidopaminergic psychotropic medications induce hyperprolactinaemia and interfere with hormonal control of erection;

- thiazide diuretics and beta-blockers are associated with erectile dysfunction, though the mechanism is unclear.

There are an increasing number of generally used treatment options for erectile dysfunction.

1 Orally active PDE-5 inhibitors reduce cyclic-GMP breakdown in the penis and are effective in reversing erectile dysfunction in approximately 60% of men with diabetes. In contrast to other treatment options, they only work if there is arousal as cyclic GMP must be generated for its breakdown to be inhibited. Currently available agents— sildenafil, tadalafil and vardenafil—differ minimally in clinical characteristics:

   - all are associated with side effects of headache, flushing, rhinitis and dyspepsia in approximately 10% of patients;

   - all are contraindicated in patients taking oral nitrates or alpha-blockers because of the risk of precipitating catastrophic hypotension;

   - sildenafil cross-reacts with retinal PDE-6 and has been associated with visual problems;[1,2]

   - sildenafil and tadalafil should not be coprescribed with potent inhibitors of cytochrome P450 isoenzyme CYP3A4 (e.g. ketoconazole and certain protease inhibitors used in treatment of human immunodeficiency virus infection) as they may prolong the half-life of the PDE-5 inhibitor;

   - tadalafil has the longest half-life, may be effective for up to 36 hours, and absorption does not seem to be slowed by a high-fat meal;

   - vardenafil should not be used in men with a genetic or acquired long QT interval as it causes minor prolongation of the QT interval.

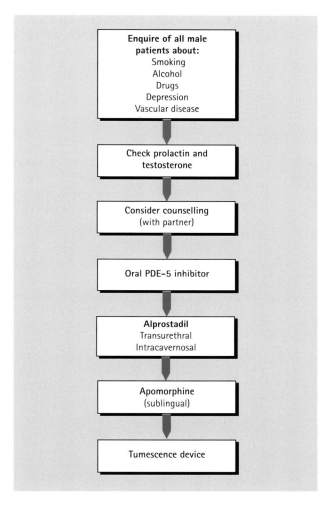

Fig. 27.1 Management of erectile dysfunction.

2 Alprostadil (prostaglandin E_1) directly relaxes vascular smooth muscle within the corpus cavernosum. When administered by injection intracavernosally into the shaft of the penis or transurethrally it is effective in approximately 65% of men. Local pain and irritation are common side effects, but are rarer with transurethral administration. Priapism is also more rare with transurethral administration, but must be treated urgently.

3 Sublingual apomorphine is a more recently licensed treatment for erectile dysfunction. It acts on central D1 or D2 receptors to stimulate an erection. The drug takes approximately 20 minutes to achieve its effect following sublingual administration. If swallowed, the drug is almost completely ineffective. In clinical trials[3,4] it is effective in approximately 40% of men, though its effectiveness in men with diabetes is uncertain. Headaches, nausea and yawning occur in over 5% of users, though these effects are dose dependent and may reduce with repeated exposure. Cardiovascular cautions for prescribing are similar to those for the PDE-5 inhibitors.

4 Vacuum tumescence devices use negative pressure to draw blood into the penis, and a constrictive band at the base of the penis restricts outflow. This prevents ejaculation and does not provide an erection along the whole shaft of the penis.

5 Penile prostheses—a malleable rod or inflatable device placed within the shaft of the penis—are very rarely used.

Recent Developments

1 There have been a number of reports of sudden death in men using sildenafil—despite the precautions outlined above. PDE-5 inhibitors are not associated with changes in coronary blood flow and their role in precipitating sudden coronary death is not certain. It is recommended that use of PDE-5 inhibitors is avoided in men with unstable coronary artery disease, recent myocardial infarction and severe hypotension.

2 Soon after sildenafil became available, there were reports of transient changes in colour vision.[1] Blue vision affects approximately 3% of men using sildenafil and does not seem to be a clinically significant problem. There have been no reports of blue vision with vardenafil and tadalafil. More recently, there have been reports of non-arteritic optic ischaemic neuropathy (NAOIN) associated with sildenafil.[2] NAOIN has been associated with permanent unilateral or bilateral reduction in visual acuity. Though the mechanism of action is uncertain, it is known that sildenafil cross-reacts with retinal PDE-6. All reported cases were in patients with an adverse cardiovascular risk profile and it may be prudent to avoid sildenafil use in such patients. However, the risk of permanent visual loss is minimal and rare side effects of the newer PDE-5 inhibitors may not yet have come to light.

Conclusion

A full history and examination must be taken to identify comorbidities—particularly cardiac status—and current treatments. This should be coupled with a frank discussion of the exact nature of the erectile dysfunction to try and determine aetiology and whether psychological assessment would be appropriate. Generally though, a chronic history of worsening erectile dysfunction not associated with excess alcohol suggests an organic diagnosis. Obesity, cigarette smoking and excess alcohol consumption are all likely to contribute to erectile dysfunction of whatever cause.

Suggested practice is to assess serum prolactin, thyroid stimulating hormone and creatinine, as well as routine biochemistry for lipid profile, liver function tests, electrolytes, a full blood count and glycosylated haemoglobin. If a hormonal aetiology is identified, it should be specifically addressed.

Otherwise, an oral PDE-5 inhibitor would be first-line therapy if there were no contraindications. Lower doses may be less effective in men with diabetes and the patient should be encouraged to persevere and try higher doses of the initial agent. If the first agent is unsuccessful, an alternative PDE-5 inhibitor can be tried but is not usually successful. Second-line treatments, such as transurethral/intracavernosal alprostadil, sublingual apomorphine or use of vacuum tumescence devices, can then be tried—usually determined by patient preference. Consulting experience suggests second-line treatments are often disappointing and it is important not to raise expectations falsely .

If treatment for erectile dysfunction is not satisfactory, it is important to broach emotional and psychological well-being in the consultation. Permanent erectile dysfunction can be devastating for some men—and for some relationships.

Further Reading

1 Jagle H, Jagle C, Serey L, Yu A, Rilk A, Sadowski B, Besch D, Zrenner E, Sharpe LT. Visual short-term effects of Viagra: double-blind study in healthy young subjects. *Am J Ophthalmol* 2004; **137**: 842–9.

2 Pomeranz HD, Bhavsar AR. Nonarteritic ischemic optic neuropathy developing soon after use of sildenafil (viagra): a report of seven new cases. *J Neuroophthalmol* 2005; **25**: 9–13.

3 von Keitz AT, Stroberg P, Bukofzer S, Mallard N, Hibberd M. A European multicentre study to evaluate the tolerability of apomorphine sublingual administered in a forced dose-escalation regimen in patients with erectile dysfunction. *BJU Int* 2002; **89**: 409–15.

4 Dula E, Bukofzer S, Perdok R, George M. Double-blind, crossover comparison of 3 mg apomorphine SL with placebo and with 4 mg apomorphine SL in male erectile dysfunction. *Eur Urol* 2001; **39**: 558–64.

28 Pre-eclampsia

Case History

At 34 weeks' gestation, proteinuria is discovered in a 24-year-old woman with type 1 diabetes in her first pregnancy. Blood pressure is recorded at 144/92 mmHg. Her urine has become dipstick-positive for protein. Her diabetic control is good (glycosylated haemoglobin, HbA1c, 6.5%) and her pregnancy to date has been uncomplicated. She has no vascular complications of diabetes.

What are the risks she faces?

How should her blood pressure be managed?

What are the implications for her obstetric care?

Will this recur in a future pregnancy?

Background

Pre-eclampsia is the development of hypertension and proteinuria after 20 weeks of gestation. It affects around 5% of pregnancies and is associated with increased risk to the mother and fetus. It is most likely to occur in the first pregnancy and risk factors include age above 40 years, obesity, family history or previous personal history of pre-eclampsia, previous hypertension, systemic lupus erythematosus and the antiphospholipid syndrome, renal disease or diabetes. Diagnostic criteria are shown in Table 28.1. When blood pressure is elevated before 20 weeks, or after 20 weeks but with no proteinuria, gestational hypertension is diagnosed. Many women are asymptomatic, underlining the need for careful screening. The most common symptoms are peripheral oedema and rapid weight gain.

The major risks of pre-eclampsia are of placental abruption, cardiac failure, acute renal failure, cerebrovascular accident and disseminated intravascular coagulation. After haemorrhage and embolism, it is the third leading cause of maternal death during pregnancy. Eclampsia is diagnosed when there is new onset of seizures in late pregnancy or in the early post-partum period in a woman with pre-eclampsia. It is rare, and occurs in less than 1% of women with pre-eclampsia. HELLP syndrome (Haemolysis, Elevated Liver enzymes, Low Platelets) is another rare complication that also occurs in less than 1% of cases.

Management prior to delivery consists of careful control of blood pressure, with monitoring of maternal and fetal health. If pre-eclampsia is suspected but there are not severe features, blood pressure measurements should be repeated after four to six hours of rest. At baseline, serum creatinine, liver tests, platelets and 24-hour urine measurements should be requested, and repeated at weekly intervals until delivery. There is no specific test to confirm the diagnosis. Admission is not always required for pre-eclampsia, although the threshold for admission is likely to be considerably lower in a patient with concurrent diabetes. Patients do not need to be confined to bed, but should be advised to

Table 28.1　Diagnostic criteria for pre-eclampsia
A: Pre-eclampsia
● Systolic blood pressure ≥140 mmHg (or increase of 30 mmHg) ● Diastolic blood pressure ≥90 mmHg (or increase of 15 mmHg) ● Proteinuria ≥0.3 g per 24 hours (1+ on dipstick) ● ≥20 weeks' gestation
B: Severe pre-eclampsia
● Systolic blood pressure ≥160 mmHg ● Diastolic blood pressure ≥90 mmHg ● Proteinuria ≥5 g per 24 hours (3+ on dipstick) ● Neurological features (hyperreflexia, clonus) ● Other features—worsening renal, cardiac or liver function, thrombocytopenia, visual disturbances, intrauterine growth restriction

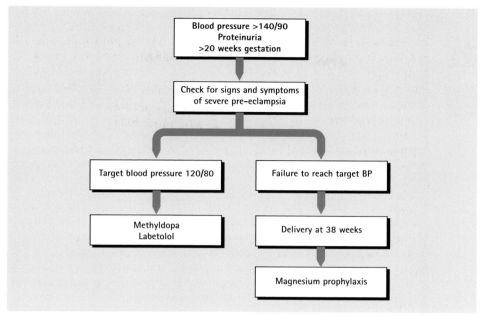

Fig. 28.1 Management of pre-eclampsia.

rest. Target blood pressure should be 120–140 mmHg systolic and 80–90 mmHg diastolic. Suitable oral agents to control blood pressure include methyldopa (initially 250 mg three times daily, increasing up to 2 g per day), or labetalol (100 mg per day, increased as necessary to 200 mg twice daily). Nifedipine or oxprenolol are suitable as adjunct or alternative therapies. Angiotensin-converting enzyme inhibitors, angiotensin II receptor blockers and diuretics are contraindicated because of risk of intrauterine growth retardation and oligohydramnios.

Severe pre-eclampsia does require admission and bed rest. In the emergency situation, oral nifedipine may be useful to lower blood pressure. For more severely affected patients, intravenous hydralazine or labetalol are the usual therapies. Hydralazine is given at a dose of 5 mg, repeated at hourly intervals as necessary. For resistant patients, infusion at an initial rate of 10 mg per hour, increased gradually as necessary, can be used. Labetalol should be given at an initial dose of 20 mg IV, with repeated or increased doses at hourly intervals. Intravenous infusion at an initial rate of 40 mg per hour is suitable for patients with severe pre-eclampsia.

Fundal height that is not consistent with pregnancy dates may indicate intrauterine growth retardation or oligohydramnios. If either of these is suspected, delivery should be considered. Delivery is generally considered at 38 weeks of gestation. Placental abruption, progressive increase in proteinuria, deterioration in renal or hepatic function, or development of thrombocytopenia (platelets less than $100 \times 10^9/l$) are also indications for early delivery, as are severe or persistent symptoms (headache, visual changes, abdominal pain, nausea and vomiting). Vaginal delivery is clearly to be preferred where possible. Regional anaesthesia is preferred if caesarean section is deemed necessary, but is contraindicated if coagulopathy is present. Magnesium is now routinely used in eclamptic patients during delivery as prophylaxis against fits. Local protocols are usually in place but are generally based around a loading dose of 6 g, followed by 2 g per hour of $MgSO_4$.

Recent Developments

1   Pre-term delivery continues to be more common in women with type 1 diabetes, reported rates being between 22% and 45%. These rates are around five-fold higher than those of the background populations. Both spontaneous and indicated pre-term deliveries are increased.[1] Pre-eclampsia is the commonest cause for indicated pre-term delivery, followed by deteriorating renal function and glycaemic control. The reasons for the increased incidence of pre-eclampsia in patients with diabetes are not known.

2   A lack of understanding of the precise underlying pathogenesis means that specific interventions do not exist. One aetiological factor is thought to be placental vascular insufficiency. Recently, Levine et al.[2] have demonstrated increased levels of soluble fms-like tyrosine kinase in patients who develop pre-eclampsia. This molecule inhibits the actions of placental growth factor and vascular endothelial growth factor. This mechanism is of interest because of recent attention to angiogenic factors in the pathogenesis of diabetic complications such as retinopathy. Other proposed aetiological factors include nitric oxide, endothelins, the renin–angiotensin system, inflammatory mediators and multiple genetic factors.[3]

3   Pre-eclampsia is associated with an unfavourable change in the balance between prostacyclin and thromboxane. In a number of studies, aspirin has been shown to decrease the risk of subsequent pre-eclampsia.[4] However, this effect is modest (odds ratio 0.86; 95% confidence interval 0.76–0.96), and may not apply to patients with diabetes. Routine use of aspirin in pregnancy for pre-eclampsia prophylaxis is not currently recommended.

4   Pre-eclampsia has been associated with long-term risk of cardiovascular disease, and a history of pre-eclampsia should be sought in patients with diabetes who are, in any case, at increased risk. Freeman et al.[5] have recently noted an association between pre-eclampsia and increased levels of inflammatory markers. Furthermore, increased interleukin-6 persisted for many years. Increased levels of this cytokine have been linked with development of insulin resistance and cardiac disease.

Conclusion

Development of pre-eclampsia in a patient with type 1 diabetes is a serious matter. The patient will need tight control of her glucose and blood pressure, and monitoring of fetal development, and this may necessitate admission to hospital. Her major risks relate to blood pressure control, and this may mean that she will face an early and interventional delivery. Her diabetes should be managed as for any other diabetic pregnancy. The level of treatment she requires for her blood pressure will depend on how this comes under control as the pregnancy progresses. The risk is greatest in first pregnancy, but pre-eclampsia itself is a risk factor for development of the condition in a subsequent pregnancy.

Further Reading

1 Lepercq J, Coste J, Theau A, Dubois LD, Timsit J. Factors associated with preterm delivery in women with type 1 diabetes: a cohort study. *Diabetes Care* 2004; **27**: 2824–8.

2 Levine RJ, Maynard SE, Qian C, Lim KH, England LJ, Yu KF, Schisterman EF, Thadhani R, Sachs BP, Epstein FH, Sibai BM, Sukhatme VP, Karumanchi SA. Circulating angiogenic factors and the risk of preeclampsia. *N Engl J Med* 2004; **350**: 672–83.

3 Pridjian G, Puschett JB. Preeclampsia. Part 2: experimental and genetic considerations. *Obstet Gynecol Surv* 2002; **57**: 619–40.

4 Coomarasamy A, Honest H, Papaioannou S, Gee H, Khan KS. Aspirin for prevention of preeclampsia in women with historical risk factors: a systematic review. *Obstet Gynecol* 2003; **101**: 1319–32.

5 Freeman DJ, McManus F, Brown EA, Cherry L, Norrie J, Ramsay JE, Clark P, Walker ID, Sattar N, Greer IA. Short- and long-term changes in plasma inflammatory markers associated with preeclampsia. *Hypertension* 2004; **44**: 708–14.

Cardiovascular Risk Factors in Diabetes

29   Smoking cessation

30   Hypertriglyceridaemia

31   Hyperlipidaemia in type 1 diabetes

32   Hyperlipidaemia in type 2 diabetes

33   Aspirin use in diabetes

34   Hypertension—uncomplicated

35   Hypertension—hard to control

PROBLEM

29 Smoking Cessation

Case History

Your 54-year-old patient with diabetes is keen to stop smoking. He has tried to give up smoking four years previously but was successful for only two months. His general practitioner recently prescribed him a nicotine gum but he did not find it effective.

Discuss briefly the pathogenesis of smoking-induced atherogenesis.

Consider the current evidence relating to the pharmacological treatment of smoking cessation within the broader context of a smoking-cessation strategy.

What new strategies are emerging?

Background

Cigarette smoking is an important risk factor for atherothrombosis. Even occasional smoking, particularly among men, is related to a higher risk of both total mortality (age-adjusted relative risk (RR) 1.6; 95% confidence interval (CI) 1.3–2.1) and cardiovascular mortality (age-adjusted RR 1.5; 95% CI 1.0–2.3). The mechanisms by which cigarette smoke exerts damage to the cardiovascular system, however, are not entirely clear due to the mixture of pharmacologically active substances contained in tobacco. Only a few of these components have been extensively studied. Nicotine and carbon monoxide, for example, are much less damaging than is whole smoke, but with the former exerting the most addictive property. Cigarette smoking, however, has been shown to induce both morphological and biochemical disturbances to the vascular endothelium, both *in vivo* and *in vitro*. This is thought to be largely mediated by increases in oxidative stress and, consequently, free radical formation.

Effective smoking-cessation strategies reduce cardiovascular events, but a systematic review from the Cochrane Tobacco Addiction Review group database showed a very low success rate in smoking cessation, especially among patients with symptomatic cardiovascular disease (secondary prevention).[1,2] Spontaneous (primary prevention) cessation rates are even lower among patients who want to give up smoking (<5% per year). The recognition that cigarette smoking is a primary disorder, in which addiction to nicotine plays a primary role, has resulted in an important change to the approach to smoking cessation. The United Kingdom and the United States guidelines on smoking cessation therapy suggest a specific action plan which integrates behavioural and pharmacological support to aid cessation as well as prevent relapse.[3] Most intensive programmes report cessation rates of about 20% with behavioural support alone, whilst quit rates are further doubled among motivated patients given various forms of nicotine replacement therapy (NRT) in combination with educational and lifestyle support. Taking regular exercise may also help people give up smoking by moderating nicotine withdrawal and cravings. Thus, pharmacological support should be provided for all smokers who are willing to use medication as part of a multi-intervention strategy. Nicotine is metabolized quickly, with a half-life of two hours. The concept behind NRT to facilitate smoking cessation is therefore to provide steady-state nicotine levels to prevent withdrawal symptoms while avoiding the reinforcing peaks associated with smoking.[4] After achieving abstinence, NRT can be tapered off and eventually discontinued. NRT is available in two forms. The transdermal systems (nicotine patches) provide a slow and steady release of nicotine with low addiction potential, and have been studied extensively and shown to be safe in patients with stable cardiovascular disease. Nicotine polacrilex (nicotine gum) should be prescribed with proper education on effective chewing strategies. It is essential, for example, to chew the gum to release the nicotine and then allow the saliva to facilitate buccal absorption. The antidepressant bupropion, a selective reuptake inhibitor of dopamine and noradrenaline, has also been shown to be effective in smoking cessation by preventing or reducing cravings and other features of nicotine withdrawal, and provides favourable outcomes on cessation-related weight gain.[5] Bupropion can also be combined with NRT to further increase cessation rates. Adverse effects of bupropion include a lowered seizure threshold, and bupropion is therefore contraindicated in those with high seizure risk. Bupropion sustained release (SR) has relatively few cardiovascular adverse effects and may be used for patients with cardiovascular disease.

Special consideration, however, is needed for hospitalized patients with acute coronary syndromes (e.g. myocardial infarction and unstable angina). Highly nicotine-dependent smokers who receive bupropion are more likely to experience a decrease in depressive symptoms during active treatment but, unfortunately, are also more likely to experience a

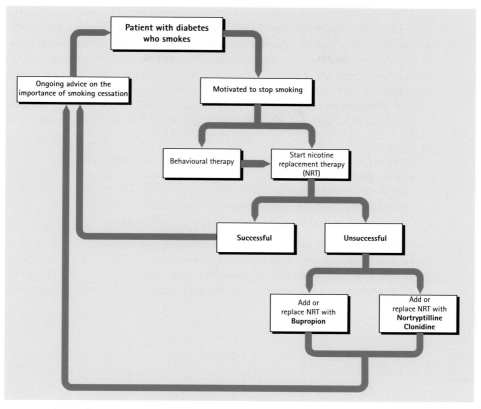

Fig. 29.1 Approach to smoking cessation in patients with diabetes.

rebound in depressive symptoms when bupropion is discontinued. The weight of evidence therefore favours NRT as the preferred first-line option for smoking cessation, with bupropion SR as a reasonable adjunct or second-line option. Other therapies where a meta-analysis has supported their efficacy in smoking cessation include the antihypertensive clonidine and the antidepressant nortriptylline, used either alone or in combination with NRT or bupropion. Finally, it is important to create a clinical and lifestyle environment that is supportive of treating patients with tobacco dependence. Simple changes in clinical routines and effective communication with the primary care physicians may help identify smokers who would like to stop smoking, and encourage intervention and links to more intensive tobacco dependence treatment programmes. These may provide patients with the stability they require in order to reduce their tobacco cravings and hopefully improve long-term success rate in smoking cessation among patients with cardiovascular disease.

Recent Developments

1   It has recently been shown that only two weeks of smoking cessation can ameliorate the enhanced platelet aggregability and intraplatelet redox imbalance in long-term smokers, largely by a reduction in oxidative stress.

2 Data have emerged to suggest that smoking is independently associated with the insulin resistance syndrome and this association may represent a major mechanistic link between cigarette smoking and cardiovascular disease. Smokers have been shown to be more insulin resistant and dyslipidaemic, and have evidence of endothelial dysfunction compared with non-smokers. Recent epidemiologic data have suggested that cardiovascular disease in smokers is primarily seen in those individuals who also have the characteristic findings of insulin resistance. This raises the intriguing possibility of treating the cardiovascular risk associated with smoking with an insulin sensitizer.

3 The role of gamma-aminobutyric acid (GABA) and metabotropic glutamate receptors as potential targets of pharmacotherapies for smoking cessation has recently been investigated. This is based on previous work which indicated a role for GABA and glutamate in the reinforcing effects of drugs of abuse. In an experimental study, compounds that increase GABAergic neurotransmission and antagonists at glutamate receptors have potential anti-smoking properties for humans.

4 Research examining the role of allelic variation in different genes which may influence smoking behaviour and nicotine dependency is also being actively pursued.[6] Dopamine receptor genes, transporter genes (serotonin and dopamine) and other genes related to metabolism of nicotine are plausible functional candidate genes.

Conclusion

The combination of smoking and diabetes is malignant, but smoking cessation rate remains low. Modern strategies to facilitate smoking cessation should incorporate behavioural therapy and pharmacological treatment as well as appropriate educational advice to individuals who are motivated to stop smoking. Research is ongoing to improve our understanding of the mechanistic link between smoking and cardiovascular disease as well as of genetic differences which might determine smoking behaviour and nicotine dependency.

Further Reading

1 Hajek P, Stead LF, West R, Jarvis M. Relapse prevention interventions for smoking cessation. *Cochrane Database Syst Rev* 2005; **1**: CD003999.

2 Critchley JA, Capewell S. Mortality risk reduction associated with smoking cessation in patients with coronary heart disease: a systematic review. *JAMA* 2003; **290**: 86–97.

3 West R, McNeill A, Raw M. Smoking cessation guidelines for health professionals: an update. Health Education Authority. *Thorax* 2000; **55**: 987–99.

4 Silagy C, Mant D, Fowler G, Lodge M. Meta-analysis on efficacy of nicotine replacement therapies in smoking cessation. *Lancet* 1994; **343**: 139–42.

5 Hurt RD, Sachs DPL, Glover ED, Offord KP, Johnston JA, Dale LC, Khayrallah MA, Schroeder DR, Glover PN, Sullivan CR, Croghan IT, Sullivan PM. A comparison of sustained-release bupropion and placebo for smoking cessation. *N Engl J Med* 1997; **337**: 1195–1202.

6 Zbikowski SM, Swan GE, McClure JB. Cigarette smoking and nicotine dependence. *Med Clin North Am* 2004; **88**: 1453–65.

PROBLEM

30 Hypertriglyceridaemia

Case History

A 57-year-old man with a strong family history of type 2 diabetes and ischaemic heart disease has a triglyceride level of 6.5 mmol/l. His cholesterol is 4.8 mmol/l. He is generally healthy, but slightly overweight, and takes no medication. Fasting blood glucose is 6.8 mmol/l and glycosylated haemoglobin (HbA1c) is in the normal range at 5.9%. He smokes ten cigarettes per day.

Is his high triglyceride level significant?

What steps might you take to manage it?

Background

Triglycerides are the predominant form of fat in the diet and in the body. The metabolic syndrome is associated with increased triglycerides, decreased high-density lipoprotein (HDL)-cholesterol and a predominance of small, dense low-density lipoprotein (LDL) particles. Each of these abnormalities is associated with increased risk of coronary heart disease. Association between hypertriglyceridaemia and coronary risk has been demonstrated in a number of studies, including the Honolulu Heart Programme, the Helsinki Heart Study and the Framingham Study. Increased triglyceride level arises because of increased hepatic production and decreased clearance of triglyceride-rich very-low-density lipoprotein (VLDL) particles.[1] Patients with very high triglyceride levels are also at risk of pancreatitis. The National Cholesterol Education Programme classifies triglyceride levels as shown in Table 30.1.

Table 30.1	National Cholesterol Education Programme guidelines for triglycerides	
	Plasma triglyceride level	
Classification	mg/dl	mmol/l
Desirable	<150	<1.7
Borderline	150–199	1.7–2.2
High	200–499	2.2–5.5
Very High	>500	>5.5
Data based on fasting plasma triglyceride levels.		

Familial (genetic) causes of hypertriglyceridaemia include:

- Type I hyperlipoproteinaemia (chylomicronaemia)—lipoprotein lipase or apolipoprotein C-II deficiency (autosomal recessive);

- Familial dysbetalipoproteinaemia —abnormal binding of apolipoprotein E;

- Familial hypertriglyceridaemia—overproduction of VLDL (autosomal dominant);

- Familial combined hyperlipidaemia—overproduction of VLDL and LDL;

- Hepatic lipase deficiency.

Most cases of hypertriglyceridaemia are secondary. Causes include obesity, high-carbohydrate diet, inactivity, oestrogen replacement and pregnancy, hypothyroidism, nephrotic syndrome, smoking and heavy alcohol intake, and hypertriglyceridaemia also occurs in diabetes/metabolic syndrome.

Management of hypertriglyceridaemia begins with lifestyle factors. The American Heart Association recommends the following to decrease triglyceride levels: if the patient is overweight, cut down on calories to reach ideal body weight; reduce saturated fat and cholesterol content of the diet; keep alcohol intake to a minimum; and increase dietary intake of fish high in omega-3 fatty acids (e.g. salmon, trout, mackerel, herring).

Drug treatment may be appropriate in an individual who is at high risk of coronary heart disease and whose triglycerides remain above 2.2 mmol/l in spite of attempts at lifestyle management. The approach to drug therapy depends on the degree of hyper-triglyceridaemia, the presence of other lipid abnormalities and the perceived risk to the patient. Nicotinic acid or related preparations (acipimox, Niaspan) can lower triglycerides and increase HDL-cholesterol. Side effects include flushing (usually self-limiting), pruritus, nausea, abdominal pain and diarrhoea, and the drugs can occasionally cause hepatic dysfunction. Fibrate drugs (e.g. gemfibrozil, bezafibrate and ciprofibrate) are peroxisome proliferator-activated receptor-α (PPAR-α) agonists and are widely used in treating combined hyperlipidaemias. They can cause muscle side effects ranging from mild aches to rhabdomyolysis, particularly when used in combination with statins. The latter group of drugs are the treatment of first choice when high LDL-cholesterol is the predominant abnormality and the patient is at high risk of heart disease. Omega-3 fatty acids, either as marine triglycerides (maxepa) or as fatty acid ethyl esters (Omacor), are often useful in isolated hypertriglyceridaemia. The relative potencies of the different drug groups are shown in Table 30.2.

Table 30.2 Triglyceride–lowering by drugs			
Drug Group	LDL–Cholesterol (Decrease)	HDL–Cholesterol (Increase)	Triglyceride (Decrease)
Statin	Up to 50%	10–20%	10–20%
Fibrate	Up to 20%	Up to 30%	35–50%
Nicotinic Acid	10–25%	15–25%	25–30%
Omega-3	—†	Up to 10%	25–30%

† = minimal effect

Recent Developments

1   There is a complex relationship between cardiovascular risk factors and the risk of developing diabetes. Recent data from the Insulin Resistance Atherosclerosis Study[2] suggest that the presence of cardiovascular risk factors including hypertriglyceridaemia and low HDL-cholesterol predict development of type 2 diabetes (Figure 30.1). The greater the number of risk factors, the greater the risk. It is uncertain whether specific interventions to improve these risk factors will prevent diabetes developing but, given the relationship between triglycerides and insulin resistance, this approach should be pursued.

2   Increased tissue levels of triglyceride are associated with insulin resistance and other features of metabolic syndrome. Magnetic resonance spectroscopy studies demonstrate hepatic lipid accumulation *in vivo* in obese patients with type 2 diabetes,[3] and the presence of elevated serum hepatic transaminase levels in the West of Scotland Coronary Prevention Study (WOSCOPS) predicted development of type 2 diabetes.[4] Also, triglyceride accumulation in skeletal muscle impairs the efficiency of substrate utilization and contributes to peripheral insulin resistance.

3   Interaction between components of the diet and genes involved in the pathogenesis of metabolic syndrome is an area of research interest. For example, polyunsaturated fatty acids and a common polymorphism of the PPAR-γ gene interact to regulate peripheral levels of triglyceride. Further study in this area may identify more effective dietary manipulations and therapies tailored to individual genotype.[5]

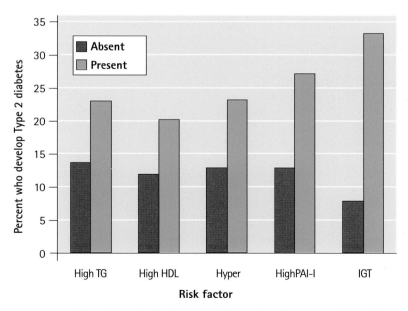

Fig. 30.1 Figure shows the development of diabetes in a four-year period in subjects with initially normal or impaired glucose tolerance (IGT) or with other cardiovascular disease (CVD) risk factors present or absent at baseline. In addition, patients with multiple risk factors were more likely to develop diabetes than those with no, or single, risk factors. TG = triglycerides; HYPER = hypertension; PAI-I = plasminogen activator inhibitor-1. *Source:* D'Agostino *et al.* 2004.[2]

Conclusion

The above patient has markedly elevated triglyceride level and a high risk of both diabetes and coronary artery disease. Attempts should be made to lower his triglyceride level. Initial management should include assessment and, if possible, improvement in diet, weight reduction, smoking cessation and reduction in alcohol intake. Given the degree of hypertriglyceridaemia, lifestyle management alone is unlikely to lower his triglyceride level into the target range. Initial drug treatment with either a nicotinic acid derivative or with omega-3 fatty acids would be first-line treatment after lifestyle intervention.

Further Reading

1   Krauss RM. Lipids and lipoproteins in patients with type 2 diabetes. *Diabetes Care* 2004; **27**: 1496–1504.

2   D'Agostino RB, Hamman RF, Karter AJ, Mykkanen L, Wagenknecht LE, Haffner SM. Cardiovascular disease risk factors predict the development of type 2 diabetes: The Insulin Resistance Atherosclerosis Study. *Diabetes Care* 2004; **27**: 2234–40.

3   Thomas EL, Hamilton G, Patel N, O'Dwyer R, Dore CJ, Goldin RD, Bell JD, Taylor-Robinson SD. Hepatic triglyceride content and its relation to body adiposity: a magnetic resonance imaging and proton magnetic resonance spectroscopy study. *Gut* 2005; **54**: 122–7.

4   Sattar N, Scherbakova O, Ford I, O'Reilly DS, Stanley A, Forrest E, Macfarlane PW, Packard CJ, Cobbe SM, Shepherd J. Elevated alanine aminotransferase predicts new-onset type 2 diabetes independently of classical risk factors, metabolic syndrome, and C- reactive protein in the West of Scotland Coronary Prevention Study. *Diabetes* 2004; **53**: 2855–60.

5   Tai ES, Corella D, Demissie S, Couples LA, Coltell O, Schaefer EJ, Tucker KL, Ordovas JM. Polyunsaturated fatty acids interact with the PPARA-L162V polymorphism to affect plasma triglyceride and apolipoprotein C-III concentrations in the Framingham Heart Study. *J Nutr* 2005; **135**: 397–403.

31 Hyperlipidaemia in Type 1 Diabetes

Case History

Your patient is 38 years old with an 11-year history of type 1 diabetes. He has no micro- or macrovascular complications of diabetes. His blood pressure is 138/78 mmHg, glycosylated haemoglogin (HbA1c) is 6.8% and lipid parameters are as follows: total cholesterol 5.1 mmol/l; high-density lipoprotein (HDL)-cholesterol 1.0 mmol/l; low-density lipoprotein (LDL)-cholesterol 3.0 mmol/l; and triglyceride 2.4 mmol/l.

Would you treat his hyperlipidaemia?

If so, which agent(s) would be most appropriate?

Background

Best management of modest hyperlipidaemia in young adults with type 1 diabetes (T1DM) is uncertain. Landmark clinical trials have demonstrated that statins are effective agents for the primary and secondary prevention of coronary heart disease (CHD) in patients with type 2 diabetes, but there are few data for the primary prevention of CHD in patients with T1DM. Moreover, since age appears to be the most important determinant of CHD risk, few trials have included patients below the age of 40 years.

However, a recognized paradox of T1DM is that, while mortality from CHD in this group of patients is three- to six-fold higher than that of the general population, their lipid and lipoprotein patterns are often generally favourable.[1] Furthermore, in patients with good glycaemic control (as is the case above), cholesterol, triglyceride and LDL levels are similar to, or even lower, than those in the general population, whereas HDL-cholesterol levels are normal or slightly increased. In the presence of CHD, although triglyceride and LDL-cholesterol levels in patients with T1DM are increased and HDL-cholesterol levels are lower than in those without heart disease, these and associated lipid and lipoprotein disturbances do not fully explain their elevated CHD risk. The risk of CHD in young patients with T1DM is likely to be an underestimate using available risk calculators and consequently treatment is often delayed.

Another factor that one should take into account when determining the cardiovascular risk of an individual with T1DM is the duration of their diabetes. Since prolonged exposure to hyperglycaemia increases an individual's vascular risk and alters their lipoprotein constituent, it is reasonable to include duration of diabetes as a further determinant to the need for statins. In light of this, the British Hypertension Society recommends that those patients with type 2 diabetes for greater than 10 years or aged over 50 years should be considered as a coronary risk equivalent and should be treated as for secondary prevention guidelines. As diabetes is considered a coronary disease equivalent, a statin should be used irrespective of lipid profile.[2]

In the absence of intervention trial data in patients with T1DM, and given the high rates of cardiovascular disease, it seems reasonable to treat as per type 2 diabetes. Young persons with T1DM exhibit abnormalities in their lipoprotein constituents and vascular wall when compared with the general population. In the Heart Protection Study (HPS), statins reduced the risk of cardiovascular events in all subgroups of patients studied, including those with pre-treatment LDL-cholesterol <3 mmol/l. It is important to note that 10% of the HPS diabetes subgroup had T1DM. When considering patients with a young onset of T1DM, approximately 20% develop diabetic nephropathy after 20 years of diabetes duration and, of those who develop diabetic nephropathy, more than 40% develop cardiovascular disease by the age of 40 years. Lipid and lipoprotein abnormalities are strongly associated with micro- and macroalbuminuria—major predictors of CHD events and risks of nephropathy progression. Preliminary evidence has also emerged to suggest that statins may slow the progression of diabetic renal disease. In light of the typically 'normal' lipid profile—which may mask their high CHD risk—adopting an aggressive cardiovascular risk-reduction strategy in young patients with T1DM should be encouraged. Clearly, the decision to start a statin in this patient should be made after appropriate discussion on risk–benefit profile with strong emphasis on the potential requirement for lifelong treatment if the drug is tolerated.

Recent Developments

1 The benefits of aggressive lipid-lowering treatment with statins in stable CHD patients were further supported in the Treating to New Target (TNT) study.[3] In this study, 10 001 patients with clinically evident CHD and LDL-cholesterol concentrations of under 130 mg/dl were randomized to daily doses of atorvastatin, 10 mg or 80 mg, for an average of 4.9 years. Over this time, a primary cardiovascular event occurred in 8.7% of individuals taking high-dose atorvastatin, compared with 10.9% taking low-dose treatment (22% relative reduction). A subanalysis of the study, involving 753 patients with diabetes, showed that high-dose statin significantly reduced the risk of individuals suffering a first major cardiovascular event by 25% compared with the low-dose (hazard ratio [HR]0.75). The 80 mg dose also reduced the time to first cerebrovascular event by 31% (HR 0.69). On the basis of these results, clinicians should consider aggressive use of lipid-lowering therapies in all patients with diabetes.

2 Teenage boys, but not girls, with T1DM have significantly higher intima–media thickness (IMT) than those without T1DM.[4] IMT is higher among boys with poor glucose control, exposure to smoke and higher total cholesterol and apolipoprotein B levels. These observations also support an aggressive approach to treating hyperlipidaemia even in young patients with T1DM, particularly in those with abnormal lipid profile and poor glycaemic control. In girls, IMT tends to be higher among those with a family history of cardiovascular disease and lower among those with favourable levels of HDL.

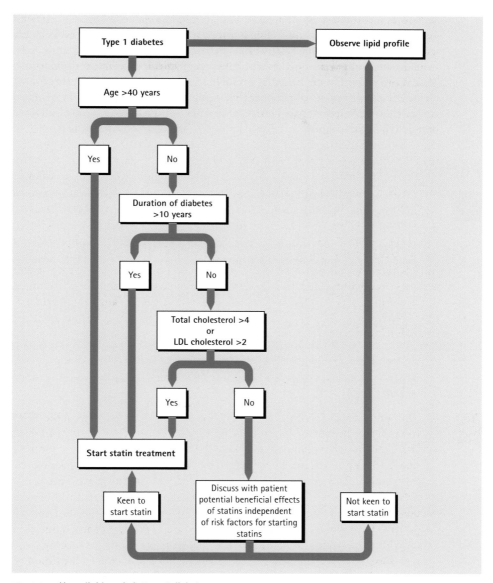

Fig. 31.1 Hyperlipidaemia in type 1 diabetes.

Conclusion

 Despite his young age and modest hyperlipidaemia, this patient has a long history of diabetes and thus a chronic exposure to hyperglycaemia and increased atherosclerotic risk.
While evidence for the use of statins has been derived largely from studies involving
middle-aged patients with type 2 diabetes,[5] evidence is emerging to support an aggressive
lipid-lowering strategy in younger patients with T1DM. Intima–media thickness and

inflammatory markers are increased—suggesting premature atherosclerosis. It is suggested that this patient is treated with a statin. However, it is important always to engage with patients in discussing the relative risk–benefits of starting statins, before embarking on what is likely to be a lifelong treatment. Given the qualitative nature of lipoprotein abnormalities in patients with T1DM, it would be conceivable in the near future for statins to be routinely prescribed to all patients (including adolescents) whose T1DM was diagnosed at least ten years previously—akin to how we approach treatment of adolescents with familial hyperlipidaemia.

Further Reading

1   Chaturvedi N, Fuller JH. Differing associations of lipid and lipoprotein disturbances with the macrovascular and microvascular complications of type 1 diabetes. *Diabetes Care* 2001; **24**: 2071–7.

2   William B, Poulter NR, Brown MJ, Davis M, McInnes GT, Potter JT, Sever PS, Thom SMcG. Guidelines for the management of hypertension 2004—BHS IV. *J Human Hypertens* 2004; **18**: 139–85.

3   LaRosa JC, Grundy SM, Waters DD, Shear C, Barter P, Fruchart J, Gotto AM, Greten H, Kastelein JJ, Shepherd J, Wenger NK. Intensive lipid lowering with atorvastatin in patients with stable coronary disease. *N Engl J Med* 2005; **352**: 1425–35.

4   Krantz JS, Mack WJ, Hodis HN, Liu CR, Liu CH, Kaufman FR. Early onset of subclinical atherosclerosis in young persons with type 1 diabetes. *J Pediatr* 2004; **145**: 452–7.

5   Haffner SM. Dyslipidaemia management in adults with diabetes. *Diabetes Care* 2004; **27**: S68–S71.

32 Hyperlipidaemia in Type 2 Diabetes

Case History

A 58-year-old woman with hypertension and type 2 diabetes for nine years has her fasting lipid profile checked. Her cholesterol is 5.4 mmol/l, triglycerides 3.4 mmol/l, and high-density lipoprotein (HDL)-cholesterol is 0.8 mmol/l. She takes oral hypoglycaemics—metformin 500 mg three times daily and gliclazide 80 mg twice daily—but her glycosylated haemoglobin (HbA1c) remains elevated at 9.2%. Blood pressure is 150/90 mmHg despite taking two antihypertensives, and she is a smoker. She admits that she does not always remember to take all of her tablets.

Does she require treatment for her dyslipidaemia?

How would you approach the management of her diabetes?

What is the most important aspect of her management to tackle first?

Background

Poorly controlled diabetes is associated with increased triglycerides, decreased HDL-cholesterol and a predominance of small, dense low-density lipoprotein (LDL) particles. Each of these three abnormalities increases the risk of vascular disease.[1] Often, total cholesterol and LDL-cholesterol are normal or near-normal. The pathogenesis of the dyslipidaemia is complex. Increased triglyceride occurs because of increased hepatic production of triglyceride-rich very-low-density lipoprotein (VLDL) particles associated with decreased clearance of these and chylomicrons due to decreased lipoprotein lipase activity. Small, dense LDL particles arise from the VLDL particles by hydrolysis and by enrichment with further triglyceride due to the action of cholesteryl ester transfer protein (CETP). The small, dense LDL particles are cleared more slowly than other LDL particles and their increased retention time in the circulation, along with their tendency to become oxidized and glycated in patients with diabetes, makes them more atherogenic. The reduction in HDL, particularly HDL-2b, particles arises because of transfer of cholesterol from these particles to triglyceride-rich VLDL particles and a reciprocal transfer of triglyceride to the HDL particles, making them more susceptible to clearance by hepatic lipase. For patients with impaired glucose utilization, including type 2 diabetes, the triglyceride and HDL abnormalities are more powerfully associated with atherosclerosis than are changes in total or HDL-cholesterol and thus should be regarded as the prime targets for treatment.

Central obesity and insulin resistance lead to increased release of free fatty acids, which in turn increase synthesis of triglycerides. Even modest weight loss of 5% of total body weight, particularly along with exercise, can decrease triglyceride levels by up to 40%, and total cholesterol by up to 15%. Modern lipid-lowering drugs are very safe. The major choice is between statins and fibrates, depending on the individual patient's pattern of dyslipidaemia and overall risk profile. Fibrates act as agonists at the peroxisome proliferator-activated receptor-α (PPAR-α) and thus increase expression of key enzymes involved in disposal of atherogenic lipoprotein particles. Although there is considerably less evidence for prevention of cardiac events than there is for statin drugs, there is still irrefutable evidence that the fibrates have a protective role.[2] For example, a secondary preventative role was demonstrated in the Veterans Affairs High-Density Lipoprotein Intervention Trial (VA-HIT), while the Helsinki Heart Study demonstrated a primary preventative effect. Both studies used gemfibrozil, and each included a small diabetic subgroup. For patients who have more marked elevations in triglycerides, treatment with nicotinic acid derivatives or omega-3 fatty acids may be considered.

For patients in whom marked reduction in LDL-cholesterol is required, the statins are the drugs of choice. Landmark trials published in the 1990s demonstrated their effectiveness and safety in secondary prevention of cardiac events. Thus, the Scandinavian Simvastatin Survival Study (4S), the Cholesterol and Recurrent Events (CARE) study and the Long-term Intervention with Pravastatin in Ischaemic Disease (LIPID) study demonstrated 25% to 32% reduction in cardiac events in patients with pre-existing coronary heart disease. The 4S and CARE studies demonstrated, in subgroup analyses, that the drugs were at least as effective in patients with diabetes. The Heart Protection Study (HPS) enrolled over 20 000 people with a total cholesterol greater than 3.5 mmol/l and who either had a previous coronary event, had other arterial occlusive disease, or had diabetes or hypertension. In a 2 × 2 factorial design, patients were randomized to receive simvastatin 40 mg per day/antioxidant vitamins or the corresponding placebos. There was no effect demonstrated with the antioxidant vitamins. Simvastatin use was associated with 18% reduction in coronary death rate. In the diabetic cohort of 5963 patients there was a 12% reduction in the incidence of a first major vascular event. The association between low-grade inflammation and risk of either diabetes or vascular disease is now well established. In addition to their action in decreasing cholesterol biosynthesis, statin drugs are now well documented to have anti-inflammatory actions and may, therefore, protect the blood vessels through multiple pathways.

For patients with severe dyslipidaemia and who are at high risk of ischaemic heart disease, statins and fibrates can be given in combination, although there is increased risk of myopathy and rhabdomyolysis, about which the patient should be warned. Muscle complications are also increased in patients with renal impairment. Ezetimibe is a relatively new drug on the market, which acts by decreasing the intestinal absorption of dietary and biliary cholesterol. It does not affect absorption of triglycerides or fat-soluble vitamins. The drug acts by binding to the Niemann-Pick C1 like protein-1, a specific cholesterol transporter protein in the gut. The drug may be given alone to patients who are intolerant of statins, but it is most effectively combined with statins to further decrease LDL-cholesterol. The drug is both safe and effective in patients with the metabolic syndrome or type 2 diabetes.

Recent Developments

1 Insulin resistance in muscle and liver may be increased by accumulation of lipid in these tissues. This accumulation may involve a transcription factor called the liver X

receptor, activation of which increases enzymes of the lipogenic pathway including fatty acid synthase.[3] The liver X receptor is also involved in the increased expression of the glucose transporter GLUT4 in response to insulin. Variations in certain key genes that regulate lipid storage in tissues may control susceptibility to metabolic syndrome to an extent. Thus, variations in the gene for lipoprotein lipase, which controls lipid storage in adipose tissue, muscle and the vascular endothelium, have been linked to insulin resistance.[4] Furthermore, variations in the gene for PPAR-α, which is partly responsible for regulating expression of lipoprotein lipase, may govern susceptibility to type 2 diabetes.[5]

2   A novel approach to increasing HDL-cholesterol is by inhibiting CETP. A recent trial with the inhibitor torcetrapib reported increased HDL-cholesterol of 46% when used alone and 61% when used with atorvastatin (Figure 32.1).[6] The drug also increased the mean size of both LDL and HDL lipoprotein particles.

3   A major theme of current nutritional research is the interaction between dietary components and the expression of genes or the activity of metabolic pathways *in vivo*. Conjugated linoleic acids have been proposed as regulators of lipid metabolism and insulin resistance.[7] There has been interest in diets that include a small amount of walnuts.[8] These contain a high proportion of polyunsaturated fats including α-linoleic acid as well as the antioxidant γ-tocopherol. Compared with a control diet, a diet that included 30 grams of walnuts per day significantly increased HDL-cholesterol and decreased LDL-cholesterol.

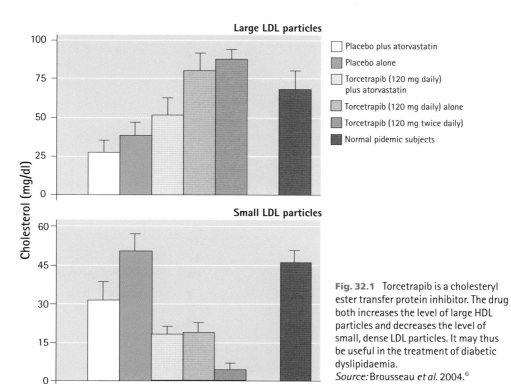

Fig. 32.1 Torcetrapib is a cholesteryl ester transfer protein inhibitor. The drug both increases the level of large HDL particles and decreases the level of small, dense LDL particles. It may thus be useful in the treatment of diabetic dyslipidaemia.
Source: Brousseau *et al.* 2004.[6]

Conclusion

The patient's risk of vascular events can be estimated using a risk calculator such as the United Kingdom Prospective Diabetes Study (UKPDS) risk engine.[9] Using this engine, her calculated ten-year risk of coronary heart disease is 31.4%, of fatal coronary heart disease 22.8%, of stroke 11.5%, and of fatal stroke 1.9%. She is at high risk and her risk parameters need to be managed vigorously. She should be strongly advised to stop smoking, as continuing to smoke would negate much of the potential benefit of therapies for the other risk factors.

Diabetes control needs improvement and every effort should be made to encourage the patient to work on diet and exercise. There is scope to increase her oral hypoglycaemic drugs, and increased metformin may be a good first step. She probably does not require insulin at this stage. A major thrust of her management should be to decrease her cardiac risk without making her drug regimen unduly complex. A fibrate drug should improve her lipid profile and may be used as a holding measure until her glycaemic control is improved.

Further Reading

1 Krauss RM. Lipids and lipoproteins in patients with type 2 diabetes. *Diabetes Care* 2004; **27**: 1496–1504.

2 Colagiuri S, Best J. Lipid-lowering therapy in people with type 2 diabetes. *Curr Opin Lipidol* 2002; **13**: 617–23.

3 Kase ET, Wensaas AJ, Aas V, Hojlund K, Levin K, Thoresen GH, Beck-Nielsen H, Rustan AC, Gaster M. Skeletal muscle lipid accumulation in type 2 diabetes may involve the liver X receptor pathway. *Diabetes* 2005; **54**: 1108–15.

4 Goodarzi MO, Guo X, Taylor KD, Quinones MJ, Saad MF, Yang H, Hsueh WA, Rotter JI. Lipoprotein lipase is a gene for insulin resistance in Mexican Americans. *Diabetes* 2004; **53**: 214–20.

5 Flavell DM, Ireland H, Stephens JW, Hawe E, Acharya S, Mather H, Hurel SJ, Humphries SE. Peroxisome proliferator-activated receptor alpha gene variation influences age of onset and progression of type 2 diabetes. *Diabetes* 2005; **54**: 582–6.

6 Brousseau ME, Schaefer EJ, Wolfe ML, Bloedon LT, Digenio AG, Clark RW, Mancuso JP, Rader DJ. Effects of an inhibitor of cholesteryl ester transfer protein on HDL cholesterol. *N Engl J Med* 2004; **350**: 1505–15.

7 Roche HM. Dietary lipids and gene expression. *Biochem Soc Trans* 2004; **32**: 999–1002.

8 Tapsell LC, Gillen LJ, Patch CS, Batterham M, Owen A, Bare M, Kennedy M. Including walnuts in a low-fat/modified-fat diet improves HDL cholesterol-to-total cholesterol ratios in patients with type 2 diabetes. *Diabetes Care* 2004; **27**: 2777–83.

9 UKPDS risk engine. http://www.dtu.ox.ac.uk

33 Aspirin Use in Diabetes

Case History

A 53-year-old woman with a four-year history of type 2 diabetes attends your clinic for annual review. She is treated with metformin and has reasonable diabetic control (glycosylated haemoglogin, HbA1c, 7.4%). For the past two years, she has taken lisinopril because of hypertension and because microalbuminuria has been noted on several occasions. Her blood pressure is well controlled.

Should she take regular aspirin?

If so, what dose should she take?

Background

Patients with diabetes have an increased risk of vascular disease that is up to four times that of the background population. Available evidence suggests that the relative risk associated with diabetes is higher in women than in men. Compared with men of comparable age, pre-menopausal women are relatively protected from risk of vascular disease. This protection appears to be lost in women who have developed diabetes.

Increased vascular risk in patients with diabetes arises from a number of factors including hyperglycaemia, dyslipidaemia, hypertension, low-grade inflammation and an increased tendency for the blood to clot. The hypercoagulable state is partly due to increased platelet aggregation under the influence of thromboxane. Aspirin irreversibly inhibits the enzyme cyclooxygenase (prostaglandin synthase), and thus decreases the production of thromboxane. Of note is that its efficacy may be diminished if it is administered with other non-steroidal anti-inflammatory drugs.

The use of aspirin for secondary prevention of vascular events is no longer controversial. Broadly speaking, the use of aspirin in a patient who has either had a vascular event or has established vascular disease will reduce the risk of subsequent myocardial infarction by one-third and the risk of stroke by one-quarter, and decrease the overall risk of death from vascular disease. These benefits apply as much to patients with diabetes as to their non-diabetic counterparts. Reviewing over 170 controlled trials in a meta-analysis involving 70 000 patients in total, the Anti-Platelet Trialists (APT) confirmed the benefits of aspirin in high-risk populations.[1] For diabetic patients, the authors estimated that around 38 vascular events were saved for each 1000 diabetic patients treated with aspirin.

There is less evidence relating to primary prevention. Recent studies suggest that risk of myocardial infarction is reduced by around one-third but it is still uncertain whether risk of stroke or overall risk of cardiovascular death is reduced. The seminal study in this area was the Early Treatment Diabetic Retinopathy Study (ETDRS),[2] in which 3711 patients with diabetes from 22 centres were randomized either to placebo or to aspirin treatment. The risk of fatal and non-fatal myocardial infarction was reduced to a degree comparable with other studies in non-diabetic cohorts. A more recent study, the Primary Prevention Project (PPP),[3] confirmed that low-dose aspirin reduced risk of vascular events in a cohort of 4495 high-risk individuals (including 1031 with diabetes), but the study suggested that the benefit of aspirin might be lower in diabetic patients.

As with all drugs, the use of aspirin is associated with a risk of side effects. Up to 25% of patients using aspirin may experience dyspepsia or other gastrointestinal side effects. These are usually mild and do not necessitate stopping the drug. Aspirin may provoke asthma, or other allergic symptoms, in a small proportion of people. The major worry is the increased risk of haemorrhage. The increased risk is probably of the order of 60% over five years with a very small risk of cerebral haemorrhage amounting to about 0.3 per 1000 patients. Caution is certainly urged in patients with haemorrhagic retinopathy, but the ETDRS trial[2] provided reassurance that aspirin was generally safe in patients with retinopathy, although there was no benefit of aspirin in preventing progression of retinopathy.

People with diabetes should have cardiovascular risk managed as vigorously as non-diabetic individuals with established vascular disease. The American Heart Association, in line with other comparable bodies, currently recommends aspirin use for individuals whose ten-year risk of a first vascular event is greater than 10%. This includes many patients with diabetes. There is evidence from a number of countries that aspirin is under-used amongst patients with diabetes. This is unfortunate since the drug is safe, cheap and effective.

The American Diabetes Association recommendations for the use of aspirin in patients with diabetes are summarized in Table 33.1. The major trials have used doses

Table 33.1	Summary of the American Diabetes Association recommendations on aspirin usage	
Number Level	Recommendation	Evidence
1	Use for secondary prevention where there is a history of ischaemic heart disease (IHD), cerebrovascular disease, peripheral vascular disease or vascular bypass procedure.	A
2	Use for primary prevention in type 2 diabetes patients over 40 years who have additional risk factors (family history of IHD, hypertension, smoking, dyslipidaemia, albuminuria).	A
3	Use for primary prevention in type 1 diabetes patients over 40 years who have additional risk factors (family history of IHD, hypertension, smoking, dyslipidaemia, albuminuria).	C
4	Not recommended for patients with aspirin allergy, bleeding tendency, those taking anticoagulant, or who have suffered a recent gastrointestinal haemorrhage. Other antiplatelet drugs may be considered.	E
5	Not recommended for patients under 21 years because of increased risk of Reye's syndrome. Patients under 30 years have generally not been studied.	

Recommendations apply equally to men and women, and the dose of aspirin recommended in each case is 75–162 mg per day.
Evidence levels:
  A = supported by multiple randomized controlled trials;
  C = incomplete or conflicting evidence
  E = expert consensus. Source: Colwell, 2004.[6]

ranging from 75 mg per day to 375 mg on alternate days. Hence, the current recommended daily dose is 75–162 mg per day.

Recent Developments

1   Other antiplatelet drugs. The suggestion from the PPP study that diabetic patients may be relatively insensitive to low-dose aspirin, because of activation of multiple pathways leading to clot formation, has stimulated interest in other antiplatelet drugs. There is a need for alternatives in any case for patients who are sensitive to aspirin. Recent work with clopidogrel, an inhibitor of ADP-induced platelet aggregation, in trials including diabetic subjects, suggests that this drug is superior to aspirin in preventing vascular events.[4] There is also interest in platelet glycoprotein IIb/IIIa antagonists, orally active forms of which have been developed, and in the drug cilostazol, a potent inhibitor of phosphodiesterase type 3. The latter drug is finding increasing usage in patients with peripheral vascular disease but its beneficial actions on platelet function may increase its use in patients at high risk of cardiovascular disease.

2   Aspirin and the metabolic syndrome. The antiplatelet and anti-inflammatory effects of aspirin contribute to its benefit in preventing macrovascular complications of diabetes. Recent evidence[5] suggests that the drug may also reduce post-prandial excursions in glucose and free fatty acids, in addition to reducing insulin resistance. The clinical significance of these observations and the optimal dose of aspirin to achieve these effects have yet to be determined.

Conclusion

Aspirin is a safe, effective and cheap drug to prevent vascular complications in patients with diabetes. Its use is recommended in diabetic patients over the age of 40 years who have other cardiovascular risk factors. On those grounds, and in the absence of contraindications, the above patient should be prescribed aspirin at a dose of 75–150 mg per day.

Further Reading

1   Antiplatelet Trialists' Collaboration. Collaborative overview of randomised trials of antiplatelet therapy– I: Prevention of death, myocardial infarction, and stroke by prolonged antiplatelet therapy in various categories of patients. *BMJ* 1994; **308**: 81–106.

2   ETDRS Investigators. Aspirin effects on mortality and morbidity in patients with diabetes mellitus. Early Treatment Diabetic Retinopathy Study report 14. *JAMA* 1992; **268**: 292–300.

3   Sacco M, Pellegrini F, Roncaglioni MC, Avanzini F, Tognoni G, Nicolucci A. Primary prevention of cardiovascular events with low-dose aspirin and vitamin E in type 2 diabetic patients: results of the Primary Prevention Project (PPP) trial. *Diabetes Care* 2003; **26**: 3264–72.

4   Hirsh J, Bhatt DL. Comparative benefits of clopidogrel and aspirin in high-risk patient populations: lessons from the CAPRIE and CURE studies. *Arch Intern Med* 2004; **164**: 2106–10.

5 Hundal RS, Petersen KF, Mayerson AB, Randhawa PS, Inzucchi S, Shoelson SE, Shulman GI. Mechanism by which high-dose aspirin improves glucose metabolism in type 2 diabetes. *J Clin Invest* 2002; **109**: 1321–6.

6 Colwell JA. Aspirin therapy in diabetes. *Diabetes Care* 2004; **27**: S72–3.

PROBLEM

34 Hypertension—Uncomplicated

Case History

A 74-year-old man with type 2 diabetes has repeated blood pressure readings of 154/90 mmHg and higher. He has no symptoms, and his diabetic control is reasonable. Dipstick urine is negative for protein.

Should he have antihypertensive therapy?

What treatment is appropriate?

Background

It is likely that blood pressure measurement has been either opportunistic or part of structured review. It is unlikely that blood pressure alone has caused referable symptoms. A clear appraisal of the potential risks of blood pressure at this level is needed to inform the consultation. This risk is partly dictated by other cardiovascular risk factors and though no absolute risk can be given for an individual, there are a number of risk calculators that can be used to give an estimate. The most commonly used Framingham, United Kingdom Prospective Diabetes Study (UKPDS) and New Zealand Cardiovascular Risk tables all give a ten-year cardiovascular risk in excess of 25% for this man, assuming he is a non-smoker with a high-density lipoprotein (HDL)-cholesterol level of 1.0 mmol/l and no prevalent cardiovascular disease.

For this discussion, there is an assumption that the patient is naïve to blood pressure treatment and that there are no clinical or biochemical features of secondary causes of hypertension. The discussion focuses on pharmacological interventions to lower blood pressure.

Intervention threshold

Data from the UKPDS,[1] HOT trial[2] (Hypertension Optimal Treatment) and MRFIT[3] (Multiple Risk Factor Intervention Trial) demonstrate that:

- hypertension affects two-thirds of people with type 2 diabetes;

- lowering elevated blood pressure reduces macro- and microvascular risk;

- there is no unequivocal threshold effect of blood pressure on macrovascular risk.

An intervention threshold of 140 mmHg systolic and/or 90 mmHg diastolic is advised by both the American Diabetes Association[4] and the Seventh Report of the Joint National Committee on Prevention, Detection, Evaluation, and Treatment of High Blood Pressure.[5] Analyses of data from UKPDS and HOT show that a 10 mmHg reduction in systolic blood pressure is associated with a reduction in:

- all cause mortality by 18%;

- microvascular disease (mainly retinopathy) by 37%;

- stroke by 44%;

- heart failure by 45%;

- major cardiovascular events by 51%.

Choice of hypotensive agent

Endpoint reduction is primarily a consequence of blood pressure reduction rather than agent selection. Where there are no comorbidities, there is little to choose between most classes of hypotensive agents—an approach supported by both the UKPDS and ALLHAT[6] (Antihypertensive and Lipid-Lowering Treatment to Prevent Heart Attack Trial) studies. The ALLHAT study demonstrated the efficacy of the cheap diuretic chlorthalidone as a first-line hypotensive agent in normoalbuminuric patients and its particular benefit in black patients where low-renin hypertension may respond less well to angiotensin-converting enzyme (ACE) inhibitors. It should be noted that the alpha-blocker arm of the ALLHAT study was terminated early because of an excess of cardiovascular events in this randomization group.

Even if there is elevated urinary albumin excretion, blood pressure reduction is still the most important factor in reducing cardiovascular events. An ACE inhibitor- or angiotensin receptor blocker-based regime may slow the progression of nephropathy—particularly when baseline creatinine is elevated.

Though studies support the need for multiple agents to control blood pressure, many patients will still not achieve optimal blood pressure control. The UKPDS, HOT and ABCD (Appropriate Blood Pressure Control in Diabetes) trials all showed that three agents were needed, on average, to achieve average diastolic blood pressure readings of 80 mmHg or so.

Finally, it is important to remember that blood pressure is not the only therapeutic target and that comorbidities and lifestyle may dictate whether a particular agent is used or not. For example, where there is left ventricular dysfunction, ACE inhibition is appropriate; beta-blockade or a calcium channel blocker may relieve anginal symptoms; if prostatic symptoms are present, alpha-blockade may provide symptomatic benefit; and where borderline erectile dysfunction is a problem, a patient may elect to avoid a thiazide diuretic or beta-blocker.

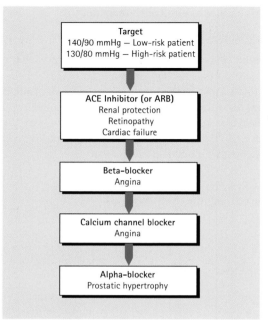

Fig. 34.1 Choice of antihypertensive drug.
ARB = angiotensin receptor blocker.

Recent Developments

1 A study by Gaede *et al.*[7] demonstrated that aggressive treatment of cardiovascular risk factors halved cardiovascular endpoints in patients with type 2 diabetes, hypertension and elevated albumin excretion. Patients were treated to a blood pressure target of 140/85 mmHg—reduced to 130/80 mmHg later in the study—in conjunction with a glycosylated haemoglobin (HbA1c) target <6.5%, total cholesterol <4 mmol/l and triglycerides <1.7 mmol/l, with near universal use of aspirin and an ACE inhibitor. However, 20% of patients did not reach the diastolic blood pressure target in the intensively treated group.

Conclusion

Evidence of prevalent cardiovascular disease should be sought, an electrocardiogram should be performed and urinary albumin excretion assessed—probably by spot urinary albumin–creatinine ratio. Assuming hypertension remains uncomplicated, a low-dose diuretic would be a reasonable first-line agent. It is difficult to be dogmatic about a blood pressure target, though a target of <130/80 mmHg is reasonable—acknowledging that the lower the target, the more difficult this will be to achieve without an unsatisfactory number of medications or side effects.

Finally, blood pressure lowering should be set within a context of aggressive cardiovascular risk reduction with smoking cessation, lifestyle intervention, antiplatelet therapy and cholesterol reduction.

Further Reading

1 UK Prospective Diabetes Study Group. Tight blood pressure control and risk of macrovascular and microvascular complications in type 2 diabetes: UKPDS 38. *BMJ* 1998; **317**: 703–13.

2 Hansson L, Zanchetti A, Carruthers SG, Dahlof B, Elmfeldt D, Julius S, Menard J, Rahn KH, Wedel H, Westerling S. Effects of intensive blood-pressure lowering and low-dose aspirin in patients with hypertension: principal results of the Hypertension Optimal Treatment (HOT) randomised trial. *Lancet* 1998; **351**: 1755–62.

3 Cupples L, D'Agostino R. Some risk factors related to the annual incidence of cardiovascular disease and death using pooled repeated biennial measurements: 30-year follow-up. In: Kannel W, Wolf P (eds). *The Framingham Study: An Epidemiological Investigation of Cardiovascular Disease*. Washington, DC: NHLBI National Printing Office, 1971; Section 34.

4 American Diabetes Association. Standards of Medical Care in Diabetes. *Diabetes Care* 2005; **28** (Suppl 1): S4–36.

5 Chobanian AV, Bakris GL, Black HR, Cushman WC, Green LA, Izzo J, Jones DW, Materson BJ, Oparil S, Wright JT, Roccella EJ. Seventh Report of the Joint Committee on Prevention, Detection, Evaluation, and Treatment of High Blood Pressure. *Hypertension* 2003; **42**: 1206–52.

6 The ALLHAT Officers and Coordinators for the ALLHAT Collaborative Research Group. Major outcomes in high-risk hypertensive patients randomized to angiotensin-converting enzyme inhibitor or calcium channel blocker vs diuretic: The Antihypertensive and Lipid-Lowering Treatment to Prevent Heart Attack Trial (ALLHAT). *JAMA* 2002; **288**: 2981–97.

7 Gaede P, Vedel P, Larsen N, Jensen GVH, Parving H-H, Pedersen O. Multifactorial intervention and cardiovascular disease in patients with type 2 diabetes. *N Engl J Med* 2003; **348**: 383–93.

PROBLEM

35 Hypertension—Hard to Control

Case History

A 54-year-old newsagent with long-standing type 2 diabetes has hypertension and a history of myocardial infarction. He takes a thiazide, angiotensin-converting enzyme (ACE) inhibitor, beta-blocker and non-dihydropyridine calcium antagonist for hypertension, but blood pressure is repeatedly recorded at 148/86 mmHg or higher. Renal function is normal and there is no fluid overload.

Should he be investigated for secondary hypertension?

Would you alter his therapy?

Background

A target blood pressure of 130/80 mmHg or lower in this situation[1] is frequently difficult to achieve. Data from the UKPDS (United Kingdom Prospective Diabetes Study)[2] support the use of multiple blood pressure agents to try and achieve good blood pressure control, though at least 20% of people with diabetes will not achieve tight blood pressure control even with intensive blood pressure management. Non-adherence to a complex treatment programme is often cited as the cause of treatment failure—particularly as aspirin, a statin and oral and injection therapy for diabetes may be prescribed in addition to the four hypotensive agents described above. However, non-adherence to treatment may be as common in patients who do respond to therapy.[3] Secondary hypertension, though relatively uncommon, should be considered when blood pressure is resistant to therapy. There are no differences in the clinical features of secondary hypertension whether a patient has diabetes or not.

The major questions are whether, and how, to:

● Investigate for white coat/office hypertension

● Investigate for secondary hypertension

  ● Renal artery stenosis

  ● Cushing's syndrome (hypercortisolism)

  ● Conn's syndrome (primary hyperaldosteronism)

  ● Phaeochromocytoma

  ● Other diagnoses

● Intensify treatment further

White coat/office hypertension

Hypertension that does not respond adequately to three or more hypotensive agents is defined as resistant and is one indication for ambulatory blood pressure monitoring (ABPM). ABPM records blood pressure away from the doctor's clinic where readings may be significantly lower. When comparing ABPM readings against clinic targets and readings, 10/5 mmHg is generally subtracted—so a clinic target of 130/80 mmHg becomes an ABPM target of 120/75 mmHg. Significant correlation between ABPM readings and cardiovascular endpoints[4] means that ABPM can be used to assess adequacy of hypotensive therapy in white coat hypertension and as a trigger to intensify treatment if blood pressure is elevated.

Secondary hypertension

It is not feasible to screen all patients with hypertension and diabetes for all causes of secondary hypertension—particularly as curable secondary hypertension in this clinical setting will be unusual. Clinical criteria are used to selectively investigate for secondary hypertension.

Renal artery stenosis

Renal artery stenosis in type 2 diabetes is the most problematic cause of secondary hypertension in diabetes and most likely to be due to atheromatous disease. There remains debate about optimal management in patients who have renal artery stenosis if there is stable, abnormal renal function and tolerably good blood pressure control. The Angioplasty and Stent for Renal Artery Lesions (ASTRAL) trial should be helpful in informing this debate. It is therefore important to investigate for renal artery stenosis only if a decision about what to do with the test result has been made. There are no definitive criteria for selecting patients for investigation, but commonly used criteria are:

● refractory hypertension with grade III retinal changes;

● sudden deterioration in control of hypertension;

● rise in creatinine >20% on starting an ACE inhibitor/angiotensin II receptor blocker;

● flash pulmonary oedema;

● asymmetric kidney size.

The gold-standard investigation is renal arteriography but this is usually reserved for use at the time of stenting, if this is indicated by less-invasive screening tests. Renal artery duplex was previously the most widely used assessment, but it is time-consuming, operator-dependent and is being superseded by magnetic resonance angiography (MRA) with paramagnetic contrast administration, or helical computed tomography (CT) with CT angiography. These techniques are reported to have sensitivity and specificity in excess of 95%.

Cushing's syndrome

Obesity and hypertension are commonly associated with type 2 diabetes and are also features of Cushing's syndrome. No screening test for Cushing's syndrome is 100% sensitive and specific, so it is important to try and raise the pre-test probability of a positive test to avoid frequent and fruitless investigation for Cushing's syndrome. There are no definitive criteria for selecting patients for investigation, but commonly used criteria are:

● simultaneous appearance of hypertension and hyperglycaemia which is resistant to treatment;

● centripetal obesity;

● new abdominal striae;

● thin skin with easy bruising.

There are pros and cons with both of the commonly used screening tests. The overnight dexamethasone suppression test (1 mg at midnight; 0900am serum cortisol <50 nmol/l) has a sensitivity of 97–100% but a specificity of only 90%. Twenty-four-hour urinary free-cortisol measurements have a sensitivity of approximately 98% and specificity of approximately 98%. However, 24-hour collections may be incomplete or intermittently normal in Cushing's syndrome.

Conn's syndrome

Up to 50% of patients with primary hyperaldosteronism are normokalaemic.[5] This may be more common in patients who have an aldosterone-secreting adenoma. There are no definitive criteria for selecting patients for investigation. Some authors recommend screening all patients with resistant hypertension who are not taking an aldosterone antagonist, using an ambulatory, 0800am plasma aldosterone concentration to plasma renin activity ratio.[5] Approximately one-quarter of patients with primary hyperaldosteronism identified following this screening test will have an adrenal adenoma. Of these, not all will be fit for surgical resection, so an oral aldosterone antagonist may be more acceptable treatment—and it may be simpler to offer this as a therapeutic trial. It is important to have considered the potential treatment outcomes and discussed them with the patient prior to doing the test.

Phaeochromocytoma and other diagnoses

Phaeochromocytoma and acromegaly may cause glucose intolerance/diabetes. The triad of headache, sweating and tachycardia is present in approximately 50% of patients presenting with phaeochromocytoma. Screening is usually with 24-hour urine collections for free catecholamines and catecholamine metabolites. Plasma metanephrine measurement is more sensitive and specific, but the assay is not universally available. Coarctation of the aorta may be identified on clinical examination for radiofemoral pulse delay.

Screening for acromegaly should be reserved for patients where the index of suspicion is high. A random growth hormone measurement of <2 ng/ml and an insulin-like growth factor-1 level in the reference range for age and sex almost certainly excludes acromegaly and precludes the need for a 75 gram oral glucose tolerance test with growth hormone testing.

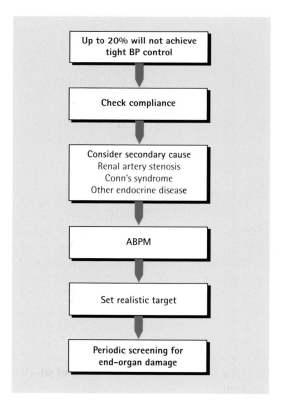

Fig. 35.1 Management of hard-to-control hypertension. BP = blood pressure.

Recent Developments

1   Obstructive sleep apnoea (OSA) is closely associated with obesity, and the prevalence is rising as it is increasingly identified by physicians. Sleep apnoea is defined as five or more apnoea/hypopnoea episodes per hour during sleep associated with daytime sleepiness. Arousal from sleep terminates apnoeic episodes and is associated with extreme hypertension, with systolic values >300 mmHg recorded. Many studies have now identified OSA as an independent predictor of systemic hypertension.[6] Effective treatment with nocturnal continuous positive airway pressure reduces mean arterial blood pressure substantially—by 10 mmHg in a recent study.[7] The diagnosis of OSA may be first suspected if excessive snoring or apnoeic events are identified by the patient's sleeping partner. Daytime somnolence presents characteristically during passive situations such as watching television, long meetings or driving. The gold-standard investigation for OSA is full polysomnography including assessment of breathing, sleeping by electroencephalogram and other physiological variables such as oxygen saturation and pulse rate. Increasing referrals for assessment have meant that many laboratories have inadequate facilities to offer full polysomnography to all those referred, and home assessment devices that record only pulse oximetry and electrocardiogram are frequently used as an initial screening test.

Conclusion

Screening for secondary hypertension will produce false-positive tests because of the high sensitivity and relatively low specificity of some of the tests outlined above. Selective testing rather than screening reduces the need for time-consuming and anxiety-provoking further investigation. The suggested practice is not to screen for secondary hypertension without a clear indication and a strategy for positive, negative and intermediate probability results.

In this case, there is little indication to screen for haemodynamically significant renal artery stenosis as renal function is normal despite use of an ACE inhibitor. MRA may reveal radiographic renal artery stenosis, but stenting of the renal arteries is associated with an uncertain risk–benefit ratio. Without other clear clinical pointers, the only other screening test to be considered would be a plasma aldosterone concentration to renin activity ratio. However, as the specificity of a positive screening test for surgically curable hypertension is so low, it may be more pragmatic to prescribe a trial of an aldosterone antagonist. This may be particularly appropriate in this case, as the patient has already suffered a myocardial infarction and a recent trial demonstrated that the use of eplerenone was associated with a 15% reduction in death following myocardial infarction associated with left ventricular failure.[8]

Suggested practice would be to ensure that the current treatment plan is acceptable to the patient and that non-adherence is not a significant problem. ABPM may identify an element of white coat hypertension. If not, a fifth hypotensive agent—probably an aldosterone antagonist—would be introduced to see if this lowered blood pressure further toward 130/80 mmHg. It is suggested to ask specifically about symptoms of OSA. Also, ensure that lipid lowering and glycaemic control are optimized, both of which may also reduce the risk of a further vascular event.

Further Reading

1 Gaede P, Vedel P, Larsen N, Jensen GVH, Parving H-H, Pedersen O. Multifactorial intervention and cardiovascular disease in patients with type 2 diabetes. *N Engl J Med* 2003; **348**: 383–93.

2 UK Prospective Diabetes Study Group. Tight blood pressure control and risk of macrovascular and microvascular complications in type 2 diabetes: UKPDS 38. *BMJ* 1998; **317**: 703–13.

3 Nuesch R, Schroeder K, Dieterle T, Martina B, Battegay E. Relation between insufficient response to antihypertensive treatment and poor compliance with treatment: a prospective case-control study. *BMJ* 2001; **323**: 142–6.

4 Redon J, Campos C, Narciso ML, Rodicio JL, Pascual JM, Ruilope LM. Prognostic value of ambulatory blood pressure monitoring in refractory hypertension: a prospective study. *Hypertension* 1998; **31**: 712–18.

5 Mulatero P, Stowasser M, Loh KC, Fardella LE, Gordon RD, Mosso L, Gomez-Sanchez CE, Veglio F, Young WF. Increased diagnosis of primary aldosteronism, including surgically correctable forms, in centers from five continents. *J Clin Endocrinol Metab* 2004; **89**: 1045–50.

6 Lavie P, Herer P, Hoffstein V. Obstructive sleep apnoea syndrome as a risk factor for hypertension: population study. *BMJ* 2000; **320**: 479–82.

7 Becker HF, Jerrentrup A, Ploch T, Grote L, Penzel T, Sullivan CE, Peter JH. Effect of nasal continuous positive airway pressure treatment on blood pressure in patients with obstructive sleep apnea. *Circulation* 2003; **107**: 68–73.

8 Pitt B, Remme W, Zannad F, Neaton J, Martinez F, Roniker B, Bittman R, Hurley S, Kleiman J, Gatlin M. Eplerenone, a selective aldosterone blocker, in patients with left ventricular dysfunction after myocardial infarction. *N Engl J Med* 2003; **348**: 1309–21.

Microvascular Complications

36 Painful neuropathy

37 Microalbuminuria

38 ACE inhibitor treatment

39 Advancing renal failure

40 Background retinopathy

41 Proliferative and pre-proliferative retinopathy

42 Macular disease

43 Autonomic neuropathy

44 The Charcot foot

PROBLEM

36 Painful Neuropathy

Case History

A 58-year-old company manager with a six-year history of type 2 diabetes complained of a persistent, sharp stabbing pain in his feet. His symptoms are worse at night and often made worse by light pressure—for example by a blanket—over his feet. On examination, he has easily palpable foot pulses and peripheral neuropathy manifesting as loss of pinprick and vibration sensation up to his ankles.

Describe the pathophysiology and clinical features of painful neuropathy.

How would you attempt to relieve his symptoms?

Background

Peripheral neuropathy is one of the most common complications of diabetes, affecting 20–50% of patients. Prolonged duration of diabetes and poor glycaemic control are major risk factors for developing peripheral neuropathy. Its precise pathogenesis is unclear but is likely to be multifactorial and include metabolic and vascular factors. Chronic hyperglycaemia results in activation of the polyol pathways and protein kinase C activation, leading to myoinositol depletion, a reduction in peripheral nerve conduction and degeneration of myelinated and unmyelinated sensory fibres. Endoneural and epineural vasculopathy have been observed, while neural hypoxia and endothelial dysfunction suggest impairment of the microcirculation.

Distal sensory peripheral neuropathy (DPN) is the most common type of diabetic neuropathy and a diagnosis of DPN can only be made after a careful clinical examination. All patients with diabetes should be screened annually for DPN by examining pinprick and vibration perception (using a 128 Hz tuning fork). Combinations of more than one test have >87% sensitivity in detecting DPN. Simple quantitative tests, using a biothesiometer for vibration sensing or a 10 g Semmes-Weinstein monofilament for pressure sense, have been shown to be useful predictors of future foot ulcer risk. Clinical presentation can be divided into 'positive' symptoms, such as painful neuropathy (as is the case for this patient), and 'negative' symptoms such as sensory loss—often in a glove and stocking distribution. Clinical examination may reveal distal muscle wasting, foot deformity, reduced (or absent) ankle reflexes, loss of vibration sense and dry skin, the latter possibly due to concurrent autonomic neuropathy. Characteristic 'positive' symptoms of painful DPN include 'burning', 'shooting', 'stabbing' or 'lancing' pain, heightened skin sensation (hyperaesthesia), pain to non-injurious stimuli (allodynia) and altered temperature sensation. Painful DPN can present in two forms: an acute and self-limiting form that resolves within a year, or a chronic form that can go on for years.[1]

Painful DPN is notoriously difficult to treat. Hence, suggested practice is to delay the initiation of treatment until the possible beneficial effect of a particular treatment is thought to outweigh its potential adverse effect. Treatment of painful neuropathy can be divided into two groups: symptom-modifying drugs (for symptom relief) and neuropathy-modifying drugs (to alter the clinical course of the nerve damage).[2]

Symptom–modifying drugs

Patients with DPN should aim for stable and optimal glycaemic control. This approach is supported by several observational studies, which suggest that neuropathic symptoms improve not only with optimization of glycaemic control but also with the avoidance of extreme blood glucose fluctuations. Most patients will still require drug treatment for painful symptoms. Simple analgesia is not effective in painful DPN. Treatment approaches that have their efficacy confirmed in randomized controlled trials include antidepressants, anticonvulsants, other drugs, acupuncture and spinal cord stimulators.

Tricyclic antidepressants, e.g. amitriptyline, have been shown to relieve pain in patients with painful DPN, independently of their antidepressant action, and are usually used as a first-line drug choice. Amitriptyline acts by blocking reuptake of norepinephrine and, if effective, would provide symptom improvement within days. The initial starting dose is 25 mg at night, with dose up-titrated until symptoms are relieved, maximum dose is achieved or side effects develop. Adverse effects include sedation, dry mouth, postural hypotension, constipation, urinary retention and, occasionally, cardiac arrhythmias. The antidepressants sertraline and trazodone have also been reported to benefit painful neuropathy, but fluoxetine (40 mg/day) did not reduce pain. Paroxetine (40 mg/day), however, has been shown in a randomized, double-blind, crossover study to significantly improve symptoms compared with placebo.

The anticonvulsant carbamazepine has traditionally been used as a second-line therapy to tricyclic antidepressants. The starting dose is usually 100 mg once or twice a day, which can be increased depending on symptoms and side effects such as blurred vision, dizziness or unsteadiness. The newer anticonvulsant, gabapentin (900–3600 mg/day), has also been shown to be effective in treating painful neuropathy. In a study involving 165 patients with painful diabetic neuropathy, gabapentin reduced mean daily pain score by 40% compared with placebo. It has been suggested that lower dosages of gabapentin (<900 mg/day) are ineffective in treating neuropathy. More recently, pregabalin (300–600 mg/day)—a developmental successor to gabapentin—was shown in three randomized, double-blind, multicentre studies of 5–8 weeks' duration to be superior to placebo in relieving pain and improving pain-related sleep interference in a total of 724 patients with painful DPN. Significant reductions in weekly mean pain scores (primary endpoint) and sleep interference scores were observed at one week and sustained thereafter. Significant reduction in pain was apparent on the first day of treatment with pregabalin 300 mg/day. In two 12-week placebo-controlled trials, twice-daily fixed doses (600 mg/day) or flexible doses (150–600 mg/day) of pregabalin were also effective in reducing pain and sleep interference in a total of 733 randomized DPN patients. Pregabalin was well tolerated in patients with painful DPN, though mild-to-moderate dizziness, somnolence and peripheral oedema were the most common adverse events. There are no data comparing different anticonvulsants or anticonvulsants in combination with antidepressants.

Other agents are used when the above drugs have failed, or in combination with traditional treatments. Tramadol is an opioid-like centrally acting, non-narcotic analgesic, which has been shown to be effective in painful DPN. The starting dose is 50 mg, increasing gradually to a maximum of 400 mg/day. Adverse effects are nausea, constipation and headaches, but these side effects are generally better tolerated than those occurring with conventional opiates. Capsaicin cream (0.75%) has also been shown to be efficacious in treating painful DPN. It acts by depleting sensory nerve terminals of the neurotransmitter substance P and blocks conduction in the type C nociceptive fibres. Other pharmacological agents, such as glyceryl trinitrate spray (a nitric oxide donor), mexiletene (antiarrhythmic agent) and amantadine (an antiviral), have also been shown in small studies to improve symptoms in patients with painful DPN. A chance observation in one patient prompted a small trial involving eight obese patients with type 2 diabetes and painful DPN. In this study, the use of the anti-obesity agent, sibutramine (15 mg/day)—a combined serotonin and noradrenaline reuptake inhibitor—resulted in a 50–100% reduction in pain within one week of treatment initiation, with pain relapse upon cessation of treatment. Larger trials are required to confirm these observations from smaller studies.

Other approaches to treatment of painful DPN include acupuncture and spinal cord stimulators. In one open-label trial, acupuncture was shown to provide significant symptomatic relief in over three-quarters of treated patients. It is thought to act by stimulating the spinal cord, midbrain and hypothalamus to release neurotransmitters with analgesic properties such as encephalins and endorphins. The effect of direct stimulation to the spinal cord has also been examined in one study. A stimulator placed in the epidural space and turned on when there was pain, was shown to provide pain relief to most patients for the duration of the study. Long-term use of spinal nerve stimulators may also provide significant pain relief over a prolonged period of time with little associated morbidity. These studies, however, were small with questionable methodology and these treatment approaches are therefore reserved for patients who do not respond to all other treatment.

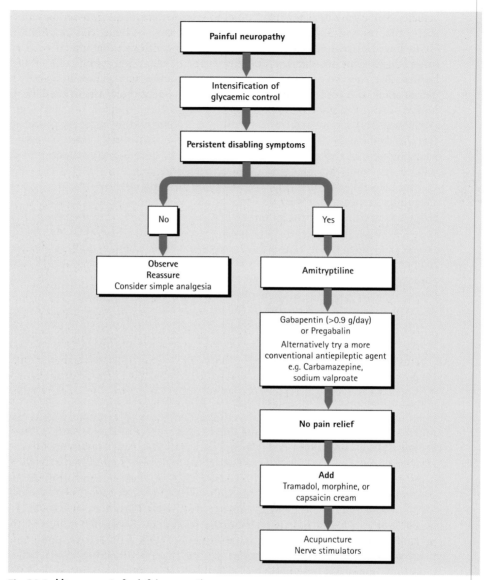

Fig. 36.1 Management of painful neuropathy.

Neuropathy-modifying drugs

The role of these agents in the treatment of painful DPN is still being investigated and does not currently form part of routine clinical practice. Alpha-lipoic acid, for example, is an antioxidant that has been shown in some trials to provide symptomatic relief. While its use is not established in most parts of the world, it has been used routinely in Germany for the past 20 years in patients with DPN. Gamma-linolenic acid has been shown in two multicentre trials to provide improvement in symptoms of DPN and nerve conduction velocity. Nerve growth factor (NGF) promotes growth of small-fibre sensory and sympto-matic neurons in peripheral nerves and is thought to be beneficial in DPN. Studies on NGF, however, have shown contradictory findings, although parenteral NGF may be of some benefit. Aldose reductase inhibitors have been extensively studied in DPN. They act by blocking the aldose reductase pathway—an important enzymatic pathway in the pathogenesis of DPN. Convincing evidence to support their efficacy is lacking due to problems with toxicity and adverse effects.

Recent Developments

1   A recent randomized, double-blind, placebo-controlled study[3] compared the efficacy of a combination of gabapentin and morphine with that of each as a single agent in patients with painful diabetic neuropathy or post-herpetic neuralgia. Patients received daily active placebo, sustained-release morphine, gabapentin, or a combination of gabapentin and morphine—each given orally for five weeks. Of 57 patients who underwent randomization (35 with diabetic neuropathy and 22 with post-herpetic neuralgia), 41 completed the trial. Mean daily pain (on a scale from 0 to 10, with higher numbers indicating more severe pain) was rated as follows: 5.72 at baseline, 4.49 with placebo, 4.15 with gabapentin, 3.70 with morphine, and 3.06 with the gabapentin–morphine combination ($P < 0.05$). Total scores on the Pain Questionnaire (on a scale from 0 to 45, with higher numbers indicating more severe pain) at a maxi-mal tolerated dose were 14.4 with placebo, 10.7 with gabapentin, 10.7 with morphine, and 7.5 with the gabapentin–morphine combination ($P < 0.05$). Gabapentin and mor-phine combined achieved better analgesia at lower doses of each drug than either as a single agent, with constipation, sedation and dry mouth as the most frequent adverse effects.

2   Recent data suggest that impaired nitric oxide (NO) synthesis may play an important role in the pathogenesis of painful DPN. In diabetic rats, impaired neuronal NO gen-eration induced hyperalgesia, whereas decreased NO production has been shown to reduce endoneurial blood flow in type 2 diabetic patients with peripheral sensory neuropathy. A preliminary study[4] reported that isosorbide dinitrate (ISDN) spray, an NO donor with potent local vasodilating properties, relieved some sensory symptoms, particularly pain and burning sensation. A subsequent pilot study showed that ISDN spray significantly reduced both neuropathic pain and burning sensation. No treat-ment difference, however, was observed with other sensory modalities (hot/cold sen-sation, tingling, numbness, hyperaesthesia and jabbing-like sensation). The potential of ISDN spray in alleviating other specific sensory symptoms associated with diabetic peripheral neuropathy merits further study.

Conclusion

The pathophysiology of painful diabetic neuropathy involves vascular and metabolic fac-tors. Treatment of painful neuropathy should be structured. Currently available agents with documented efficacy in clinical trials for symptomatic relief of neuropathic pain include anticonvulsant drugs (such carbamazepine, gabapentin and pregabalin), tricyclic antidepressants, opiates and other treatment options such as mexiletene, tramadol, capsaicin cream, acupuncture and spinal cord stimulators.[1,2]

Further Reading

1 Boulton AJM, Vinik AI, Arezzo JC, Bril V, Feldman EL, Freeman R, Malik RA, Maser RE, Sosenko JM, Ziegler D. Diabetic Neuropathies: A statement by the American Diabetes Association. *Diabetes Care* 2005; **28**: 956–62.

2 Singleton JR. Evaluation and treatment of painful peripheral polyneuropathy. *Semin Neurol* 2005; **25**: 185–95.

3 Gilron I, Bailey JM, Tu D, Holden RR, Weaver DF, Houlden RL. Morphine, gabapentin, or their combination for neuropathic pain. *N Engl J Med* 2005; **352**: 1324–34.

4 Yuen KC, Baker NR, Rayman G. Treatment of chronic painful diabetic neuropathy with isosorbide dinitrate spray: a double-blind placebo-controlled cross-over study. *Diabetes Care* 2002; **25**: 1699–1703.

PROBLEM

37 Microalbuminuria

Case History

A 36-year-old teacher underwent microangiopathy screening at his general practitioner's surgery. He has evidence of background retinopathy, no evidence of peripheral neuropathy and no proteinuria on urine analysis. Urinary albumin–creatinine ratio was 5.2, 5.9 and 5.5 mg/mmol on three separate sample assessments. His blood pressure was controlled at 132/74 mmHg. He was referred to your clinic for advice.

Outline the natural history of diabetic renal disease.

How would you further investigate this patient?

How would you manage this patient?

Background

Diabetic nephropathy is the most common cause of end-stage renal disease in the western world and is associated with greatly increased cardiovascular morbidity and mortality as well as the presence of other microvascular complications. Increased understanding of the natural history of diabetic renal disease (described below) has supported therapeutic intervention much earlier in the course of the disease.

Stage 1. Hyperfiltration—increased glomerular filtration rate (GFR) reflecting under-lying glomerular hyperfiltration and hyperperfusion.

Stage 2. Silent phase—normalization of GFR associated with early histological abnor-malities in the kidney such as glomerular hypertrophy and subtle thickening of glomerular basement membrane.

Stage 3. Microalbuminuria—defined as a urinary albumin excretion rate (AER) of 20–200 μg/min (30–300 mg/24 h); equivalent to a urine albumin–creatinine ratio (ACR) of 10–25 mg/mmol, or ACR of >2.5 for males and >3.5 for females, confirmed over three separate occasions within a three-month period, in the absence of a urinary tract infec-tion. The onset of stage 3 predicts the development of overt renal disease and is associated with an increased risk of cardiovascular events.

Stage 4. Overt nephropathy—defined as AER above 200 μg/min or 300 mg/24 h (equivalent to ACR of >25 mg/mmol or protein–creatinine ratio of >0.3 from a spot morning urine sample). Urine dipstick is positive for protein and, untreated, this stage is associated with a relentless loss of GFR (by 1–24 ml/min/year) until end-stage renal failure supervenes.

The patient described above should have microalbuminuria confirmed with three posi-tive ACR tests over a three-month period. AER assessment is more precise and can be for-mally measured using an overnight (8 hours) urine collection, which is more practicable for the patient than a 24-hour collection. Albumin excretion may vary by as much as 40% and clinicians should be aware of potential confounding factors and non-diabetic causes of albuminuria. Upon confirmation of microalbuminuria, serum urea and creatinine should be measured at baseline and then every six months. Risk factors associated with the progression of renal disease and cardiovascular disease should be identified and treated (Figure 37.1). If microalbuminuria is left untreated, the trend is one of increasing protein-uria until overt nephropathy develops. The rate of progression of microalbuminuria is heavily influenced by blood pressure control, blood glucose control and the use of agents which block the activation of the renin–angiotensin system.

The beneficial effect of lowering blood pressure in reducing progression of diabetic renal disease and overall cardiovascular mortality is well established. Blood pressure reduction also reduces AER and retards progression from micro- to macroalbuminuria. Various blood pressure targets have been assessed, as have different classes of antihyper-tensive agents, alone and in combination. Although appropriate blood pressure targets have not been clearly established, it seems reasonable to suggest a target of 130/80 mmHg for patients with microalbuminuria, with a lower target of 125/75 mmHg suggested for patients with heavy proteinuria (>1 g/day). In practice, evidence from clinical trials has illustrated the difficulty in achieving such targets, which require multiple antihypertensive therapies.

While blood pressure reduction (rather than the choice of antihypertensive agent *per se*) should be the paramount aim of therapy, inhibitors of the renin–angiotensin system (RAS) may exert renoprotective effects beyond their antihypertensive properties. In the EUCLID study (EURODIAB Controlled Trial of Lisinopril in Insulin-Dependent Diabetes Mellitus),[1] involving 530 patients, angiotensin-converting enzyme (ACE) inhibition with lisinopril slowed the progression of nephropathy in normotensive patients with type 1 dia-betes, with the greatest effect being seen in those with microalbuminuria. A meta-analysis

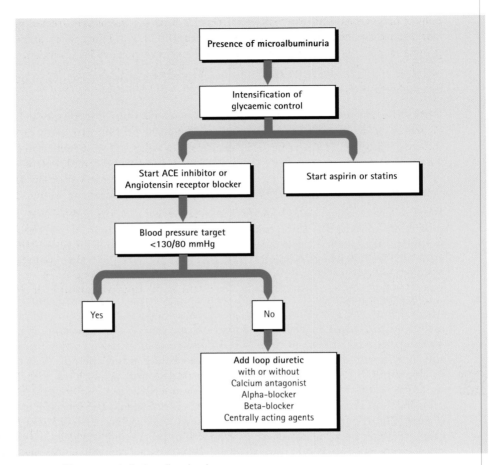

Fig. 37.1 Management of microalbuminuria.

of individual patient data (698 patients) examining the effect of ACE inhibition compared to placebo in microalbuminuric type 1 diabetes followed for at least two years, confirmed that ACE inhibitors reduced the risk of developing proteinuria by 60% and increased the likelihood of reverting to normal albumin excretion three-fold over two years.[2] The beneficial effect of ACE inhibition, however, appeared to wane after the first year of treatment, suggesting delay rather than prevention of proteinuria. Several small, short-term studies in type 1 diabetes have also shown similar reduction in AER with angiotensin II receptor blockers. The role of RAS inhibitors in normoalbuminuric, normotensive patients with type 1 diabetes, however, remains unproven. For patients with microalbuminuria and hypertension, a combination of an ACE-inhibitor and a loop diuretic is often used as the first-line antihypertensive treatment.

The strongest evidence for preventing microalbuminuria progression in patients with type 1 diabetes by means of tight glucose control comes from the Diabetes Control and Complications Trial (DCCT). Intensive therapy achieved a mean reduction of 2% in glycosylated haemoglobin (HbA1c) compared with the conventionally treated group. In the cohort of patients with microalbuminuria, 5.2% of the intensively treated group developed overt proteinuria at nine years compared with 11.3% of the conventionally treated group—a risk reduction in developing proteinuria of 56% (95% confidence interval 18–76). Thus, the United Kingdom and United States recommendations are to establish and maintain tight blood glucose control, with a HbA1c target of <7% if this can be achieved safely.

The presence of microalbuminuria signifies a major risk of cardiovascular death. Aggressive management of cardiovascular risk factors is thus essential.[3] A study involving patients with type 2 diabetes and microalbuminuria reported a 50% reduction in cardiovascular morbidity and mortality and 60% reduction in progression to proteinuria in the group allocated intensive, multifactorial intervention according to a target-driven protocol. Aspirin, statins and ACE inhibitors were prescribed for everyone in the intensively treated group, with lifestyle advice to encourage weight loss and smoking cessation and definition of strict targets for HbA1c. Although similar data in patients with type 1 diabetes are not yet available, the benefit of lipid lowering and antiplatelet treatment in patients with high cardiovascular risk is overwhelming. Moreover, there is strong evidence to suggest that hyperlipidaemia is associated with a more rapid progression of renal disease. It is thus suggested practice to initiate statins and aspirin treatment for all patients with microalbuminuria, targeting towards an optimal lipid profile.

Recent Developments

1   Recent studies have suggested a favourable, changing trend in the natural history of diabetic nephropathy among patients with type 1 diabetes. It is estimated that over a lifetime of diabetes, 50% of patients will develop microalbuminuria. Of these, 20–30% may progress to proteinuria, but a further 40% will remain microalbuminuric and, importantly, 20–30% of patients may revert to normoalbuminuria.[4] This may be explained by improved management of blood pressure and blood glucose control.

2   Increased understanding of the biochemical mechanisms involved in the pathogenesis of diabetic nephropathy has led to research in developing future therapeutic strategies to prevent the progression of microalbuminuria by limiting glucose-mediated renal damage. This includes development of advanced glycation end product inhibitors (e.g. aminoguanidine), aldose reductase inhibitors and, more recently, protein kinase C-β inhibitors (ruboxistaurin). The role of complete renin–angiotensin–aldosterone system blockade by combining an ACE inhibitor, an angiotensin II receptor blocker and an aldosterone antagonist (e.g. eplerenone) for patients with microalbuminuria is being investigated.

3   More recently, molecular studies have focused on the role of the glomerular epithelial cells (or podocytes) in mediating albuminuria in patients with diabetes. Longitudinal data show an association between podocyte loss and albuminuria.[5] Abnormalities in podocyte proteins have been shown to cause proteinuric renal disease in humans and morphological changes in the podocyte's foot processes (broadening and effacement) lead to slit spaces between podocytes allowing the passage of protein into Bowman's space. Preliminary experimental work has suggested that abnormalities in podocyte morphology and structure may be reversed therapeutically.

Conclusion

The detection of microalbuminuria identifies a group of patients with a high risk of cardiovascular morbidity and mortality as well as increased risk of diabetic renal disease. Aggressive management of patients' blood pressure (which should include therapy with a RAS inhibitor) and blood glucose, and the use of statins and aspirin may improve clinical outcome. Further studies are underway to determine new therapeutic strategies to retard progression of renal disease in patients with diabetes.

Further Reading

1 The EUCLID study group. Randomised placebo-controlled trial of lisinopril in normotensive patients with insulin-dependent diabetes and normoalbuminuria or microalbuminuria. *Lancet* 1997; **349**: 1787–92.

2 The ACE Inhibitors in Diabetic Nephropathy Trialist Group. Should all patients with type 1 diabetes mellitus and microalbuminuria receive angiotensin-converting enzyme inhibitors? A meta-analysis of individual patient data. *Ann Intern Med* 2001; **134**: 370–9.

3 Arun C, Stoddart J, Mackin P, MacLeod JM, New JN, Marshall SM. Significance of microalbuminuria in long-duration type 1 diabetes. *Diabetes Care* 2003; **26**: 2144–9.

4 Perkins B, Ficociello LH, Silva KH, Finkelstein DM, Warram JH, Krolewski AS. Regression of microalbuminuria in Type 1 diabetes. *N Engl J Med* 2003; **348**: 2285–93.

5 White KE, Bilous RW, Marshall SM, El Nahas M, Remuzzi G, Piras G, De Cosmo S, Viberti G. Podocyte number in normotensive type 1 diabetic patients with albuminuria. *Diabetes* 2002; **51**: 3083–9.

38 ACE Inhibitor Treatment

Case History

A 36-year-old lady with type 1 diabetes is noted to have microalbuminuria and mild hypertension. Her baseline serum creatinine is 80 μmol/l. She is started on lisinopril 10 mg per day. Creatinine rises to 110 μmol/l six weeks later. Serum potassium is normal, and her blood pressure is 144/92 mmHg.

Should her angiotensin–converting enzyme (ACE) inhibitor be discontinued?

Would treatment with another antihypertensive drug be more appropriate?

When should angiotensin receptor blocker (ARB) treatment be considered in type 1 diabetes?

What is the present evidence relating to dual ACE inhibition and ARB use?

How should this patient be monitored?

Background

Diabetes is now the leading cause of end-stage renal failure. Diabetic nephropathy affects up to 40% of patients with diabetes and is associated with increased risk of other microvascular, as well as macrovascular, complications of diabetes. Microalbuminuria occurs when urinary protein excretion is between 30 mg and 300 mg per 24 hours, and is the earliest stage of diabetic nephropathy. Tight glycaemic and blood pressure control is recommended to prevent diabetic nephropathy, both in type 1 and type 2 diabetes.[1] It is not certain that blockade of the renin–angiotensin system (RAS) has a specific role in preventing nephropathy in type 1 diabetes. There is no evidence to support RAS inhibition in patients with type 1 diabetes who are not hypertensive and do not have albuminuria. RAS inhibition does appear to be protective in similar patients with type 2 diabetes. Effective treatment of hypertension both slows progression of diabetic renal disease and reduces risk of a cardiovascular event. Numerous trials with diuretics, beta-blockers and ACE inhibitors have shown benefits in patients with diabetes. There does appear to be a specific role, over and above decreasing blood pressure, of RAS blockade in slowing the progression of established nephropathy, both in type 1 and type 2 diabetes. It is uncertain whether RAS blockade reduces risk of cardiovascular disease over and above its effects on blood pressure. Results of the HOPE (Heart Outcomes Protection Evaluation) and LIFE (Losartan Intervention For Endpoint reduction in hypertension) studies suggested that RAS blockade may be superior, but the studies do not allow that conclusion to be firmly drawn.

Antagonists of the angiotensin II type 1 receptor (ARBs) have recently become available for patients with hypertension with or without nephropathy. These agents have a good side-effect profile, as they are highly selective AT_1 receptor blockers, and may benefit vascular tone and modelling because of unopposed AT_2 receptor-mediated action. A recent meta-analysis[2] suggested that ARBs are not superior to other available antihypertensives in terms of blood pressure reduction. There are limited long-term data and a beneficial effect on cardiovascular morbidity and mortality has yet to be convincingly demonstrated. The most compelling argument for their use is in patients with type 2 diabetes and nephropathy, where at least three recent studies have demonstrated retarded progression of nephropathy.

Increased serum creatinine after starting ACE inhibitors or ARBs is common, but increases of >50% only occur in around 5% of patients. The agents can also impair potassium excretion, leading to hyperkalaemia. Monitoring urea and electrolytes within two

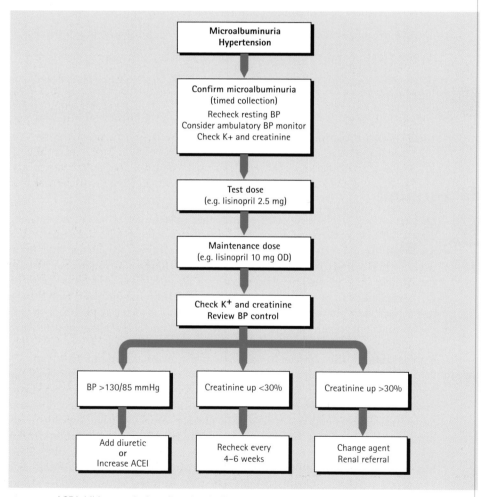

Fig. 38.1 ACE inhibitors and microalbuminuria. The above scheme is for a patient with type 1 diabetes. BP = blood pressure; OD = once daily; ACEI = angiotensin converting enzyme inhibitor.

weeks of starting RAS blockade and at two-monthly intervals, at least for the first year, is recommended. Glomerular filtration rate (GFR) is maintained by a pressure gradient (normally around 35 mmHg) across the renal ultrafiltration surface. This gradient relies on adequate perfusion pressure in the afferent arterioles and vasoconstriction in the efferent arterioles. The former is reduced by renal artery stenosis and the latter maintained by angiotensin II, and so is decreased by RAS blockade. Renal artery stenosis has been reported in up to 17% of patients with type 2 diabetes and macrovascular disease, and would be a contraindication to RAS blockade. In these patients, decreased renal perfusion led to a worsening of creatinine clearance and may precipitate acute renal failure. Renal artery stenosis should be considered in all patients who have disseminated atherosclerosis, and should be suspected in patients who have renal impairment without proteinuria and in those whose kidneys are asymmetrical on ultrasound examination. The investigation of choice for renal artery stenosis is now magnetic resonance angiography, but the diagnosis can also be made with Doppler ultrasonography and captopril renography.

Recent Developments

1   Many patients with hypertension or heart failure have insulin resistance. The question of whether treatment with ACE inhibitors or ARBs can prevent, or delay the onset of, type 2 diabetes has recently been addressed by Scheen[3] in a meta-analysis. He reviewed eight hypertension (including HOPE and ALLHAT [Antihypertensive and Lipid-Lowering Treatment to Prevent Heart Attack Trial]) and two heart failure trials. Of 36 167 patients treated with RAS blockade, 7.4% developed diabetes compared with 9.6% of 39 902 patients treated with other agents. This was a relative risk reduction of 22%, and was highly statistically significant.

2   Genetic factors play an important part in the development of diabetic nephropathy. Polymorphisms in the RAS are important determinants of the variable activity of the system between individuals.[4] Thus, different forms of the genes for angiotensinogen, ACE and the angiotensin II type 1 receptor have been identified. Genotyping could be helpful to identify patients at risk of progressive renal disease, and also to target therapies that block the RAS.

3   There is now considerable evidence that ACE inhibitors have a beneficial effect on all-cause mortality in patients with diabetes and renal disease.[5] While ARBs have comparable benefits in terms of blood pressure, proteinuria and renal function, their long-term mortality benefits in this group of patients remain to be established.

4   There are theoretical benefits of blocking both the production and the action of angiotensin II by concurrent administration of an ACE inhibitor and an ARB.[6,7] The CALM (Candesartan And Lisinopril Microalbuminuria) study, published in 2000, demonstrated benefits of dual blockade in blood pressure reduction and micro-albuminuria. Other studies, both in diabetic and non-diabetic cohorts, have confirmed the potential benefits of dual blockade, but this is not currently routinely recommended, although it should be considered in high-risk individuals.

Conclusion

This patient has diabetic nephropathy and available evidence suggests that blockade of the RAS is the treatment of choice for management of her hypertension. Blood pressure control is generally more important than tight glucose control in slowing the advance of nephropathy. There is no indication to stop this patient's ACE inhibitor at present, but her renal function should be closely monitored—every six weeks or so. An angiotensin receptor blocker would not offer an advantage in this case. The case for routinely using dual blockade with an ACE inhibitor and ARB is not strong enough at present. If this patient's blood pressure remained imperfectly controlled while taking an ACE inhibitor, the next stage would be to prescribe a diuretic along with the ACE inhibitor. General measures should include limiting sodium and protein intake, management of dyslipidaemia and considering aspirin use if the patient is at high risk of a cardiovascular event.

Further Reading

1   Gross JL, de Azevedo MJ, Silveiro SP, Canani LH, Caramori ML, Zelmanovitz T. Diabetic nephropathy: diagnosis, prevention, and treatment. *Diabetes Care* 2005; **28**: 164–76.

2   Siebenhofer A, Plank J, Horvath K, Berghold A, Sutton AJ, Sommer R, Pieber TR. Angiotensin receptor blockers as anti-hypertensive treatment for patients with diabetes mellitus: meta-analysis of controlled double-blind randomized trials. *Diabet Med* 2004; **21**: 18–25.

3   Scheen AJ. Reninangiotensin system inhibition prevents type 2 diabetes mellitus. Part 1. A meta-analysis of randomised clinical trials. *Diabetes Metab* 2004; **30**: 487–96.

4   Jacobsen P, Tarnow L, Carstensen B, Hovind P, Poirier O, Parving HH. Genetic variation in the renin–angiotensin system and progression of diabetic nephropathy. *J Am Soc Nephrol* 2003; **14**: 2843–50.

5   Strippoli GFM, Craig M, Deeks JJ, Schena FP, Craig JC. Effects of angiotensin converting enzyme inhibitors and angiotensin II receptor antagonists on mortality and renal outcomes in diabetic nephropathy: systematic review. *BMJ* 2004; **329**: 828.

6   Andersen NH, Mogensen CE. Dual blockade of the renin angiotensin system in diabetic and nondiabetic kidney disease. *Curr Hypertens Rep* 2004; **6**: 369–76.

7   Wolf G, Ritz E. Combination therapy with ACE inhibitors and angiotensin II receptor blockers to halt progression of chronic renal disease: pathophysiology and indications. *Kidney Int* 2005; **67**: 799–812.

PROBLEM

39 Advancing Renal Failure

Case History

A 28-year-old chef has had type 1 diabetes from age 11. Glycosylated haemoglobin (HbA1c) has rarely been below 10%. Proteinuria was identified at age 23 and he subsequently failed to attend out-patient appointments. He has been referred back as his serum creatinine is now 186 μmol/l.

How should he be managed?

Does he require referral to a renal physician?

Will tightening glycaemic control improve his outlook?

Background

Long-standing proteinuria and poor glycaemic control make diabetic nephropathy (increased urinary albumin excretion in the absence of other causes) the most likely diagnosis. However, alternative diagnoses such as structural renal disease, childhood reflux nephropathy, membranous nephropathy, immunoglobulin A nephropathy or glomerulonephritis should be considered. The stage of renal disease should be identified so that appropriate action can be taken to treat complications of renal failure and plan for renal replacement therapy. Nephropathy in type 1 diabetes is almost invariably associated with retinopathy and frequently associated with neuropathy, so these should be specifically identified.

Diabetic nephropathy is marked by progression from normal urinary albumin excretion (UAE), through increased UAE, to reduced glomerular filtration rate (GFR) and finally, end-stage renal failure. Approximately one in three people who have had type 1 diabetes for 20 years will develop persistent microalbuminuria (UAE 30–300 mg/24 h), of whom half will already have gone on to develop persistent macroalbuminuria (>300 mg/24 h).[1] The DCCT/EDIC (Diabetes Control and Complications Trial/Epidemiology of Diabetes Interventions and Complications) study cohort[2] demonstrated that poor glycaemic control is the major modifiable risk factor associated with increased UAE in type 1 diabetes. Studies in the 1980s suggested that progression from microalbuminuria to macroalbuminuria occurred eventually in approximately 80% of patients. However, aggressive intervention, as described below, can halt or reverse progression of microalbuminuria in up to 60% of patients.[3] Where macroalbuminuria or reduced GFR are already established, aggressive intervention can substantially slow progression of renal disease. However, at least one in five people receiving renal replacement in industrialized nations have diabetes.

Table 39.1 Advancing renal failure

GFR (ml/min/1.73m²)	Stage	Interpretation	Action
≥90	1	Renal damage with normal or raised GFR	Make diagnosis and slow progression
60–89	2	Mild	Estimate speed of progression
30–59	3	Moderate	Evaluate complications
15–29	4	Severe	Prepare for renal replacement
<15 (or dialysis)	5	Renal failure	Renal replacement

GFR = glomerular filtration rate.

GFR is the best guide to the stage of renal disease and is a prompt for appropriate action to be taken. The Cockcroft–Gault formula has been modified following the publication of the Modification of Diet in Renal Disease (MDRD) study and the MDRD calculation of GFR is now preferred—particularly as it performs better as GFR declines.[4] Serum creatinine is a poor guide to GFR because it is dependent upon many variables including sex, weight, age, race and diet. Creatinine clearance measured by urinary collection overestimates GFR because of tubular secretion of creatinine. Direct measurement of GFR is too cumbersome for general use.

In macroalbuminuric patients with type 1 diabetes, projected decline in renal function is approximately 1 ml/min/month. Only blood pressure reduction has a proven effect in reducing the decline in renal function, though multifactorial intervention to treat dyslipidaemia and improve glycaemic control and the use of low-dose aspirin may all benefit microvascular and macrovascular disease elsewhere.

Lowering blood pressure[5] using an angiotensin-converting enzyme (ACE) inhibitor-based regime slows loss of GFR by approximately two-thirds and halves the risk of death, dialysis or transplantation over four years.[6] Dual blockade of the renin–angiotensin system (RAS) with an ACE inhibitor and angiotensin receptor blocker may have synergistic effects.[7] A target blood pressure of <125/75 mmHg is reasonable, but this will require more than two antihypertensive agents in at least 65% of patients. Suggested practice is to use a diuretic in combination with RAS blockade; then a long-acting calcium antagonist or cardioselective beta-blocker as a third-line agent and other agents as tolerated beyond that. A rise in serum creatinine of 20% with initial inhibition of the RAS would be tolerated in this situation, but a continuing rapid rise should prompt withdrawal of RAS blockade and consideration of renal artery stenosis.

Intensive blood glucose control has little positive effect on the decline of renal function once GFR is reduced. However, intensification of glycaemic control is good practice because of effects on retinopathy and neuropathy—which are almost universal in this clinical setting. Similarly, the use of statin therapy to drive low-density lipoprotein (LDL) cholesterol below 2.6 mmol/l and low-dose aspirin may not preserve renal function but may reduce the risk of a cardiovascular event—the likeliest ultimate cause of death.

Recent Developments

1   It is unlikely that therapy will become available that can universally prevent established decline of GFR in moderate renal disease. However, ever-lower blood pressure
targets and novel treatments show promise in reducing the rate of this decline.

2   A meta-analysis[8] of the effect of statin therapy on decline of GFR in patients with diabetic and non-diabetic nephropathy suggested that statin treatment could slow GFR
decline by approximately 0.15 ml/min/month. Observations of positive effects of
statin therapy on decline of GFR have also been reported in the Heart Protection
Study. The mechanism by which this occurs is unclear. It may simply be preservation
of renal arterial calibre, or may be by preserving vascular endothelial function and a
more haemodynamically advantageous balance between endothelium-derived
vasodilators, such as nitric oxide, and vasoconstrictors, such as angiotensin II and
endothelin.

3   Novel agents directed at earlier nephropathy also show some promise in reducing
albumin excretion rate in human subjects and in experimental diabetes:

- A four-month study of oral sulodexide,[9] an orally available glycosaminoglycan,
reduces albumin excretion rate in micro- and macroalbuminuric patients with
type 1 and type 2 diabetes. Its effects seem to be mediated in part by a reduction in
the activity of transforming growth factor-β, acting directly on the mesangial
matrix and basement membrane to improve selectivity of the glomerular ultrafil-
trate without affecting renal haemodynamics.

- Ruboxistaurin, an inhibitor of protein kinase C-β, has been shown to reduce albumin excretion, normalize GFR and reverse glomerular lesions in experimental diabetes in rodents,[10] though it remains untested in this situation in humans.

Conclusion

This man has stage 3 (moderate) renal disease with MDRD GFR of 40 ml/min/1.73m². He
is very likely to require renal replacement therapy in the future as it is unlikely that deterioration in renal function can be reversed, though it could be slowed. It is likely that he will
require referral to the nephrology team as he has moderate renal damage with clear progression of disease. These points should be explained to the patient.

Assessment of the renal disease should include a careful history, examination and laboratory and radiological investigations. Microscopy of urinary sediment, urine culture,
24-hour urine collection (or urine spot protein–creatinine ratio) and ultrasound of the
renal tract will help exclude glomerulonephritis and structural renal disease and coinci-
dent urinary infection and quantify albumin excretion rate. Urinary albumin excretion
<500 mg/24 h should prompt re-evaluation for non-diabetic renal disease. Renal biopsy
would not usually be undertaken unless it is clear that there has been very rapid decrease in
GFR or no retinopathy or unexplained haematuria.

A careful retinal examination and foot examination are mandatory. Risk factors for
visual loss in this patient include poor glycaemic control and non-attendance for screening examination of the retina. Efforts to intensify glycaemic control should be made—
ideally to an HbA1c of <7%, though this seems an unlikely goal. Blood pressure should be

treated to <125/75 mmHg using an ACE inhibitor-based regime, statin therapy initiated aiming for an LDL <2.6 mmol/l, low-dose aspirin started and tobacco consumption stopped. Haemoglobin and iron status should be checked. Hepatitis B status should be ascertained and vaccination commenced in preparation for haemodialysis, as serological conversion rates drop as GFR declines. Finally he should be advised to avoid cannulation or venepuncture to his non-dominant arm. This precaution will preserve the veins for a potential future haemodialysis fistula.

Further Reading

1 Hovind P, Tarnow L, Rossing P, Jensen BR, Graae M, Torp I, Binder C, Parving HH. Predictors for the development of microalbuminuria and macroalbuminuria in patients with type 1 diabetes: inception cohort study. *BMJ* 2004; **328**: 1105.

2 The Diabetes Control and Complications Trial/Epidemiology of Diabetes Interventions and Complications Research Group. Retinopathy and nephropathy in patients with type 1 diabetes four years after a trial of intensive therapy. *N Engl J Med* 2000; **342**: 381–9.

3 Perkins BA, Ficociello LH, Silva KH, Finkelstein DM, Warram JH, Krolewski AS. Regression of microalbuminuria in type 1 diabetes. *N Engl J Med* 2003; **348**: 2285–93.

4 Levey AS, Bosch JP, Lewis JB, Greene T, Rogers N, Roth D. A more accurate method to estimate glomerular filtration rate from serum creatinine: A new prediction equation. *Ann Intern Med* 1999; **130**: 461–70.

5 Parving HH, Andersen AR, Smidt UM, Svendsen PA. Early aggressive antihypertensive treatment reduces rate of decline in kidney function in diabetic nephropathy. *Lancet* 1983; **1**: 1175–9.

6 Lewis EJ, Hunsicker LG, Bain RP, Rohde RD. The effect of angiotensin-converting-enzyme inhibition on diabetic nephropathy. *N Engl J Med* 1993; **329**: 1456–62.

7 Mogensen CE, Neldam S, Tikkanen I, Oren S, Viskoper R, Watts RW, Cooper ME. Randomised controlled trial of dual blockade of renin-angiotensin system in patients with hypertension, microalbuminuria, and non-insulin dependent diabetes: the candesartan and lisinopril microalbuminuria (CALM) study. *BMJ* 2000; **321**: 1440–4.

8 Fried LF, Orchard TJ, Kasiske BL. Effect of lipid reduction on the progression of renal disease: a meta-analysis. *Kidney Int* 2001; **59**: 260–9.

9 Gambaro G, Kinalska I, Oksa A, Pont'uch P, Hertlova M, Olsovsky J, Manitius J, Fedele D, Czekalski S, Perusicova J, Skrha J, Taton J, Grzeszczak W, Crepaldi G. Oral sulodexide reduces albuminuria in microalbuminuric and macroalbuminuric type 1 and type 2 diabetic patients: the Di.N.A.S. randomized trial. *J Am Soc Nephrol* 2002; **13**: 1615–25.

10 Kelly DJ, Zhang Y, Hepper C, Gow RM, Jaworski K, Kemp BE, Wilkinson-Berka JL, Gilbert RE. Protein kinase C beta inhibition attenuates the progression of experimental diabetic nephropathy in the presence of continued hypertension. *Diabetes* 2003; **52**: 512–18.

40 Background Retinopathy

Case History

A 36-year-old housewife with long-standing type 1 diabetes attends your clinic for routine diabetic review. Two weeks prior, she underwent retinopathy screening at her local optician. The report showed evidence of scattered microaneurysm and no other abnormalities.

How common is retinopathy in patients with diabetes?

How severe is her retinopathy?

How would you prevent the retinopathy from progressing?

When would you refer her to the ophthalmologist?

Background

Diabetic retinopathy is a major cause of preventable visual loss amongst the 25–65 years age group. After 15 years of diabetes, almost all persons with type 1 diabetes will have some evidence of retinopathy, with about 50% developing proliferative retinopathy. Patients with type 2 diabetes, meanwhile, have a lower risk of developing retinopathy; however, the presence of retinopathy may be their first clinical manifestation of diabetes. In the United Kingdom Prospective Diabetes Study (UKPDS), approximately 37% of patients with type 2 diabetes were reported to have retinopathy at diagnosis. After 15 years from diagnosis, 5–10% of patients with type 2 diabetes will develop proliferative retinopathy and about 10–15% will have clinically significant macular oedema (MO). Patients with type 2 diabetes are more likely to develop earlier and more severe MO compared with type 1 diabetes. Blindness occurs not only as a result of complications of diabetic retinopathy (e.g. vitreous haemorrhage or retinal detachment) and MO, but also due to an increased risk of cataracts and glaucoma. Prevention of retinopathy progression and early detection of sight-threatening retinopathy is therefore the best approach to reduce the risk of blindness. Hence, the implementation of an efficient screening programme should be a high priority for all organizations providing diabetes health care.

Clinical lesions in diabetic retinopathy

Diabetic retinopathy is a disease of the retinal vasculature and is characterized by loss of pericyte cells, retinal capillary closure, thrombosis, non-perfusion and capillary leakage. Classification of diabetic retinopathy is shown in Table 40.1.

Table 40.1 Classification of diabetic retinopathy

Classification	Clinical findings
Non-proliferative diabetic retinopathy	
Minimal	Microaneurysms (MA) only
Mild	MA + [intraretinal haemorrhage ± hard exudates away from fovea ± cotton-wool spots (CWS)]
Moderate	MA one/more quadrant + [CWS ± venous beading ± intraretinal microvascular abnormality (IRMA)]
Severe	Any one of the following (4-2-1 rule): Intraretinal haemorrhage in 4 quadrants or venous beadings in 2 quadrants or IRMA in 1 quadrant
Very severe	Any two of the above
Proliferative diabetic retinopathy	
Early	New vessels at disc (NVD)(<1/4 disc diameter) ± New vessels elsewhere (NVE) without bleeds ± Pre-retinal bleeds or vitreous haemorrhage and NVE <1/2 disc diameter without NVD
Late	NVD >1/4 disc diameter ± NVD with haemorrhage ± NVE >1/2 disc diameter with haemorrhage

Prevention

The Diabetes Control and Complications Trial (DCCT)[1] and the UKPDS[2] have clearly shown that good glycaemic control is important in reducing the development and progression of retinopathy in patients with type 1 and type 2 diabetes. In the DCCT, patients assigned to tight glycaemic control (mean glycosylated haemoglobin, HbA1c 7%), achieved a 47% reduction in the risk of developing pre-proliferative and proliferative retinopathy and 56% reduction in the need for photocoagulation when compared with the conventionally treated group (mean HbA1c 8.9%). In the UKPDS, a reduction of HbA1c by 0.9% resulted in a 25% reduction in microvascular endpoint, largely driven by reductions in retinopathy endpoints. Studies on retinopathy progression, however, have demonstrated a paradoxical worsening of retinopathy within the first year of intensive glycaemic control. This paradoxical worsening, however, did not amount to visual loss in those with mild to moderate retinopathy and the long-term benefits of intensive treatment should counterbalance this early worsening. Nevertheless, when intensive glycaemic control treatment is initiated in those with severe retinopathy, patients should ideally be referred to an ophthalmologist.

Hypertension is a major risk factor for retinopathy progression and in the UKPDS, tight blood pressure control reduces the risk of retinopathy progression by approximately one-third. Whilst both captopril and atenolol were equally effective in reducing retinopathy in the UKPDS, evidence is emerging that agents that modulate the renin–angiotensin system (RAS) may have specific retinal-protective effects, independent of blood pressure reduction. The EUCLID study (EURODIAB Controlled Trial of Lisinopril in Insulin-Dependent Diabetes Mellitus) showed that lisinopril treatment in normotensive patients with type 1 diabetes was associated with a reduction in the risk of retinopathy progression (by at least one level on the EURODIAB scale) and the risk of progression to proliferative retinopathy. Despite a difference in the baseline glycaemic control between the two treatment groups, due to inadequate randomization, results from EUCLID form the basis of further studies to clarify the role of RAS inhibitors in reducing retinopathy progression. Potential mechanisms of RAS inhibitors in reducing retinopathy include reducing angiogenic growth factor expression, as well as inhibiting the direct and indirect effects of angiotensin II on angiogenesis and increasing endothelial permeability.

The role of aspirin in modulating retinopathy progression was investigated in The Early Treatment Diabetic Retinopathy Study (ETDRS). Aspirin (650 mg/day) was not shown to have any effect in preventing visual loss in patients with advanced retinopathy, but in patients with mild to moderate retinopathy, the role of aspirin is unclear. Patients with diabetes with high serum lipid concentrations also have an increased risk of developing proliferative retinopathy, clinically significant MO and retinal hard exudates. Studies investigating the role of statins in reducing retinopathy progression, however, have so far been confined to small, under-powered studies, albeit with favourable outcomes.

Screening for diabetic retinopathy is therefore essential and has been shown to be cost effective and result in reduced risk of visual disability. Current recommendations suggest that patients with mild non-proliferative diabetic retinopathy should be screened annually and if more severe changes develop, screening should be arranged on a three-monthly basis. Diabetic retinopathy may worsen in pregnancy and screening is therefore recommended at each trimester. Direct ophthalmoscopy as a screening modality is extremely operator-dependent and is associated with high error rates and low sensitivity and specificity. An effective high-quality screening programme should encompass high population coverage, sensitivity >80% and specificity >95%, with agreed referral process and criteria, as well as locally agreed system of governance.[3] The UK national screening committee has advocated the use of digital retinal photography, conducted and evaluated by trained personnel.

Recent Developments

1   The DIabetic Retinopathy Candesartan Trial (DIRECT)[4] is an ongoing large, randomized, double-blind control study involving more than 4000 patients, to determine the impact of treatment with candesartan (an angiotensin receptor blocker) for primary and secondary prevention of diabetic retinopathy.

2   Extensive experimental and clinical data have supported the potential benefit of a protein kinase C-β inhibitor[5] (ruboxistaurin) in attenuating retinopathy progression. Two large, multicentred trials—Diabetic Retinopathy Study (DRS) and protein kinase C-Diabetic Macular Edema (DME)—are ongoing to evaluate whether oral treatment with ruboxistaurin will delay progression in patients with moderate to severe retinopathy. Results should be announced in 2006.

Conclusion

Diabetic retinopathy is very common and affects nearly all patients with type 1 diabetes after 20 years of having diabetes. Reassuringly, this patient's retinopathy is mild and does not currently require ophthalmological referral. She requires annual screening and referral

Table 40.2 Criteria for referral to ophthalmology
Patients should be referred to the ophthalmologist for any of the following criteria:
• An unexplained drop in visual acuity
• There are hard exudates within 1 disc diameter of the fovea
• Macular oedema is present
• There are unexplained retinal findings
• Pre-proliferative or more advanced (severe) retinopathy is present

to an ophthalmologist should be made if she fulfils any of the points listed on Table 40.2. Treatment to achieve tight blood sugar and blood pressure control will reduce the risk of retinopathy progression.

Further Reading

1 Diabetes Control and Complications Trial Research Group. The effect of intensive treatment of diabetes on the development and progression of long term complications in insulin-dependent diabetes. *N Engl J Med* 1993; **329**: 977–86.

2 UK Prospective Diabetes Study Group. Tight blood pressure control and risks of macrovascular and microvascular complications in type 2 diabetes: UKPDS 38. *BMJ* 1998; **317**: 703–13.

3 Hutchinson A, McIntosh A, Peters J, O'Keefe C, Khunti K, Baker R, Booth A. Effectiveness of screening and monitoring tests for diabetic retinopathy—a systematic review. *Diabet Med* 2000; **17**: 495–506.

4 Chaturvedi N, Sjoelie AK, Svensson A. DIRECT Programme Study Group. The DIabetic Retinopathy Candesartan Trials (DIRECT) programme, rationale and study design. *J Renin Angiotensin Aldosterone Syst* 2002; **3**: 255–61.

5 Idris I, Gray S, Donnelly R. Protein kinase C activation: isozyme-specific effects on metabolism and cardiovascular complications in diabetes. *Diabetologia* 2001; **44**: 659–73.

41 Proliferative and Pre-proliferative Retinopathy

Case History

A 26-year-old mechanic has failed to attend his last three diabetes clinic appointments. He attends for review, and his visual acuity in both eyes is 6/24. Fundoscopy revealed widespread microaneurysms in both eyes, and hard and soft exudates in both eyes but most prominently in the upper temporal quadrant of his left eye and near the right macular region. There is also evidence of venous beading, intraretinal microvascular abnormality and new vessels near the left optic disc.

What is the significance of his fundoscopy findings?

What is the prognosis of his eyes if left untreated?

Discuss the medical and ophthalmic management of his advanced retinopathy.

Background

Proliferative diabetic retinopathy is defined as the presence of new vessels on the surface of the retina or optic disc. New vessels often arise in the posterior pole of the retina and are associated with retinal ischaemia. If untreated, 50% of patients with retinal new vessels are blind within five years. Where new vessels are within one disc diameter of the optic disc, prognosis is often worse, with 50% of patients becoming blind within two years. When new vessels are seen, patients should be referred urgently (by fax or telephone) to an ophthalmologist. The natural history of diabetic new vessels is of initial proliferation followed by regression. Adherence of fibrous tissue to the new vessels and contraction of the surrounding vitreous can cause traction on the new vessels leading to haemorrhage, retinal detachment and subsequent visual loss. The prevalence of proliferative retinopathy is directly related to the duration of diabetes and degree of hyperglycaemia. Meticulous control of glycaemia and blood pressure level is therefore the most effective approach to preserving vision. In patients with established proliferative retinopathy, the mainstay of treatment is retinal laser photocoagulation with or without operative procedures.

The observation that extensive retinal photocoagulation had unexplained beneficial effects on both new vessel formation and macular oedema prompted the organization of the Diabetic Retinopathy Study (DRS)[1] followed by the Early Treatment Diabetic Retinopathy Study (ETDRS).[2] Both studies, which included a total of approximately 5400 patients, form the basis for current approaches to treatment of advanced retinopathy (pre-proliferative and proliferative retinopathy, as well as macular oedema) using photocoagulation therapy.[3] The principal form of treatment for proliferative retinopathy is panretinal laser photocoagulation, usually by argon laser. Laser photocoagulation works by ablating ischaemic inner retinal tissues and oxygen-consuming photoreceptors, as well as by destroying retinal pigment epithelium resulting in the release of anti-angiogenic factors. Panretinal photocoagulation is beneficial in patients with new vessels at the disc and vitreous haemorrhage, and possibly in patients with new vessels elsewhere or those with severe non-proliferative retinopathy. A more recent analysis of the ETDRS data suggests that early treatment with panretinal photocoagulation may be effective in reducing visual loss, particularly in patients with type 2 diabetes. Complications of laser treatment include transient macular oedema, constriction of visual fields, retinal haemorrhage, uveitis, retinal vein occlusion and, rarely, retinal detachment. Headaches may also follow laser treat-

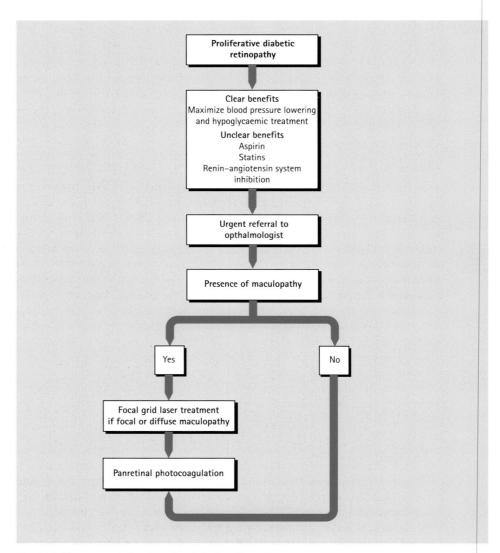

Fig. 41.1 Management of proliferative diabetic retinopathy.

ment, and if severe, glaucoma should be excluded. The risks of these complications are reduced by using low-energy levels and by applying the treatment over several sessions. ETDRS showed that aspirin did not affect the progression of retinopathy, risk of visual loss or the risk of vitreous haemorrhage among patients with proliferative retinopathy, although aspirin did reduce the risk of morbidity and death from cardiovascular disease by 17%. Patients with persistent vitreous haemorrhage, persistent severe proliferative retinopathy or macular retinal detachment will benefit from pars plana vitrectomy. The Diabetic Retinopathy Vitrectomy Study showed that patients with type 1 diabetes benefit from early rather than late vitrectomy,[4] whilst deferment of vitrectomy did not appear to affect visual outcomes in patients with type 2 diabetes. Unfortunately, vitrectomy is associated with a variety of complications and rates of no light perception have been reported to be more than 20%.

For practical purposes, clinically significant macular oedema (CSMO) is defined as any retinopathy lesion within half a disc diameter of the centre of the macula. Diagnosis of macular oedema is made clinically and sometimes with the aid of fluorescein angiography. Macular disease should be suspected in patients with reduced visual acuity, reduced colour vision and/or reduced contrast sensitivity. Whilst patients with ischaemic maculopathy are not responsive to treatments, laser treatment is often effective in patients with focal and diffuse exudative maculopathy. In focal maculopathy, treatment is applied directly at the area of leakage (e.g. microaneurysms at the centre of a circinate exudate), whilst diffuse macular oedema is often treated with grid macular treatment, commencing 500 mm from the centre of the macula with sparing of the fovea. Patients should be reviewed about 2–4 months after treatment. Data from ETDRS suggest that a combination of focal and grid photocoagulation reduced the risk of moderate loss of visual acuity in patients with CSMO by about 50%. Immediate photocoagulation is beneficial if oedema involves the centre of the macular, but treatment may be deferred if this is not the case. Where CSMO exists with proliferative retinopathy, ETDRS recommended that the macula should be treated first, as panretinal photocoagulation may lead to a worsening of the maculopathy. Similarly, cataract extraction may also worsen maculopathy and thus macular laser treatment should be applied first, prior to cataract surgery.

Recent Developments

1   Increased understanding of the pathophysiological mechanisms of diabetic retinopathy has led to the identification of new pharmacological approaches in attenuating retinopathy progression. Activation of protein kinase C (PKC), specifically the β isoform of PKC, is implicated in both the early- and late-stage manifestations of retinopathy.[5] Studies are ongoing to determine the effectiveness of an orally administered PKC-β inhibitor in ameliorating retinopathy progression, proliferation and retinal vascular leakage.

2   Two potential mediators of retinal angiogenesis and vascular leakage have recently been identified. Pigment Epithelial-Derived Factor (PEDF) inhibits both angiogenesis and vascular leakage, whilst Angiopoietin-1 (ANG-1) is pro-angiogenic but inhibits vascular leakage and its action is regulated by Angiopoietin-2 (ANG-2). Experimental studies are ongoing to improve our understanding of the factors which regulate PEDF, ANG-1 and ANG-2 action.

3　Preliminary evidence has suggested that vitreal injection of triamcinolone acetonide, a minimally water-soluble steroid injected in suspension form, is well-tolerated and decreased the progression of diabetic macular oedema as assessed by optical coherence tomography and fluorescein angiography. It may therefore be a potential treatment of diabetic macular oedema and warrants extensive investigation in a randomized, prospective clinical trial.

Conclusion

This patient has proliferative retinopathy at the optic disc. Untreated, 50% of such patients will become blind within two years of presentation. Urgent referral to an ophthalmologist is, therefore, mandatory. Treatment includes retinal photocoagulation therapy with aggressive blood sugar and blood pressure control to prevent retinopathy progression. He will undergo panretinal photocoagulation treatment over several sessions to reduce the discomfort of high-intensity laser treatment given over fewer sessions.

Further Reading

1　Diabetic Retinopathy Study Research Group. Photocoagulation treatment of proliferative diabetic retinopathy: clinical application of Diabetic Retinopathy Study (DRS) findings, DRS report number 8. *Ophthalmology* 1981; **88**: 583–600.

2　Early Treatment Diabetic Retinopathy Study Research Group. Early photocoagulation for diabetic retinopathy. ETDRS report number 9. *Ophthalmology* 1991; **98**: 766–85.

3　Ferris FL, Davis MD, Aiello LM. Treatment of diabetic retinopathy. *N Engl J Med* 1999; **341**: 667–78.

4　The Diabetic Retinopathy Vitrectomy Study Research Group. Early vitrectomy for severe vitreous haemorrhage in diabetic retinopathy. *Arch Ophthalmol* 1990; **108**: 958–64.

5　Frank RN. Potential new medical therapies for diabetic retinopathy: Protein kinase C inhibitors. *Am J Opthalmol* 2002; **133**: 693–8.

42 Macular Disease

Case History

A 74-year-old woman with a ten-year history of type 2 diabetes and hypertension has noted deterioration in vision. She has numerous haemorrhages and exudates around both maculae. Diabetes is reasonably well controlled (glycosylated haemoglobin, HbA1c 7.4%) on 80 mg gliclazide per day. Blood pressure was 145/95 mmHg at her most recent visit, and she takes bendrofluazide 2.5 mg per day for hypertension. Her cholesterol level is 5.6 mmol/l.

What is the prognosis for her vision?

How should she be managed?

Would she benefit from tighter diabetic control?

Background

Diabetic retinopathy is the commonest cause of blindness in the working-age population. However, visual handicap is much more common in the elderly and, amongst older patients with diabetes, macular disease is a much more common cause of visual loss than is classical diabetic retinopathy. Diabetic maculopathy (DMa), characterized by retinal thickening due to oedema and exudates within two disc diameters of the macula, is due to poor retinal perfusion and excessive capillary leakage. Retinal thickening at the posterior pole may cause early loss of colour vision and is associated with high risk of visual impairment amongst elderly patients with diabetes. Although present in up to 50% of patients with diabetic retinopathy, DMa has been much less intensively studied than classical retinopathy. It is associated with poor control and long duration of diabetes, with neuropathy and nephropathy, and with risk factors for atherosclerotic disease. The prevalence of DMa is increasing as the number of elderly patients with type 2 diabetes in the population increases.

In the Liverpool Diabetic Eye Study,[1] the cumulative incidence of sight-threatening maculopathy was 4.8% over six years among patients with type 2 diabetes. The corresponding figure for sight-threatening retinopathy was 6.1%. Jeppesen and Bek[2] recently documented the causes of blindness in Århus County, Denmark; 0.6% of patients with type 1 diabetes and 1.5% of patients with type 2 diabetes were blind. Proliferative diabetic retinopathy accounted for 66.2% of blindness in type 1 diabetes, but only 18% of blindness in type 2 diabetes. DMa was the cause of blindness in 18.5% of type 2 patients, and age-related macular degeneration (AMD) accounted for 21.9% of cases.

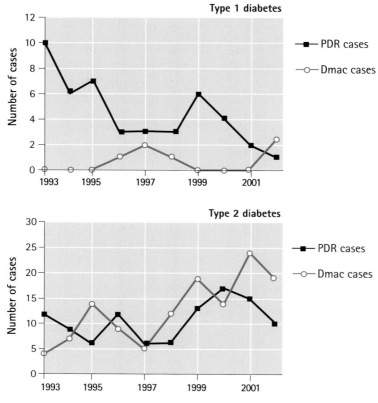

Fig. 42.1 Sight loss due to macular disease and proliferative retinopathy. Dmac, diabetic macular disease; PDR, proliferative diabetic retinopathy. Blindness from proliferative diabetic retinopathy is decreasing in type 1 diabetes as detection and treatment become more effective. In type 2 diabetes, Dmac is a more common cause of blindness than proliferative retinopathy. *Source:* Jeppesen & Bek, 2004.[2]

AMD affects up to 25 million people worldwide, and an estimated 300 000 people in the United Kingdom are either blind or partially sighted because of the condition.[3] The condition is associated with age, hypertension, smoking and family history. Slow degeneration of the retinal pigment membrane cells in dry AMD leads to gradual deterioration in vision over many years. In the wet form, there is choroidal neovascularization, oedema and leakage of blood and lipid materials. This form is often associated with rapid deterioration in vision. Photocoagulation using a thermal laser was the treatment of choice for wet AMD until recently. Photodynamic therapy using the photosensitizer verteporfin and a non-thermal laser is now the treatment of choice.

There has been debate about whether AMD is more common amongst patients with diabetes, although a recent study has suggested that neovascular AMD is associated with diabetes.[4] Vascular factors are almost certainly important determinants of deterioration in AMD and it is no surprise that deteriorating vision in subjects with AMD appears to be more rapid when diabetes is present.[5] The role of nutritional factors is also of interest. Antioxidant vitamin (A, C and E) levels are often decreased in patients with either AMD or diabetes. There has been recent interest in AMD in the potential protective role of the carotenoids lutein and zeaxanthin, levels of which are decreased in obese subjects.[3]

Recent Developments

1 A recent study from the United Kingdom Prospective Diabetes Study (UKPDS) Group[6] has investigated progression of retinopathy in relation to tight blood pressure control in 1148 patients with hypertension and type 2 diabetes followed for a mean of 2.6 years. Patients allocated to tight blood pressure control developed fewer micro-aneurysms, hard exudates and cotton wool spots. They were less likely to have progressive retinopathy and to require photocoagulation. The investigators did not detect any difference in those whose blood pressure was controlled with an angiotensin-converting enzyme inhibitor or with a beta-blocker.

2 A very significant predisposition to AMD associated with modifiable risk factors is emerging: thus, smoking appears to be a potent risk factor with smokers being around twice as likely to develop AMD.[7] There is also a strong association with obesity,[4] and this may relate to the pro-oxidant state that exists in obese subjects.

Conclusion

The patient is at high risk of developing severe visual impairment and requires urgent referral to an ophthalmologist for consideration of photocoagulation. Both diabetic maculopathy and age-related macular degeneration are leading causes of visual loss among older patients with diabetes. The pathogenesis of these conditions is less well understood than that of diabetic retinopathy. Control of blood pressure is probably the most important aspect of this lady's management and, if she has persistently increased pressure, consideration should be given to stepping up her antihypertensive therapy. Tighter glycaemic control may be obtained with an increased dose of gliclazide or change to another hypoglycaemic drug or combination therapy. Change to insulin is probably not warranted, particularly if her vision is deteriorating. Consideration should be given to lowering her cholesterol pharmacologically, as cardiovascular risk factors are associated with progression of macular disease.

Further Reading

1 Younis N, Broadbent DM, Vora JP, Harding SP. Incidence of sight-threatening retinopathy in patients with type 2 diabetes in the Liverpool Diabetic Eye Study: a cohort study. *Lancet* 2003; **361**: 195–200.

2 Jeppesen P, Bek T. The occurrence and causes of registered blindness in diabetes patients in Arhus County, Denmark. *Acta Ophthalmol Scand* 2004; **82**: 526–30.

3 Chopdar A, Chakravarthy U, Verma D. Age related macular degeneration. *BMJ* 2003; **326**: 485–8.

4 Clemons TE, Milton RC, Klein R, Seddon JM, Ferris FL. Risk factors for the incidence of Advanced Age-Related Macular Degeneration in the Age-Related Eye Disease Study (AREDS) AREDS report no. 19. *Ophthalmology* 2005; **112**: 533–9.

5 Voutilainen KRM, Teräsvirta ME, Uusitupa MI, Niskanen LK. Age-related macular degeneration in newly diagnosed type 2 diabetic patients and control subjects: a 10-year follow-up on evolution, risk factors, and prognostic significance. *Diabetes Care* 2000; **23**: 1672–8.

6 Matthews DR, Stratton IM, Aldington SJ, Holman RR, Kohner EM. Risks of progression of retinopathy and vision loss related to tight blood pressure control in type 2 diabetes mellitus: UKPDS 69. *Arch Ophthalmol* 2004; **122**: 1631–40.

7 Evans JR, Fletcher AE, Wormald RPL. 28,000 cases of age related macular degeneration causing visual loss in people aged 75 years and above in the United Kingdom may be attributable to smoking. *Br J Ophthalmol* 2005; **89**: 550–3.

PROBLEM

43 Autonomic Neuropathy

Case History

A 52-year-old man with long-standing type 1 diabetes complains that he feels light-headed when he stands up. He has been losing weight recently and also complains of nausea, constipation and erectile dysfunction. There is a postural drop in his systolic blood pressure of 30 mmHg. His glycosylated haemoglobin (HbA1c) is 9.1% and he takes Mixtard insulin 36 units twice daily.

What is the differential diagnosis for his symptoms?

How should he be investigated?

What treatment options are available?

Background

Diabetes is the commonest cause of autonomic neuropathy, which usually occurs in patients with long-standing diabetes and is generally accompanied by peripheral sensori-motor diabetic neuropathy. Even in a patient with diabetes, other causes of autonomic neuropathy should be considered. These include amyloidosis, a paraneoplastic syndrome, post-infection, toxins including heavy metals and drugs including vincristine and amiodarone.[1] Apart from orthostatic hypotension, patients with autonomic neuropathy may suffer from: gastric paresis, which may give rise to nausea, vomiting and loss of appetite; altered bowel habit, usually presenting predominantly with constipation; bladder dysfunction, with incomplete emptying and increased residual volume; loss of sweating, particularly peripherally, and sometimes excess sweating meditated centrally, often in response to food intake (gustatory sweating); and men may suffer from erectile dysfunc-tion, although vascular and psychological factors frequently contribute to this symptom.

Cardiac autonomic neuropathy impairs heart rate response to exercise and leads to an increase in resting heart rate due to loss of vagal tone—and so, no heart rate response to the Valsalva manoeuvre. Diabetic autonomic neuropathy (DAN) increases the risk of sudden death, although other factors such as the presence of coronary artery disease and nephropathy are also important predictors.[2] DAN is an important complication of diabetes, not only because of the symptoms it produces, but also because of its relationship with sudden death, decreased hypoglycaemic awareness, risk of silent myocardial ischaemia and increased perioperative risk.

Orthostatic hypotension is defined as a decrease in systolic blood pressure of greater than 20 mmHg, or a diastolic fall of greater than 10 mmHg, on standing or head-up tilt, and is frequently one of the most disabling symptoms of DAN. Efferent sympathetic denervation leads to decreased vasoconstriction of splanchnic, skeletal and other vascular beds. This leads to decreased cerebral blood flow in circumstances where peripheral blood flow increases. Before drug treatment is considered, non-pharmacological measures

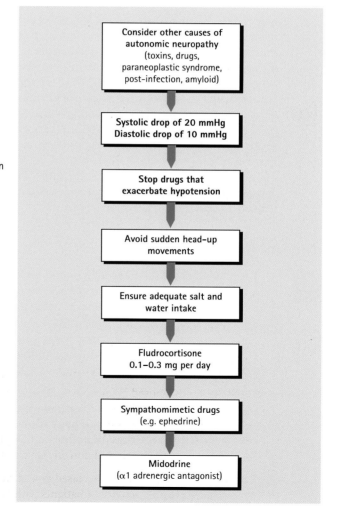

Fig. 43.1 Orthostatic hypotension

should be used where possible. Drugs that exacerbate hypotension should be stopped or the dose reduced. Patients should be instructed that situations associated with sudden head-up posture or straining may exacerbate symptoms of orthostatic hypotension. The symptoms are often worse early in the morning because of nocturnal natriuresis. Exercise increases skeletal muscle blood flow and food or alcohol increase splanchnic blood flow—both may increase symptoms of orthostatic hypotension. Ensure adequate salt and fluid intake. With severe symptoms and in acute illness, this may require intake of up to 10 litres of fluid per day and up to 10 grams of salt. Where symptoms are particularly disabling in the morning, head-up tilt of the bed activates the renin–angiotensin system overnight and decreases overnight salt and water loss. Atrial overpacing has been used by some to compensate for decreased blood pressure. This is not generally recommended but demand cardiac pacing may be beneficial in patients with carotid sinus hypersensitivity.

When drug treatment is necessary, 9α-fluorohydrocortisone (fludrocortisone), a potent mineralocorticoid, is the drug of first choice. Doses of 0.1–0.3 mg/day may be effective. Where symptoms are worse early in the morning, taking the drug before bed may reduce nocturnal natriuresis. Side effects of overdosing include hypertension, fluid retention and hypokalaemia. Sympathomimetic drugs such as ephedrine (15–45 mg three times daily) may reduce symptoms. Side effects include tremor, reduced appetite, mood disturbances and nightmares, and urinary retention. The specific α_1-adrenoreceptor antagonist midodrine at a dose of 2.5–10 mg three times daily has been used widely, but is not available in all countries. Release of vasodilatory peptides after food intake may contribute to symptoms. The short-acting somatostatin analogue octreotide may alleviate such symptoms at a dose of 25–100 μg three times daily. There is no specific evidence relating to the use of long-acting somatostatin analogues. Loss of salt and water overnight may exacerbate symptoms in the early morning. Desmopressin—either subcutaneously or orally—may alleviate symptoms at this time. Finally, erythropoietin has been used for autonomic symptoms in patients with renal failure and anaemia as it may improve oxygen delivery to neural tissues.

Recent Developments

1   Recent studies are shedding light on the epidemiology of DAN, and its importance as a complication of diabetes. Prevalence varies from 2% in patients with diabetes of recent onset to 35% in patients with long-standing type 1 diabetes. Recent evidence form the EURODIAB study[3] confirms that glycaemic exposure (duration of diabetes and poor control) is a risk factor, along with age, hypertension and the presence of retinopathy. The presence of microalbuminuria, independent of hypertension, also predicts development of DAN in patients with diabetes.[4]

2   DAN can be diagnosed by simple bedside tests. However, even with tests in neurophysiological laboratories, the condition may be under-diagnosed. A semiquantitative imaging test using the radiopharmaceutical ^{123}I-metaiodobenzylguanidine has been used to demonstrate reduced catecholamine uptake in patients with DAN, and could form the basis for a simple and non-invasive clinical test.[5]

3   Patients with diabetes are at increased risk of carotid artery stenosis (CAS). Impaired afferent baroreceptor activity in patients with CAS may lead to postural hypotension

and decreased heart rate responses to lowering of blood pressure.[6] Thus, orthostatic hypotension may occur as a symptom of macrovascular disease rather than of generalized autonomic failure.

4   There is an association between autonomic neuropathy and the production of erythropoietin, and decreased production of the peptide may underlie the association between autonomic neuropathy and diabetic nephropathy. Erythropoietin has been suggested as a potential treatment for neuropathy in diabetes and may protect against neuropathic symptoms, including those caused by failure of the autonomic nervous system.[7]

Conclusion

The patient has symptoms strongly suggestive of diabetic autonomic neuropathy. Treatment of this condition is difficult and is usually directed towards management of individual symptoms. Empirically, his diabetes control should be improved. There is no direct evidence that this will improve his neuropathy but, as with other types of neuropathy, tight glycaemic control may prevent it advancing. Large doses of insulin can have a vasodilator effect, and attempts should be made to optimize control while keeping the insulin dose as low as possible. Education may help the patient to rationalize his symptoms and avoid situations that provoke postural hypotension. If pharmacological treatment proves necessary, fludrocortisone is the usual drug of first choice. Symptoms are often worse in the morning, in which case the drug is best given at night to minimize sodium loss in the urine overnight. If symptoms persist, or fludrocortisone is not tolerated, consider sympathomimetic drugs, octreotide, desmopressin or erythropoietin.

Further Reading

1   Freeman R. Autonomic peripheral neuropathy. *Lancet* 2005; **365**: 1259–70.

2   Suarez GA, Clark VM, Norell JE, Kottke TE, Callahan MJ, O'Brien PC, Low PA, Dyck PJ. Sudden cardiac death in diabetes mellitus: risk factors in the Rochester diabetic neuropathy study. *J Neurol Neurosurg Psychiatry* 2005; **76**: 240–5.

3   Witte DR, Tesfaye S, Chaturvedi N, Eaton SEM, Kempler P, Fuller JH. Risk factors for cardiac autonomic neuropathy in type 1 diabetes mellitus. *Diabetologia* 2005; **48**: 164–71.

4   Moran A, Palmas W, Field L, Bhattarai J, Schwartz JE, Weinstock RS, Shea S. Cardiovascular autonomic neuropathy is associated with microalbuminuria in older patients with type 2 diabetes. *Diabetes Care* 2004; **27**: 972–7.

5   Scott LA, Kench PL. Cardiac autonomic neuropathy in the diabetic patient: does 123I-MIBG imaging have a role to play in early diagnosis? *J Nucl Med Technol* 2004; **32**: 66–71.

6   Akinola A, Mathias CJ, Mansfield A, Thomas D, Wolfe J, Nicolaides AN, Tegos T. Cardiovascular, autonomic, and plasma catecholamine responses in unilateral and bilateral carotid artery stenosis. *J Neurol Neurosurg Psychiatry* 1999; **67**: 428–32.

7   Lipton SA. Erythropoietin for neurologic protection and diabetic neuropathy. *N Engl J Med* 2004; **350**: 2516–17.

44 The Charcot Foot

Case History

A 53-year-old unemployed man with long-standing type 1 diabetes is referred to hospital because his foot is painful and his left ankle is swollen. An X-ray of the foot and ankle shows fractures of the 4th and 5th metatarsals.

What causes these changes?

How should he be managed?

Background

The differential diagnosis of a unilaterally swollen lower limb is broad. It is important to reach a positive diagnosis so that appropriate treatment is offered—particularly where the integrity of the limb is threatened by delay in treatment. Deep vein thrombosis, ankle sprain, cellulitis or simple fracture are all possible diagnoses, but the finding of metatarsal fractures is key in ensuring that an acute (Charcot) neuroarthropathic joint is considered.

Jean-Marie Charcot described the neuroarthropathic joint in syphilis in 1883. In 1936, Jordan described similar changes as a 'neuritic manifestation [of] diabetes mellitus'. The (Charcot) neuroarthropathic joint of diabetes is now recognized as a potentially devastating late complication that affects 1 in 700 patients, though this is probably an underestimate.

The pathophysiology of neuroarthropathy is imperfectly understood but involves synergistic abnormalities of both the joints and vascular supply of the limb.

- Sensorimotor neuropathy in the affected limb is universal. Proprioceptive loss puts abnormal stresses through joints made lax by motor neuropathy. Inappropriate signalling of pain means that chronic low-grade trauma is under-recognized.

- Glycation of connective tissues may reduce flexibility of the foot and also induce abnormal stresses through small joints.

- Autonomic neuropathy causes abnormal shunting of blood resulting in osteopaenia, bounding foot pulses and inadequate resolution of chronic minor trauma.

- These factors increase the risk of low-trauma fracture and impair normal healing. The consequences of a minor fracture can then be potentially devastating: instability, further fracture, subluxation/dislocation of the tarsus/ankle, permanent deformity, plantar ulceration, infection and amputation are all recognized.

A long history of diabetes (usually >15 years) and profound peripheral neuropathy are universal, though pain is often a feature of acute neuroarthropathy. In a non-ulcerated foot, the diagnosis is frequently missed on first presentation and late diagnosis can be responsible for permanent disability. A high index of suspicion is needed. Plain X-ray may demonstrate only minimal changes of osteopaenia or loss of joint space. Vascular calcification is a frequent finding, but is not specific to neuroarthropathy. A stress fracture may be invisible on plain X-ray and a careful history, supported by bone scintigraphy or magnetic resonance imaging (MRI), may be needed. Resorption of phalanges, subluxation/dislocation, bone fragmentation and sclerosis are characteristic late changes of neuroarthropathy, but can be indistinguishable from changes associated with osteomyelitis. If there is ulceration/infection, then bone scintigraphy and MRI are often unhelpful in differentiating between neuroarthropathy and osteomyelitis. In this case it is pragmatic to treat both—though using a bisphosphonate would be unusual.

There are three potential treatments for the non-infected, acutely neuroarthropathic foot: offloading, bisphosphonates and surgery (Figure 44.1).

Offloading

If acute neuroarthropathy is suspected, the limb should be promptly offloaded and immobilized. This will usually require a removable, non-weight-bearing cast with crutches/wheelchair for mobility. This limits further disruption of the architecture of the foot and allows healing to commence. This is the mainstay of treatment and may require immobilization for many weeks or months until there is radiological evidence of stabilization and repair and the foot is cool.

Once the initial episode has resolved, considerable care should be taken to find appropriate footwear. Residual deformity should be accommodated in bespoke orthotic footwear. Where there is no or minimal residual deformity, precautions should be taken to protect the neuropathic foot from future trauma.

Bisphosphonates

The objective, clinical evidence of benefit from bisphosphonates is modest. One prospective, randomized study of 39 patients has been published.[1] This studied the effects of 90 mg pamidronate or placebo on clinical and biochemical measures of activity in a 'hot' neuroarthropathic foot. Symptom score, foot temperature and markers of bone turnover were lower in the foot treated with pamidronate during the initial weeks of treatment, though longer-term outcomes were not different between the two groups. Bisphosphonates are now used as adjunctive treatment. Oral bisphosphonates are likely to take the place of intravenous bisphosphonates.

Surgery

There are many small studies of primary surgical treatment—particularly where the ankle is involved or there has been substantial subluxation/dislocation at the talo-navicular joint or of the whole tarso-metatarsal complex (the Lisfranc dislocation). Surgery should generally be avoided in the acute phase, unless late presentation means that limb salvage cannot be achieved in any other way.[2] Surgery also has a role in selected patients following resolution of the acute episode. Collapse of the arch can cause deformities such as a 'rocker-bottom' foot or medial bony protuberance, which may cause skin ulceration due to abnormal pressure loading. Surgical intervention to realign the affected joint can be helpful, but usually only if there is no associated infection.

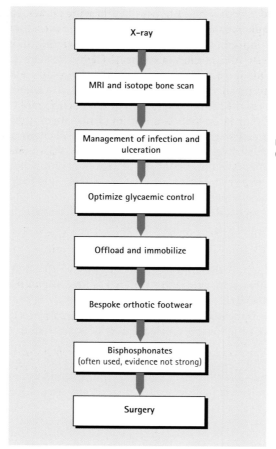

Fig. 44.1 Management of the Charcot foot.

Recent Developments

1 A link between vascular calcification and osteopaenia in neuroarthropathy has recently been proposed.[3] The receptor activator of nuclear factor kappa B ligand (RANKL)/osteoprotegerin signalling pathway regulates bone turnover in various diseases and is thought to mediate the calcification of vascular smooth muscle cells in coronary and peripheral vascular disease. Peptides such as calcitonin gene-related peptide, produced by nerves and other tissues, normally exert control over the activation of this pathway. The author postulates that this links neuropathy, unregulated vascular calcification and calcium resorption from bone in diabetic neuroarthropathy.

Conclusion

In a patient with long-standing diabetes with a swollen foot and metatarsal fractures, a positive diagnosis and treatment plan are essential. Diagnoses such as thrombosis and infection are possible, but would not usually be associated with metatarsal fracture. If there is peripheral neuropathy, it would be prudent to treat this as an acute neuroarthropathy and immobilize the affected lower limb in a non-weight-bearing plaster. Suggested practice is also to administer a bisphosphonate in the acute phase—intravenously if possible or orally if this cannot be managed. The plain X-ray should be repeated after two weeks to determine if there has been deterioration or healing. Weight-bearing should not recommence until there is clear radiological evidence of healing and the temperatures of the affected and unaffected limb are equal.[4]

Once healed, it is important to assess the shape of the foot. If there is deformity, consideration should be given to bespoke, orthotic footwear. The incidence of recurrence, contralateral neuroarthropathy or foot ulceration is in excess of 40% and the patient should be encouraged to seek prompt medical advice if either foot becomes warm, swollen or painful in the future.

Further Reading

1 Jude EB, Selby PL, Burgess J, Lillystone P, Mawer EP, Page SR, Donohoe M, Foster AV, Edmonds ME, Boulton AJ. Bisphosphonates in the treatment of Charcot neuroarthropathy: a double-blind randomised controlled trial. *Diabetologia* 2001; **44**: 2032–7.

2 Bono JV, Roger DJ, Jacobs RL. Surgical arthrodesis of the neuropathic foot. A salvage procedure. *Clin Orthop Relat Res* 1993; **296**: 14–20.

3 Jeffcoate W. Vascular calcification and osteolysis in diabetic neuropathy-is RANK-L the missing link? *Diabetologia* 2004; **47**: 1488–92.

4 Saltzman CL, Hagy ML, Zimmerman B, Estin M, Cooper R. How effective is intensive nonoperative initial treatment of patients with diabetes and Charcot arthropathy of the feet? *Clin Orthop Relat Res* 2005; **435**: 185–90.

Macrovascular and Other Complications

45   Angina in patients with type 2 diabetes

46   Advances in management of peripheral vascular disease

47   Renal artery stenosis

48   Foot ulceration

49   Transient ischaemic attack

PROBLEM

45 Angina in Patients with Type 2 Diabetes

Case History

A 52-year-old smoker with type 2 diabetes is referred with myocardial-sounding exertional chest pain. He is normotensive. Glycaemic control is reasonable (glycosylated haemoglobin, HbA1c 7.2%), and he is treated with oral hypoglycaemic drugs.

How should he be managed?

Should he be immediately referred for coronary angiography?

What are the most appropriate anti-anginal agents?

Background

Ischaemic heart disease, type 2 diabetes and smoking are factors independently associated with an increased risk of cardiovascular disease and death. Diabetes is now regarded as a coronary risk equivalent following work by Haffner and others.[1] The history, examination and diagnostic testing—targeted toward ischaemic heart disease—should clarify the prognosis of coronary disease, optimal medical management and timing of appropriate coronary intervention.

All patients with diabetes and ischaemic heart disease should have aggressive risk factor reduction. Smoking cessation, low-dose aspirin, statin therapy (target low-density lipoprotein [LDL] at least <2.6 mmol/l),[2] blood pressure lowering (target at least <130/80 mmHg) and intensification of glycaemic control is usual. There is debate about whether angiotensin-converting enzyme (ACE) inhibitors should be used routinely and whether intensification of glycaemic control has an appreciable effect on macrovascular disease progression. However, microalbuminuria and microvascular complications of diabetes often coexist with coronary heart disease.

A resting electrocardiogram (ECG), blood tests for fasted lipid levels, renal function and HbA1c, and urine testing to determine urinary albumin excretion will contribute to overall risk stratification in advance of exercise ECG testing. Exercise ECG testing helps determine both diagnosis and prognosis in patients who are able to exercise adequately and do not have left bundle branch block, resting ST-T wave abnormalities or digitalis effect on the resting ECG. If the exercise ECG is positive, it will be used to help determine whether coronary intervention is warranted. If exercise ECG testing is negative, the high pre-test probability in this case means that angina is still a likely diagnosis. Consideration should be given to coronary angiography if symptoms warrant this or further non-invasive testing with exercise or pharmacological stress imaging using echocardiography, thallium-201 or sestamibi-technetium-99m radionuclide imaging.

Exercise ECG testing identifies the amount of ischaemic but viable myocardium and whether revascularization may be beneficial. Indications for coronary angiography in patients fit for revascularization include:

- poor exercise capacity due to coronary ischaemia;

- angina at low workload;

- low peak systolic blood pressure or a fall in blood pressure during exercise;

- flat or downsloping ST segment depression of >1 mm during exercise/recovery;

- ST segment elevation during exercise/recovery;

- significant ventricular dysrhythmia (tachycardia/couplets), particularly at low workload or during recovery.

Coronary angiography provides anatomical information to select patients for revascularization by coronary artery bypass grafting (CABG) or percutaneous coronary intervention (PCI). The BARI trial (Bypass Angioplasty Revascularization Investigation)[3] demonstrated that five-year survival in patients with diabetes was better in those who received CABG (81%) than those who received PCI (66%). This may be because the prevalence of complex cardiac disease—three vessel disease with left ventricular dysfunction—is greater in the presence of diabetes and less amenable to PCI. However, these data do not reflect current practice: CABG in early trials was frequently performed using saphenous vein rather than internal mammary artery grafts, and PCI was performed without aggressive cardiovascular risk factor reduction, clopidogrel, heparin, glycoprotein IIb/IIIa inhibitors and, most recently, drug-eluting coronary stents. The current choice between CABG or PCI is tilting toward PCI.[4,5]

Very-long-term follow-up data from new stenting protocols and techniques are not yet available, but these practices are in regular use and have displaced conventional tech-

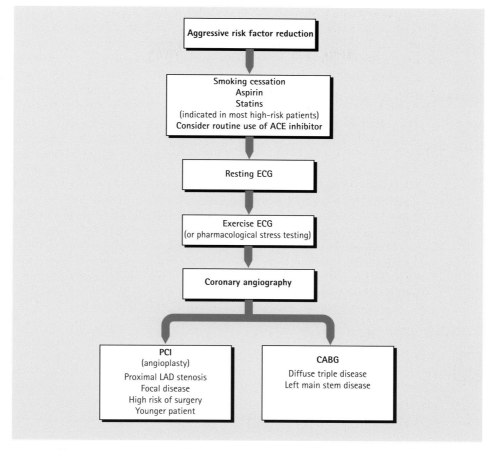

Fig. 45.1 Management of angina.

niques in certain situations. Some centres now prefer to carry out PCI with drug-eluting stents rather than CABG if technically possible. The American College of Cardiology/ American Heart Association guidelines[6] do not yet reflect preferred current practice.

PCI preferred:

● Proximal, isolated left anterior descending (LAD) stenosis, particularly if there is left ventricular dysfunction or medical treatment has failed

● Focal coronary disease with good left ventricular function

● Young patients who may require repeat CABG in their lifetime

● Older patients with comorbidities that preclude surgery

CABG preferred:

● Significant left main stem disease

- Diffuse triple vessel disease
- Two vessel disease with significant LAD disease
- Patients with diabetes

Recent Developments

1 The risk of restenosis requiring repeated intervention following PCI in patients with diabetes is approximately double that of patients without diabetes. Restenosis rates are halved by coronary stenting after balloon angioplasty, but 10–15% of patients without diabetes still suffer restenosis—usually within the first nine months of placement. Sirolimus (an immunosuppressant) and paclitaxel (an antineoplastic agent) are now used in polymer-coated drug-eluting stents to inhibit growth of vascular intima during the first few weeks following stent deployment. Both have demonstrated superior efficacy to bare metal stents in clinical trials—further halving restenosis rates to 3–5% in patients without diabetes. Comparative trials suggest that sirolimus may be superior to paclitaxel.[4] A recent trial comparing sirolimus- and paclitaxel-coated stents in patients with diabetes demonstrated angiographic restenosis rates of 12% with paclitaxel and 6.4% with sirolimus.[7]

Conclusion

A middle-aged male smoker with diabetes and exertional chest pain is likely to die of atheromatous vascular disease. Strenuous efforts should be made to reduce cardiovascular risk factors. Dietary counselling, exercise and smoking cessation should support pharmacological intervention to achieve treatment targets consistent with the Steno Trial[8] (blood pressure <130/80 mmHg, HbA1c <6.5%, LDL-cholesterol <2.6 mmol/l and low-dose aspirin). The use of an ACE inhibitor if urinary albumin excretion is normal is controversial but is likely to form part of the treatment regimen for blood pressure.

If the resting ECG provides no contraindication, an exercise ECG following withdrawal of negatively chronotropic drugs is indicated for diagnosis and prognosis. A positive exercise ECG should support intervention as outlined above. If the exercise ECG is negative, further non-invasive testing may be appropriate—depending upon local expertise and availability. However, if activity is significantly limited by anginal symptoms despite medical treatment of angina (beta-blocker/calcium antagonist/potassium channel opener/nitrate as tolerated), coronary angiography with a view to revascularization is indicated. The mode of revascularization will depend on coronary anatomy, availability of local expertise and advances in revascularization techniques.

Further Reading

1 Haffner SM, Lehto S, Rönnemaa T, Pyörälä K, Laakso M. Mortality from coronary heart disease in subjects with type 2 diabetes and in nondiabetic subjects with and without prior myocardial infarction. *N Engl J Med* 1998; **339**: 229–34.

2 Collins R, Armitage J, Parish S, Sleigh P, Peto R. Study of cholesterol-lowering with simvastatin in 5963 people with diabetes: a randomised placebo-controlled trial. *Lancet* 2003; **361**: 2005–16.

3 The Bypass Angioplasty Revascularization Investigation (BARI) Investigators. Comparison of coronary bypass surgery with angioplasty in patients with multivessel disease. *N Engl J Med* 1996; **335**: 217–25.

4 Kastrati A, Dibra A, Eberle S, Mehilli J, Suarez de Lezo J, Goy JJ, Ulm K, Schomig A. Sirolimus-eluting stents vs paclitaxel-eluting stents in patients with coronary artery disease: meta-analysis of randomized trials. *JAMA* 2005; **294**: 819–25.

5 Subramanian VA, Patel NU, Patel NC, Loulmet DF. Robotic assisted multivessel minimally invasive direct coronary artery bypass with port-access stabilization and cardiac positioning: paving the way for outpatient coronary surgery? *Ann Thorac Surg* 2005; **79**: 1590–6.

6 Eagle KA, Guyton RA, Davidoff R, Edwards FH, Ewy GA, Gardner TJ, Hart JC, Herrmann HC, Hillis LD, Hutter AM Jr, Lytle BW, Marlow RA, Nugent WC, Orszulak TA. ACC/AHA 2004 guideline update for coronary artery bypass graft surgery: a report of the American College of Cardiology/American Heart Association Task Force on Practice Guidelines Guideline Update for Coronary Artery Bypass Graft Surgery. *Circulation* 2004; **110**: e340–437.

7 Dibra A, Kastrati A, Mehilli J, Pache J, Schuhlen H, von Beckerath N, Ulm K, Wessely R, Dirschinger J, Schomig A. Paclitaxel-eluting or sirolimus-eluting stents to prevent restenosis in diabetic patients. *N Engl J Med* 2005; **353**: 663–70.

8 Gaede P, Vedel P, Larsen N, Jensen GVH, Parving H-H, Pedersen O. Multifactorial intervention and cardiovascular disease in patients with type 2 diabetes. *N Engl J Med* 2003; **348**: 383–93.

PROBLEM

46 Advances in Management of Peripheral Arterial Disease

Case History

A retired 61-year-old man is beginning to develop symptoms of intermittent claudication affecting his right calf. Foot examination reveals loss of dorsalis pedis and posterior tibial pulses on his right foot. His ankle–brachial pressure index (ABPI) is 0.72 taken in his affected limb. He does not smoke and you encourage him to continue to walk to stimulate collateral circulation. He is not keen for surgical intervention.

Discuss lifestyle measures that he should adopt.

What is the medical management for his problem?

Discuss emerging treatment for the management of peripheral vascular disease

Background

Measurement of ABPI is a non-invasive method to assess peripheral arterial disease (PAD). Patients with intermittent claudication typically have an ABPI ratio of 0.6–0.8. The mainstay of treatment for intermittent claudication is smoking cessation and regular exercise. A meta-analysis of randomized controlled trials of physical exercise has confirmed the benefits of regular exercise in improving walking distance.[1] Walking programmes should be supervised and involve 30 minutes per session, at least three times per week for six months. The beneficial effects may arise from improvement in patients' cardiovascular fitness, increased production of nitric oxide and/or modification of cardiovascular risk factors. Patients should be told to 'walk through the pain' during exercise programmes, rather than to stop at the point when the pain begins since this helps increase collateral blood supply. Raising the heel of the shoe by 1 cm will also increase walking distance by reducing the workload on calf muscles.

Large randomized trials have shown that aspirin, as monotherapy or in combination with dipyridamole, delays the progression of established PAD, as determined by serial angiography and need for surgical revascularization. In the CAPRIE study (Clopidogrel versus Aspirin in Patients at Risk of Ischaemic Events), clopidogrel resulted in a significant reduction in cardiovascular events, particularly in the subgroup of patients with PAD. Combination antiplatelet therapy may be preferred in patients with PAD who undergo angioplasty or stenting procedures. The phosphodiesterase type 3 inhibitor, cilostazol, also has effects on platelet function as well as on vasodilation and lipid levels. Double-blind, placebo-controlled trials in over 2000 patients have shown that cilostazol improves exercise tolerance, and evidence from subgroup analyses of multicentre trials suggests that patients with diabetes also respond favourably to cilostazol. This drug has been approved in the United Kingdom for improvement in pain-free and maximum walking distances. Blood pressure should also be lowered in patients with diabetes and PAD.[2] In the United Kingdom Prospective Diabetes Study (UKPDS) cohort, a 10 mmHg lowering in systolic blood pressure produced a non-significant 16% reduction in risk of lower limb amputation or peripheral vascular disease-related mortality. The Appropriate Blood Pressure Control in Diabetes (ABCD) study showed that in patients with type 2 diabetes with established PAD and a baseline diastolic blood pressure of 80–89 mmHg, intensive blood pressure control (mean blood pressure over four years 128/75 mmHg) cancelled out the excess risk of a cardiovascular event associated with PAD. In the 4046 subjects with PAD in the Heart Outcomes Protection Evaluation (HOPE) study, ramipril conferred a more significant reduction in morbidity and mortality compared with the total study cohort. Beta-blockers can be used safely in patients with diabetes particularly if a strong indication exists. Controlled studies have shown that beta-blockers do not adversely affect walking capacity or symptoms of intermittent claudication.

Cholesterol lowering with statins and aggressive management of hyperglycaemia may also have disease-modifying effects on atherosclerosis in the lower limb. In the Scandinavian Simvastatin Survival (4S) study, 4% of the participants had intermittent claudication. The number of cases of new or worsening claudication during the trial was significantly less in the statin treatment group. The Heart Protection Study (HPS) showed a significant 24% reduction in vascular events with simvastatin, which was consistent in all subgroups, including patients with PAD. A Cochrane meta-analysis of lipid-lowering therapy in patients with PAD showed that active therapy reduces disease progression, the

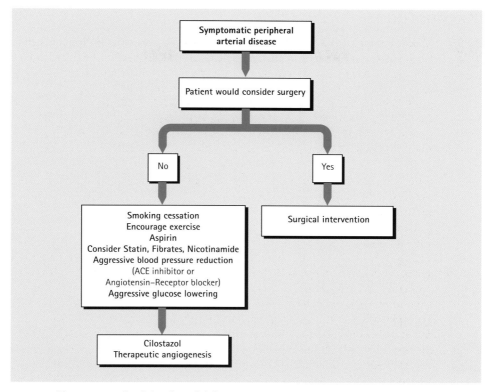

Fig. 46.1 Management of peripheral arterial disease.

severity of claudication and mortality. Hyperglycaemia, meanwhile, precedes the development of PAD and lower extremity amputation in patients with diabetes. A 1% increase in glycosylated haemoglobin (HbA1c) was associated with a 35–42% increased risk for ABPI <0.9 or obstructed crural arteries. In the UKPDS, patients who were allocated to tight glycaemic control showed a trend towards a reduction in deaths from PAD and fewer amputations (relative risk 0.61; $P = 0.099$).[3]

Recent Developments

1   It is now recognized that the severity of symptoms in PAD and treatment outcomes are related to the degree of occlusive arterial disease and to the extent of collateral vessel formation. Therapeutic angiogenesis[4] by local administration of angiogenic growth factors, such as vascular endothelial growth factor (VEGF), in the form of gene transfer using viral or plasmid vectors or recombinant protein delivery, may stimulate collateral circulation through growth and proliferation of new blood vessels. Gene transfer allows prolonged expression of the protein, reduced systemic exposure to growth factors and ease of delivery to peripheral tissues, which may be advantageous. Although pre-clinical studies of VEGF delivered via gene transfer have been able to induce collateral blood flow and arteriogenesis, results from phase 1 and phase II 'proof of concept' clinical studies have been inconsistent. These inconsistencies may be explained by

differences in VEGF isoforms (e.g. VEGF121 and VEGF165), utilization of non-optimal doses and duration of VEGF expression, as well as uncertainties about the efficiency of gene transfer in adult skeletal muscles due to low concentrations of adenoviral receptors and physical barriers to transfection.

2   Advances in the understanding of the pathophysiology of glycaemic vascular injury have also identified pathways which have potential for therapeutic modulation.[5] These include: (1) increased oxidative stress and free radical-mediated damage; (2) formation of advanced glycosylation end-products; (3) diversion of glucose into the aldose reductase pathway; and (4) activation of one or more isozymes of protein kinase C. Experimental studies in targeting these pathways have focused on developing agents to restore normal vasorelaxation, stabilize plaques, reduce intercellular adhesion and enable regression of inflammatory mediators. In addition, further understanding of anti-atherosclerotic properties of currently available agents has also widened the scope of use of these agents. For example, recent ultrasonography evidence has shown that angiotensin-converting enzyme inhibitor may retard the progression of atherosclerosis as demonstrated by carotid intima–media thickness; statins improve endothelial function independent of their lipid-lowering effects, whilst cilostazol inhibits neo-intimal hyperplasia and increases VEGF-mediated collateral vessel formation.

Conclusion

Lifestyle measures should include regular exercise and smoking cessation. His medical management should be based not only in the context of lower limb salvage but also in terms of cardiovascular risk protection. Thus, antiplatelet agents and statins should be initiated with aggressive blood pressure reduction using a regimen which includes agents that block the renin–angiotensin system. There is evidence to support the use of cilostazol for symptom relief although long-term outcome remains unclear. Research into future therapies has focused on the role of therapeutic angiogenesis via VEGF gene therapy as well as therapeutic modulation of mediators of glycaemic vascular injury.

Further Reading

1   Gardner AW, Poehlman ET. Exercise rehabilitation programs for the treatment of claudication pain. A meta analysis. *JAMA* 1995; **274**: 975–80.

2   MacGregor A, Price J, Hau C, Lee A, Carson M, Fowkes F. Role of systolic blood pressure and plasma triglycerides in diabetic peripheral arterial disease. The Edinburgh Artery Study. *Diabetes Care* 1999; **22**: 453–8.

3   Adler A, Stevens R, Neil A, Stratton I, Boulton A, Holman R. UKPDS 59: Hyperglycaemia and other potentially modifiable risk factors for peripheral arterial disease in type 2 diabetes. *Diabetes Care* 2002; **25**: 894–9.

4   Collinson DJ, Donnelly R. Therapeutic angiogenesis in peripheral arterial disease: can biotechnology produce an effective collateral circulation? *Eur J Vasc Endovasc Surg* 2004; **28**: 9–23.

5   Idris I, Gray S, Donnelly R. Protein Kinase C activation: isozyme-specific effects on metabolism and cardiovascular complications in diabetes. *Diabetologia* 2001; **44**: 659–73.

47 Renal Artery Stenosis

Case History

A 54-year-old man presented with hypertension (blood pressure 160/92 mmHg). He is known to have stable angina and previously underwent angioplasty of his right femoral circulation for intermittent claudication. He stopped smoking three years ago. Renal function was impaired, with plasma urea 6.8 mmol/l and creatinine 130 μmol/l. Urine dipstick showed no proteinuria. He has no evidence of retinopathy or peripheral neuropathy.

What is the likely cause of his renal impairment?

How would you investigate him?

How would you treat his high blood pressure and abnormal renal function?

Background

This patient clearly has widespread atherosclerosis with abnormal renal function. In the absence of proteinuria, diabetic nephropathy is less likely to be the cause of his renal impairment. In view of his medical history, it is highly likely that he has some degree of atherosclerotic renovascular disease with bilateral renal artery stenosis (RArtS) contributing to his renal impairment.

Radiologically significant RArtS (>50% stenosis) is common and has been found in approximately 42% of patients with peripheral vascular disease. It is a common cause of chronic renal failure and constitutes about 15% of patients undergoing haemodialysis programmes for end-stage renal failure in the United Kingdom. In view of the accelerated nature of atherosclerosis in patients with diabetes, it is unsurprising that patients with diabetes constitute a large proportion of those found to have RArtS. Whilst accurate long-term epidemiological data for patients with diabetes and RArtS is lacking, it is estimated from smaller studies that radiologically significant RArtS occurs in approximately 15% of patients with diabetes and hypertension.[1] There should be a high index of suspicion for RArtS in patients with diabetes as many will be treated with an angiotensin-converting enzyme (ACE) inhibitor or an angiotensin receptor blocker (ARB), and these agents may induce an acute decline in renal function. The degree of RArtS, however, does not predict patients at risk of acute renal dysfunction after an ACE inhibitor or ARB challenge. RArtS should be considered in patients with diabetes who have unexplained renal impairment (particularly in the absence of proteinuria), a history of atherosclerosis, asymmetric kidney size at ultrasound examination, and in patients who develop an acute rise in creatinine (by >30%) within ten days of ACE inhibitor or ARB therapy.[2]

Obstruction to the renal blood flow induces chronic ischaemia—predominantly of the renal tubules. Renal perfusion is then dependent on angiotensin II-induced vasoconstriction of the efferent arteriole. Failure to maintain glomerular filtration occurs when renal perfusion pressure drops below 70–85 mmHg. This is not likely to be observed until arterial luminal narrowing exceeds 50%.

When RArtS is suspected, imaging studies can support and confirm the diagnosis. These techniques include:

- Ultrasound—helpful to determine the presence of a solitary kidney or obstructive nephropathy as a cause of renal impairment. Ischaemic nephropathy is suggested when there is significant asymmetry of the kidney size (i.e. size discrepancy of >1.5 cm).

- Radionuclide scanning—scanning following a single dose of captopril is only useful in patients with normal renal function. The sensitivity and specificity of this test is low.

- Duplex ultrasound scanning—obtains flow velocity data and can be used in patients with any level of renal function. Although the test is very sensitive and specific (98%), it is extremely labour intensive and technician-dependent.

- Magnetic resonance angiography (MRA)—non-invasive technique of choice. Provides useful information on renal vascular anatomy, and allows direct measurement of the blood flow rate, glomerular filtration rate and renal perfusion rate. Sensitivity of MRA is 90% for proximal RArtS and 80–100% for main RArtS, with a positive predictive value of 58%, and a negative predictive value of 100% for detecting stenosis of the main renal artery.

- Conventional arteriography—gold standard for diagnosing RArtS. An invasive technique with risk of bleeding from an arterial puncture and risk of contrast nephropathy.

Treatment

Cardiovascular risk should be aggressively managed. This may require the use of statins and aspirin as well as antihypertensive agents, aiming for a blood pressure below 125/75 mmHg. In the absence of long-term data, indications for treatment by renal artery revascularization (angioplasty for non-ostial lesions and stenting for ostial lesions) remain unclear. Most nephrologists, however, would agree that renal revascularization is indicated if:[3]

1 Stenosis >80%

2 Stenosis >50% but with a documented rise in creatinine (by >30%) after starting an ACE inhibitor/ARB, or a single functioning kidney

3 Absence of chronic ischaemic nephropathy (kidney length >8 cm)

4 Renal impairment is potentially reversible (creatinine <350 μmol/l)

5 Episodes of flash pulmonary oedema (acute left ventricular failure in the absence of myocardial ischaemia)

6 Severe hypertension resistant to aggressive medical therapy

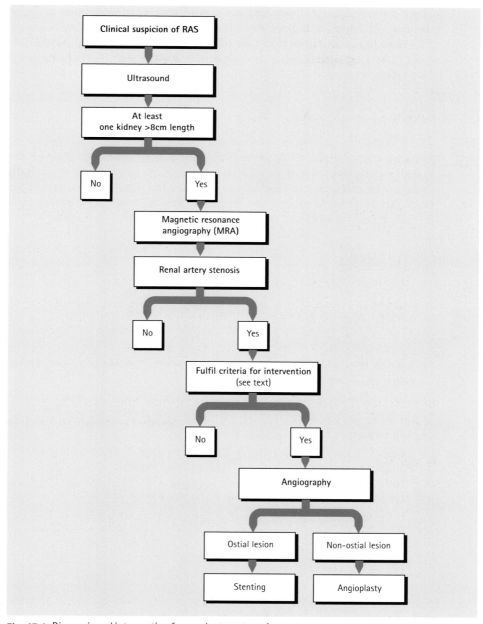

Fig. 47.1 Diagnosis and intervention for renal artery stenosis.

Recent Developments

1 The ASTRAL (Angioplasty and Stent for Renal Artery Lesions) trial[4] is a multicentre study in the United Kingdom involving 1000 patients with atherosclerotic RArtS, including many with diabetes. This is the largest interventional trial in atherosclerotic

RArtS and is designed to address the issue of whether renal artery revascularization with balloon angioplasty and/or endovascular stenting can safely prevent progressive renal failure among patients with RArtS. Results of the trial should be available in 2006 and will hopefully dictate appropriate treatment options for patients with significant RArtS.

Conclusion

RArtS is common in patients with diabetes and should be suspected if there is evidence of progressive renal dysfunction, particularly if associated with peripheral vascular disease, lack of retinopathy or absence of significant proteinuria. MRA is the investigation of choice, while conventional arteriography remains the gold-standard technique for diagnosis. Treatment of the patients should include the use of statins, aspirin, aggressive blood pressure reduction and renal artery revascularization where appropriate.[5]

Further Reading

1 Valabhji J, Robinson S, Poulter C, Robinson AC, Kong C, Henzen C, Gedroyc WM, Feher MD, Elkeles RS. Prevalence of renal artery stenosis in subjects with type 2 diabetes and coexistant hypertension. *Diabetes* 2000; **23**: 539–43.

2 Main J. When should atheromatous renal artery stenosis be considered? A guide for the general physician. *Clin Med* 2003; **3**: 520–5.

3 Krijnen P, Van Jaarsveld BC, Deinum J. Which patients with hypertension and atherosclerotic renal artery stenosis benefit from immediate intervention? *J Hum Hypertens* 2004; **18**: 91–6.

4 ASTRAL trial. http://www.astral.bham.ac.uk/.

5 Salifu MO, Haria DM, Badero O, Aytug S, McFarlane SI. Challenges in the diagnosis and management of renal artery stenosis. *Curr Hypertens Rep* 2005; **7**: 219–27.

48 Foot Ulceration

Case History

A 67-year-old woman with long-standing type 2 diabetes has a foot ulcer on the plantar surface of her right foot, underneath her 1st and 2nd metatarsal. There was evidence of infection but no clinical suspicion of underlying osteomyelitis. The ulcer has been an ongoing problem over the previous ten months.

Discuss the clinical course of a diabetic foot ulcer.

Describe the biology of a chronic diabetic ulcer.

Discuss the multidisciplinary management of diabetic foot ulcer.

Background

Diabetic foot ulcers affect up to 15% of people with diabetes and account for approximately 24 000 hospital-bed days in the United Kingdom (UK)and 300 000 hospitalizations in the United States annually. They are a major source of mortality, disability and distress to patients, many of whom suffer from other comorbidities. Treatment cost is high and creates an enormous financial burden to healthcare providers and affected individuals.[1,2] Ulcers generally do not respond well to treatment.[3] Current data suggest that only a third of those managed in secondary care in the UK heal by three months, and half at six months. Amputation rates are increasing in patients with diabetes, while decreasing in those without diabetes. Ultimately, between 15% and 27% of patients with non-healing ulcers will require some form of amputation.

The normal healing process involves secretion of collagen and other factors to facilitate wound closure followed by the production of cytokines, fibroblasts and growth factors which induce proliferation and eventual scar formation. Chronic diabetic ulcers exhibit specific abnormalities in their biology which impairs this healing process. Important differences, for example, exist in the cellular infiltrate and expression of extracellular matrix in chronic diabetic ulcers compared with normal healing ulcers. Fibroblasts derived from diabetic ulcers show diminished proliferative capacity *in vitro* and abnormal morphology when compared with control fibroblasts. Hyperglycaemia is also associated with impaired glucose utilization by skin keratinocytes as well as reduced skin proliferation and differentiation *in vitro*. Lack of sensation, poor infection healing and abnormalities in the micro- and macrocirculation all contribute to worse outcomes of diabetic ulcers. The pathophysiological relationship between diabetes and impaired ulcer healing is thus complex. Vascular, neuropathic and biochemical parameters and immune responses may all contribute to defective tissue repair.

The mainstays of diabetic foot ulcer treatment are:

1 Wound debridement

2 Control of infection

3 Revascularization

4 Offloading and foot pressure redistribution

Wound debridement

Debridement of all necrotic, callus and fibrous tissue forms a major part of foot ulcer management and should only be performed by an accredited podiatrist. Chronic ulcers produce elastase, collagenase and proteases which interfere with the normal reparative properties of locally produced cytokines and growth factors. Appropriate ulcer debridement will clear proteases and bacterial products producing a clean wound which facilitates healing. Application of platelet-derived growth factor (PDGF), for example, has been shown to promote ulcer healing but only in ulcers that have undergone adequate debridement.

Control of infection

The majority of diabetic foot ulcers have mild to moderate degrees of infection. Because all ulcers are contaminated, culture of non-infected ulcers is not generally recommended. Organisms found range from non-pathogenic skin commensals (diphtheroids) to pathogenic organisms such as *Staphylococcus aureus* (the most important pathogen), Pseudomonas, gram-negative bacteria and anaerobes. An ulcer can be considered to be infected if an organism is isolated from a pure culture, is repeatedly isolated or is isolated from deep tissue, or if there is an inflammatory response and purulent secretion. Bacterial load may also provide a definite answer to infection status. A bacterial count of $>10^5$ colonies/ml is considered to be an indication for antibiotic treatment. Radiographs should be obtained in most patients with deep or long-standing ulcers to rule out osteomyelitis. Gentle probing may detect sinus tract formation, and a positive probe-to-bone finding has a high predictive value for underlying osteomyelitis ($>90\%$). Failure to diagnose underlying osteomyelitis often results in failure of wound healing. Commonly used antibiotics are amoxicillin/clavulanate (Augmentin), flucloxacillin, cephalosporins, quinalones, metronidazole and clindamycin. Surgical drainage, deep debridement or local, partial foot amputations are necessary adjuncts to antibiotic treatment for infections that are deep or limb-threatening.

Revascularization

Peripheral arterial disease is a major predisposing factor for foot ulceration and poor healing. While most diabetic ulcers are neuroischaemic in origin, purely ischaemic ulcers are typically 'punched out', painful and are located at pressure areas such as the heel, in-between toes and distally. Gangrene of the extremities is common and may be compounded by the presence of infection. The most important physical finding is the absence of palpable pulses. Decreased bleeding during ulcer debridement is also a sign of arterial insufficiency. Referral to a vascular surgeon is indicated in patients with non-healing ulcer and evidence of lower limb ischaemia.

Offloading and foot pressure redistribution

The maximal pressure exerted on a deformed foot when walking is twice that exerted on a normal foot. In addition, 75% of patients with neuropathy have much wider feet than normal. Thus, pressure reduction and appropriate footwear are essential components of treatment and must be pursued to promote ulcer healing and to reduce ulcer recurrence.[4] The latter is particularly relevant given that the recurrence rate of an ulcer is as high as 70% over three years. Ill-fitting footwear should be replaced with pressure-relieving footwear. This comes in the form of postoperative shoes, half shoes (which limit weight-bearing to the heel or the forefoot) or 'scotch-cast boots'. Insertion of Plastazote insoles with excavation at an ulcer site may further facilitate ulcer healing. Crutches or wheel-chair use might also be recommended to totally offload pressure from the foot. Greater use of total contact casting (TCC) should also be encouraged, as cast walls carry 30% of the pressure load and help to protect the ulcer. In a randomized controlled trial, TCC healed a higher proportion of neuropathic ulcers, in a shorter time, compared with two other modalities of offloading: removable cast walkers and half shoes.[5] A previous meta-analysis of 526 ulcers in 493 patients reported 88% healing in a mean time of 43 days. Improper use of TCC may, however, predispose patients to infection or development of additional ulceration. More recently, a study showed that ulcers with moderate ischaemia or infection can also be treated effectively with casting, although the healing rate was lower for ulcers with infection. Technique for applying a TCC is therefore important.

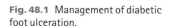

Fig. 48.1 Management of diabetic foot ulceration.

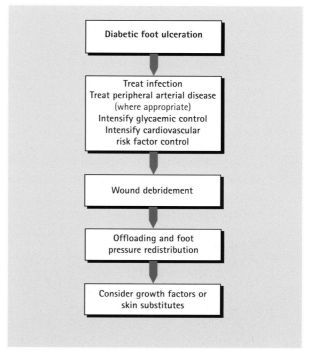

Recent Developments[6]

1. Novel approaches using 'skin substitutes' and growth factors may revolutionize the management of diabetic foot ulcer in the future. Bioengineered graftskin (Apligraf) and human dermis (Dermagraft) are cultivated from human fibroblasts and secrete cytokines and growth factors which enhance ulcer healing. While preliminary studies have suggested that these products may be useful, results from large, randomized clinical trials using these products have been less convincing. Results from further trials are awaited.

2. PDGF stimulates ulcer healing by promoting fibroblast and smooth-muscle proliferation, enhancing collagen production and promoting angiogenesis. The genetically engineered PDGF, becaplermin (Regranex gel), is approved for use on neuropathic diabetic foot ulcers. Studies of this treatment involving more than 1000 patients have shown that this product is effective in promoting ulcer healing, provided that ulcers are adequately debrided and are of moderate size. The major limitation to the routine use of this product is cost.

Conclusion

Diabetic foot ulcers are a major source of distress, disability and cost. They do not respond well to treatment and only a third of unselected ulcers heal within three months. The recurrence rate is high and up to one-third of patients require some form of amputation. The most frequent underlying aetiologies are neuropathy, peripheral arterial disease and foot deformity. Chronic diabetic ulcers exhibit specific differences in the cellular infiltrate and rate of expression of extracellular matrix proteins compared with normal healing ulcers. Thus prevention of ulcer should be emphasized during routine diabetes consultation. The main aim in the treatment of diabetic foot ulcers is to obtain ulcer closure. A multidisciplinary approach should include pressure offloading, frequent wound debridement, treatment of infection and appropriate intervention to improve lower limb blood supply.

Further Reading

1. Bloomgarden ZT. The diabetic foot. *Diabetes Care* 2001; **24**: 946–51.

2. Jeffcoate WJ, Harding KG. Diabetic foot ulcers. *Lancet* 2003; **361**: 1545–51.

3. Margolis DJ, Kantor J, Berlin JA. Healing of diabetic foot ulcers receiving standard treatment. A meta-analysis. *Diabetes Care* 1999; **22**: 692–5.

4. Rathur HM, Boulton AJ. Pathogenesis of foot ulcers and the need for offloading. *Horm Metab Res* 2005; **37** (Suppl 1): 61–8.

5. Armstrong DG, Nguyen HC, Lavery LA, van Schie CH, Boulton AJ, Harkless LB. Off-loading the diabetic foot wound: a randomized clinical trial. *Diabetes Care* 2001; **24**: 1019–22.

6. Bennett SP, Griffiths GD, Schor AM, Leese GP, Schor SL. Growth factors in the treatment of diabetic foot ulcers. *Br J Surg* 2003; **90**: 133–46.

PROBLEM

49 Transient Ischaemic Attack

Case History

A 58-year-old man with type 2 diabetes developed transient left-sided weakness with slurring of speech lasting for four hours. On clinical examination, he is in sinus rhythm, blood pressure is 142/84 mmHg and there is an audible right-sided carotid bruit on auscultation. He has no history of ischaemic heart disease and does not smoke. He currently takes low-dose aspirin and an angiotensin-converting enzyme (ACE) inhibitor at night.

How should he be managed?

What investigations should be carried out?

What is his prognosis?

Background

The risk of transient ischaemic attack (TIA) is, surprisingly, the same (or slightly lower) in patients with diabetes compared with patients without diabetes. This observation may be explained by the fact that diabetes induces a higher likelihood of developing a full stroke when exposed to an equivalent cerebrovascular insult. The combination of diabetes and TIA is, however, particularly malignant, with patients at very high risk of future disabling cardiovascular events.

Large randomized trials have shown that aspirin, at doses of 75–150 mg/day, reduces stroke risks in patients with diabetes.[1] There is, however, theoretical evidence that patients with diabetes may require slightly higher doses of aspirin to achieve similar antiplatelet effects, and this may explain the surprisingly non-significant reductions of stroke risks in some studies with aspirin conducted in the diabetic cohort of larger trials. Clopidogrel is superior to aspirin for stroke prevention, particularly in patients with diabetes, but aspirin and clopidogrel in combination conferred no further benefits in patients with recent TIA and was associated with increased risks of bleeding complications. Similarly, the addition of dipyridamole to aspirin treatment in diabetic patients resulted in a non-significant reduction in stroke recurrence. Antithrombotic therapy, aiming at international normalized ratio (INR) of 2–3, reduces stroke risk in patients with atrial fibrillation.[2] A meta-analysis of antithrombotic therapy in atrial fibrillation showed that warfarin reduced stroke by about 60%, with numbers needed to treat for one year to prevent one stroke of 13; aspirin reduced stroke by about 20%, with numbers needed to treat of 40 for secondary prevention. There is no evidence to support the routine use of warfarin for patients in sinus rhythm.

Meta-analysis of various antihypertensive trials has confirmed the benefits of intensive blood pressure control in stroke prevention.[3] When these trials were considered individually, the evidence supporting aggressive blood pressure reduction seemed to be largely derived from patients with diabetes. In the UKPDS (United Kingdom Prospective Diabetes Study), a 10 mmHg reduction of mean systolic blood pressure in patients with type 2 diabetes led to a 44% reduction in stroke incidence. Systolic hypertension and 'non-dipping' nocturnal blood pressure are also both associated with a higher risk of stroke and cardiovascular mortality. The ideal first-line antihypertensive agent is still uncertain. A meta-analysis comparing different antihypertensive agents has shown a small but significant benefit in favour of calcium channel blockers in preventing stroke, while other comparative studies involving patients with diabetes have been less favourable to calcium antagonists. The ALLHAT trial (Antihypertensive and Lipid-Lowering treatment to prevent Heart Attack), which enrolled more than 12 000 participants with type 2 diabetes, showed no significant difference for either drug class for stroke risk reduction, although the overall cardiovascular outcomes were slightly in favour of a diuretic. Recent trials have also highlighted the vasculoprotective effects of agents which block the renin–angiotensin system, possibly independent of blood pressure lowering. The HOPE study (Heart Outcomes Protection Evaluation) showed that ramipril (compared to placebo) reduced the risks of any stroke by 32% and fatal stroke by 61%. A further substudy, however, suggested that the favourable outcome seen with ramipril in HOPE may in fact have been due to a significantly lower nocturnal blood pressure in the ramipril-treated group. PROGRESS (the Perindopril PROtection aGainst REcurrent Stroke Study) showed a reduction in the risk of recurrent strokes using the perindopril plus indapamide combination. Importantly, PROGRESS showed no benefit from perindopril monotherapy despite modest antihypertensive actions (5/3 mmHg), whereas indapamide alone may have reduced stroke by as much as 38%. Thus, effective blood pressure reduction rather than the choice of initial agent is the most important issue in reducing stroke risks. The British Hypertension Society has produced the AB/CD guideline for choosing appropriate initial treatment and for deciding how to combine antihypertensives effectively.

Statins may also prevent strokes in patients with diabetes. The recent CARDS[4] trial (Collaborative Atorvastatin Diabetes Study) randomized 2338 patients with type 2 diabetes to placebo or atorvastatin 10 mg daily. Atorvastatin significantly reduced the incidence of new stroke by 48%, independent of patient's age, gender or baseline cholesterol or blood pressure levels. This confirmed findings from the LIPID trial (Long-term Intervention with Pravastatin in Ischaemic Disease), which showed a 39% stroke reduction with pravastatin in patients with diabetes. The Heart Protection Study (HPS) showed a 25% reduction in stroke with simvastatin irrespective of baseline cholesterol. In the 4S study (Scandinavian Simvastatin Survival Study), treatment with simvastatin reduced stroke in the diabetic cohort by 62% compared with 23% in people without diabetes. Treatment with statins, however, did not seem to eliminate the excess cardiovascular risk associated with a low baseline level of high-density lipoprotein (HDL)-cholesterol. The VA-HIT study (Veterans Affairs High-Density Lipoprotein Intervention Trial) included 769 patients with diabetes with normal low-density lipoprotein (LDL) but low HDL-cholesterol levels; gemfibrozil, an agent which specifically increases HDL-cholesterol but has negligible effect on LDL-cholesterol levels, resulted in a 39% reduction in coronary heart disease. Little data is available on the effect of raising HDL on the incidence of stroke, but it is unlikely that the protective effect of raising HDL levels is confined to the coronary

Table 49.1 Multi–interventional package for the treatment of TIA and prevention of stroke in patients with diabetes

Symptoms/risk factors	Intervention
Hypercoagulability/atrial fibrillation	Aspirin, dipyridamole, clopidogrel, warfarin
Smoking cessation therapy, bupropion	Behavioural therapy, nicotine replacement
Hyperglycaemia	Sulphonylurea, metformin, glitazones, insulin
Insulin resistance	Weight loss, glitazones, metformin
Dyslipidaemia	Statins, fibrate, nicotinic acid
Hypertension	ACE inhibitor, angiotensin AT1 receptor blocker, diuretic (and other agents including beta-blockers)
Microalbuminuria/proteinuria	ACE inhibitor, angiotensin AT1 receptor blocker, aggressive blood pressure reduction
Screening for diabetes-related vasculopathy	Eye screening, foot examination, assessment for coronary artery disease

Source: Idris et al. Int J Clin Pract (in press).

circulation. A large study specifically targeting HDL-cholesterol in patients with diabetes is underway.

Patients with haemodynamically significant carotid artery stenosis should be considered for carotid endarterectomy if they are fit for surgery. Evidence from two large trials, the Asymptomatic Carotid Atherosclerosis Study (ACAS)[5] and the North American Symptomatic Carotid Endarterectomy Trial (NASCET),[6] showed that surgical revascularization for asymptomatic and symptomatic haemodynamically significant carotid artery stenosis resulted in fewer strokes during follow-up compared with medical therapy alone. Patients with diabetes constituted 23% and 19%, respectively, of the total study participants and seemed to benefit equally. In the European Carotid Surgery Trial (ECST),[7] the benefits of carotid endarterectomy in reducing stroke became significant only in those with more than 70% carotid artery stenosis, but not in those with carotid near-occlusion. Peri- and post-endarterectomy outcomes in patients with diabetes are variable—some suggest an increased rate of coronary heart disease, whilst others report more favourable outcomes. Surgical risk, however, is inversely related to surgical experience and patients should thus be referred to centres with extensive experience in performing endarterectomy.

Recent Developments

1   Early trials of carotid artery stenting were stopped prematurely due to poor outcomes in stented patients. Recent advances in stent designs, delivery systems and devices to protect the brain from embolization during stenting have improved clinical outcomes. Further studies are underway to determine whether carotid artery stenting is a true alternative to carotid endarterectomy as the treatment of choice for carotid artery stenosis.

Conclusion

Patients with diabetes and TIA are at great risk of developing future stroke and cardiac events. Management strategies should therefore target aggressive cardiovascular risk factor reduction, which includes lifestyle changes, and pharmacological and surgical treatment. Clopidogrel is superior to aspirin for stroke prevention, while blood pressure reduction should be achieved with the most appropriate agent tailored to the patient's age, ethnic group, concurrent medications and comorbid state. Recent evidence has also supported the use of statins to prevent stroke occurrence. Finally, in patients with haemodynamically significant carotid artery stenosis, carotid endarterectomy has been shown to improve clinical outcomes.[6]

Further Reading

1   Sivenius J, Laakso M, Riekkinen P Sr, Smets P, Lowenthal A. European stroke prevention study: effectiveness of antiplatelet therapy in diabetic patients in secondary prevention of stroke. *Stroke* 1992; **23**: 851–4.

2   Stroke Prevention in Atrial Fibrillation Investigators. Warfarin versus aspirin for prevention of thromboembolism in atrial fibrillation: Stroke prevention in Atrial Fibrillation II study. *Lancet* 1994; **343**: 687–91.

3   MacMahon S, Peto R, Cutler J, Collins R, Sorlie P, Neaton J, Abbott R, Godwin J, Dyer A, Stamler J. Blood pressure, stroke, and coronary heart disease. Part 1, Prolonged differences in blood pressure: prospective observational studies corrected for the regression dilution bias. *Lancet* 1990; **335**: 765–74.

4   Colhoun HM, Betteridge DJ, Durrington PN, Hitman GA, Neil HA, Livingstone SJ, Thomason MJ, Mackness MI, Charlton-Menys V, Fuller JH. Primary prevention of cardiovascular disease with atorvastatin in type 2 diabetes in the Collaborative Atorvastatin Diabetes Study (CARDS): multicentre randomised placebo-controlled trial. *Lancet* 2004; **364**: 685–96.

5   Executive Committee for the Asymptomatic Carotid Atherosclerosis Study. Endarterectomy for asymptomatic carotid artery stenosis. *JAMA* 1995; **273**: 1421–8.

6   North American Symptomatic Carotid Endarterectomy Trial Collaborators. Beneficial effect of carotid endarterectomy in symptomatic patients with high-grade carotid stenosis. *N Engl J Med* 1991; **325**: 445–53.

7   Rothwell PM, Gutnikov SA, Warlow CP. Reanalysis of the final results of the European Carotid Surgery Trial. *Stroke* 2003; **34**: 514–23.

Diabetes in Special Groups of Patients

50   Diabetes and respiratory disease
51   Diabetes and cystic fibrosis
52   Diabetes and dialysis
53   Diabetes and coeliac disease

PROBLEM

50 Diabetes and Respiratory Disease

Case History

A 42-year-old obese man with no history of diabetes complained of overwhelming daytime lethargy to the extent that he sometimes falls asleep at traffic lights. His wife mentioned that he snores heavily at night. His fasting glucose is 6.9 mmol/l on two separate occasions. He has normal thyroid function.

What is his most likely diagnosis?

How does his diagnosis relate to diabetes and his cardiovascular risk?

How would you treat him?

Background

This patient has clinical features of sleep apnoea. The condition is characterized by recurrent episodes of upper airway collapse and obstruction during sleep, leading to recurrent oxyhaemoglobin desaturation and arousals from sleep. Anatomical factors, such as enlarged tonsils, macroglossia and abnormal positioning of the maxilla or the mandible, are major predisposing factors to airway collapse. The site of obstruction in most patients is the soft palate, extending to the region at the base of the tongue. Sleep apnoea can be caused by either complete airway obstruction (obstructive apnoea) or partial obstruction (obstructive hypopnoea—i.e. slow, shallow breathing), both of which can induce sleep arousal. The frequent arousals and the inability to achieve or maintain the deeper stages of sleep lead to excessive daytime sleepiness, personality changes, memory loss and depression. Other physical signs and symptoms that support a likely diagnosis of obstructive sleep apnoea include loud snoring, witnessed apnoeic episodes, waking up not feeling refreshed, morning headaches and obesity. Polysomnography (overnight sleep study) with an Apnoea–Hypopnoea Index (AHI) score of >5–10/h—derived from the total number of apnoeas and hypopnoeas divided by total sleep time—is generally used as a cut-off level for the diagnosis of sleep apnoea.

Obstructive sleep apnoea (OSA) is recognized to be associated with increased cardiovascular morbidity and mortality. Untreated, OSA is associated with a significant 2–4-fold increase of developing fatal and non-fatal cardiovascular events. Whilst the higher cardiovascular risk was previously thought to be due to its link with obesity, recent evidence has suggested that OSA may be independently associated with the metabolic syndrome. This syndrome consists of a cluster of risk factors which includes hypertension, microalbuminuria, dyslipidaemia, insulin resistance, glucose intolerance, central obesity and increased proatherogenic proteins. In a study by Coughlin et al.,[1] metabolic syndrome was found to be nine times more likely to exist in patients with OSA compared with those without and occurs independently of obesity, smoking and age. Using mathematical models and the euglycaemic hyperinsulinaemic clamp technique to determine insulin sensitivity index, obese patients with OSA have been shown to be more insulin resistant than patients with simple obesity, independently of the degree and distribution of adiposity. Hypoxic state associated with OSA has been postulated to account for the increased vascular risk seen in patients with OSA.

More recently, data from the Sleep Heart Health Study (SHHS) have shown that sleep-disordered breathing (SDB) is independently associated with glucose intolerance and insulin resistance and may lead to type 2 diabetes mellitus. Conversely, diabetes mellitus might be a cause of SDB, mediated through autonomic neuropathy that may alter ventilatory control mechanisms. Further data from the same patient cohort showed that participants with sleep duration of less than five hours per night have a 2.5- and 1.3-fold increased risk of developing type 2 diabetes and impaired glucose tolerance.[2] Because this effect was present in subjects without insomnia, voluntary sleep restriction was thought to contribute to the large public health burden of type 2 diabetes. A study involving more than 8000 subjects who participated in one of the three MONICA Augsburg surveys between 1984 and 1995 showed that difficulty in maintaining sleep was also associated with an increased risk of type 2 diabetes in both men and women from the general population. Meanwhile, results from the Nurses Health Study cohort, which followed 69 852 United States female nurses aged 40–65 years without diabetes at baseline, showed that snoring is independently associated with increased risk of developing diabetes.[3] Similarly, in a Finnish population-based cohort study involving 593 subjects, habitual snoring was found to be more common in subjects with diabetes than in subjects with impaired glucose regulation or normal glucose tolerance. In this study, impaired insulin sensitivity, type 2 diabetes and smoking were all associated independently with habitual snoring, whilst high body mass index and male sex were associated independently with OSA. Epidemiological data have also shown a link between OSA and hypertension. For example, untreated OSA predisposes to an increased risk of new hypertension, whilst treatment of OSA has been shown to lower blood pressure. Possible mechanisms whereby OSA may

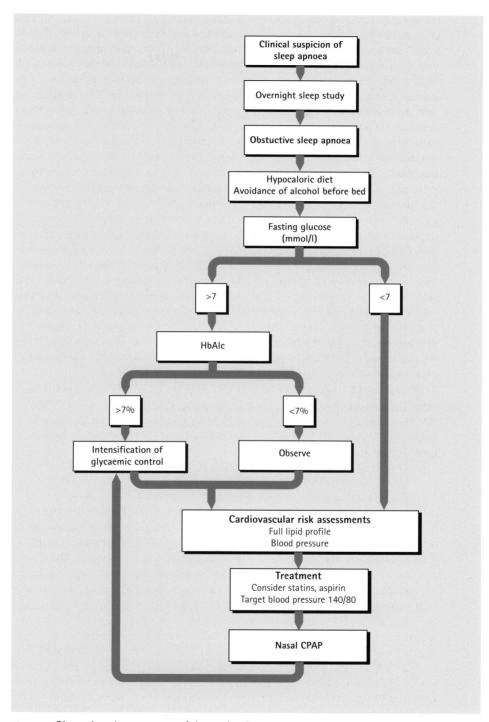

Fig. 50.1 Diagnosis and management of obstructive sleep apnoea.

contribute to hypertension in obese individuals include sympathetic activation, insulin resistance, elevated angiotensin II and aldosterone levels and endothelial dysfunction.

Conservative measures such as weight loss, avoidance of alcohol 4–6 hours before bed and sleeping on one side are reasonably effective in patients with mild apnoea. In patients with moderate to severe apnoea, nasal continuous positive airway pressure (CPAP) has become the standard treatment for OSA. CPAP works by splinting the upper airway, preventing the soft tissues from collapsing. By this mechanism, it effectively eliminates the apnoeas and/or hypopnoeas, decreases the arousals, and normalizes the oxygen saturation. Emerging data suggest that this form of treatment is not only effective in improving patients' symptoms but has also been shown to improve insulin resistance, glucose metabolism and patients' cardiovascular risks.[4] Flow-mediated vasodilation has been shown to improve after four weeks of nasal CPAP treatment, suggesting improvement in endothelial function due to CPAP treatment. In a study involving nine obese patients with type 2 diabetes, three months of CPAP treatment was shown to improve insulin sensitivity without any changes in body mass index. Another study, involving 40 patients, showed more rapid improvement in insulin sensitivity (after day two of CPAP treatment), with improved CPAP efficacy seen in subjects who are less obese. In a recent study involving 25 patients with type 2 diabetes, CPAP treatment (mean treatment duration of 83 ± 50 days) significantly reduced 1-hour post-prandial glucose levels, and in 17 patients with a baseline glycosylated haemoglobin (HbA1c) level greater than 7%, there was a significant reduction in HbA1c level (9.2% ± 2.0% to 8.6% ± 1.8%). The reduction in HbA1c level was more prominent in subjects who used CPAP for more than four hours per day. These studies suggest that SDB is pathophysiologically related to impaired glucose homeostasis, and that CPAP can be an important therapeutic approach for patients with diabetes and SDB. In a further prospective study of 54 patients with coronary artery disease (≥70% coronary artery stenosis) and OSA (AHI ≥15), CPAP treatment was associated with a decrease in the occurrence of new cardiovascular events, and an increase in the time to such events, compared with the group who declined CPAP treatment despite comparable baseline parameters.

Recent Developments

1   Further study is required to investigate the epidemiological evidence linking sleep-related disorders to risks of developing diabetes as well as cardiovascular and microvascular disorders. The SHHS is a multicentre cohort study implemented by the National Heart Lung and Blood Institute to determine the cardiovascular and other consequences of SDB. Further data analysis and collaborative study with the SHHS investigators is expected to improve our understanding on the metabolic complications of sleep-related disorders.

2   A broader link has recently emerged between diabetes and abnormal lung function. A recent study, using data from the Third National Health and Nutrition Examination Survey (1988–1994),[5] showed that plasma glucose level two hours after oral administration of 75 grams of glucose was inversely related to forced expiratory volume in one second (FEV(1)) and forced vital capacity. In the total study population, persons with previously diagnosed diabetes had an FEV(1) 119.1 ml (95% confidence interval

−161.5 to −76.6) lower than persons without diabetes. This effect was greater in those with poorly controlled diabetes. These findings suggest that impaired glucose autoregulation is associated with impaired lung function. The mechanism for this remains unclear.

Conclusion

This patient most likely has obstructive sleep apnoea. Sleep-related disorders, OSA and abnormal lung function have been shown to be important predictors of developing glucose intolerance, insulin resistance, diabetes and cardiovascular complications. For patients with OSA, treatment with nasal CPAP has been shown to not only improve patients' symptoms but also their glucose homeostasis and cardiovascular risks. The routine use of statins and aspirin for all patients with OSA may also be merited. The role of insulin sensitizers in patients with OSA has not been studied yet.

Further Reading

1   Coughlin SR, Mawdsley L, Mugarza JA, Calverley PMA, Wilding JPH. Obstructive sleep apnoea is independently associated with an increased prevalence of metabolic syndrome. *Eur Heart J* 2004; **25**: 735–41.

2   Gottlieb DJ, Punjabi NM, Newman AB, Resnick HE, Redline S, Baldwin CM, Nieto FJ. Association of sleep time with diabetes mellitus and impaired glucose tolerance. *Arch Intern Med* 2005; **165**: 863–7.

3   Al-Delaimy WK, Manson JE, Willett WC, Stampfer MJ, Hu FB. Snoring as a risk factor for type II diabetes mellitus: a prospective study. *Am J Epidemiol* 2002; **155**: 387–93.

4   Babu AR, Herdegen J, Fogelfeld L, Shott S, Mazzone T. Type 2 diabetes, glycemic control, and continuous positive airway pressure in obstructive sleep apnea. *Arch Intern Med* 2005; **165**: 447–52.

5   McKeever TM, Weston PJ, Hubbard R, Fogarty A. Lung function and glucose metabolism: an analysis of data from the Third National Health and Nutrition Examination Survey. *Am J Epidemiol* 2005; **161**: 546–56.

PROBLEM

51 Diabetes and Cystic Fibrosis

Case History

A 24-year-old woman with cystic fibrosis is found to have a random glucose level of 15 mmol/l. She has no thirst or polyuria, and her weight is steady (body mass index 18 kg/m²). She has not been in hospital with an infective exacerbation for 18 months. Her forced expiratory volume in one second (FEV(1)) is 75% of predicted. She has regular treatment with bronchodilators (salbutamol and atrovent), recombinant human DNase (Pulmozyme) and pancreatic enzyme supplements, but does not require continuous prophylactic antibiotic therapy. She is in a stable relationship and would like to consider starting a family in the foreseeable future.

What is the cause of her diabetes?

Does it have any bearing on her prognosis?

How should her diabetes be managed?

Is it realistic or desirable that she become pregnant?

Background

Cystic fibrosis (CF) is the commonest life-threatening inherited genetic disorder. It occurs in one in every 2000–3000 Caucasian births, but is less common in other racial groups. Inheritance is autosomal recessive, and up to 1 in 20 Caucasians are genetic carriers. The responsible gene is the cystic fibrosis transmembrane conductance regulator gene located on the long arm of chromosome 7 (7q31.2), and over one thousand different mutations of this gene have been described. The gene is an ATP-binding cassette (subfamily C, member 7), the products of which, along with a cyclic-AMP dependent chloride channel, regulate efflux of salt and water from cells. Reduced water content of secretions including sweat, saliva, mucus and digestive enzymes leads to thick, viscid secretions causing bronchopulmonary infection and exocrine pancreatic insufficiency.

The adult cystic fibrosis population is growing. Life expectancy for CF patients has increased in the past 30 years from 16 years to 32 years. This is largely due to improved medical care but also because there is considerable phenotypic variation and increased numbers of patients with less severe disease are being recognized. As a consequence of the demographic change in the CF population, cystic fibrosis-related diabetes (CFRD) is becoming increasingly diagnosed.[1,2] CFRD is currently diagnosed by standard blood glucose criteria, although it is possible that disease-specific criteria should be considered. It is an important complication as there is a strong correlation with poor and deteriorating health, and a significant incidence of microvascular complications. Microalbuminuria may be detected, particularly during infectious exacerbations. Undernutrition may lead to low creatinine levels in blood and urine. Urine albumin–creatinine ratio, therefore, may be of limited use in screening for renal disease. Limited life expectancy means that macrovascular complications are not currently a problem for CF patients although low-grade inflammation and hypertriglyceridaemia, both common in CF, might mean that patients are at risk.

Up to 15% of CF patients have diabetes. This proportion is increasing, and up to 50% of patients have abnormalities in carbohydrate tolerance. The major underlying abnormality is decreased insulin secretion as a result of fatty infiltration and fibrosis of the pancreas. Patients are not generally entirely insulin deficient and, as a consequence, fasting glucose may be relatively normal with the major abnormality being in the post-prandial period. An element of insulin resistance may be present in some patients because of the effects of chronic illness and concurrent use of steroids, but this is not the major mechanism for hyperglycaemia.[3] However, this is usually offset by the fact that most patients are underweight. The peak incidence of CFRD is in the late teens, and it is recommended that all teenagers and adults with CF be screened for diabetes annually.[1] The optimal screening method has yet to be determined.

The nutritional requirements of patients with CF are complex, and may have a bearing on diabetes management. Even a toddler with CF may require up to 2000 kcal/day, compared with 3500 kcal/day for a child, and up to 5000 kcal/day for an adult. In general, energy requirements are 150% of normal, but may be greater in those who are severely malnourished or have severe malabsorption. The recommended dietary composition (40% fat, 40% carbohydrate, 20% protein) is very different to that recommended for diabetes (30% fat, 55% carbohydrate, 15% protein). The lower carbohydrate intake makes for easier control of glycaemia but the total amount may be much higher than for a non-CF diabetic patient of comparable weight. A diet high in milk, cheese, eggs, meat and fish can provide the necessary protein and fat intake. In addition, supplementation with calcium, iron, zinc and fat-soluble vitamins (A, D, E and K) should be considered. Most patients have exocrine pancreatic failure and require pancreatic enzyme supplements. Severely malnourished patients may require nutritional supplements or enteral tube feeding in some cases.

There are no long-term outcome studies demonstrating benefit of tight glycaemic control, but tight control is almost certainly warranted in view of the striking relationship between hyperglycaemia and physical deterioration in CF patients. Insulin resistance is not a major problem and insulin-sensitizing drugs are not, therefore, indicated. Also, metformin could increase gastrointestinal symptoms, which are already prevalent in CF, and hypoxia may increase risk of lactic acidosis. Glitazones should only be used with caution because of the high prevalence of liver abnormalities in CF. Sulphonylureas and post-prandial glucose regulators may be of use for some patients, but insulin is usually the treatment of choice in CFRD. Because the major glucose abnormality is in the post-prandial period, short-acting analogues are the mainstay of treatment if the patient is willing and able to have three or four injections a day. The high-calorie intake and the rapid increase in glucose after eating are further reasons for choosing short-acting insulin analogues, supplemented if need be by long-acting background insulin.

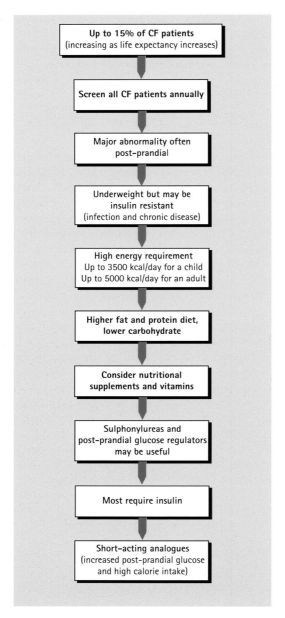

Fig. 51.1 Cystic fibrosis-related diabetes.

Recent Developments

1 In the largest ever epidemiological study of CFRD in adolescents and adults, Marshall *et al.*[4] reported a prevalence of 17.1% in females and 12.0% in males. The reason for this gender difference is not known. Exocrine pancreatic insufficiency was associated with CFRD, and this may account for the higher prevalence of CFRD with some genotypes. The incidence of CFRD is related to age. It was associated with liver disease,

poorer nutritional status, more severe pulmonary compromise and more frequent infective exacerbations.

2   Increasing numbers of patients with CF are reaching adult life with reasonable health. The proportion that seeks fertility advice or achieves pregnancy is relatively low. A recent United Kingdom study confirms that the outlook for pregnancy in a CF patient is relatively good.[5] Poor nutrition and poor respiratory function are the major factors that decrease the likelihood of pregnancy being achieved amongst women with CF. Men with CF are generally infertile because of impaired development of the vas deferens. However, sperm recovery techniques can be used to achieve pregnancy.

3   Less than 10% of patients with CF are diagnosed in adult life.[6] Such patients often have a much more benign course with lesser degrees of pulmonary pathology. The fact that they are diagnosed later, and may survive longer, means that diabetes may become an increasing problem in this group. CF is often harder to diagnose when onset is late as the typical multiorgan pathology is often absent, the genetic mutations are different and the sweat test is not always positive.

Conclusion

This woman appears to have reasonable functional status in spite of her cystic fibrosis. Her diabetes is likely to be caused by relative insulin deficiency as a result of pancreatic damage. Generally, diabetes is more likely to occur in CF patients who are severely malnourished and have severe pulmonary disease. This lady is in reasonable health for an adult patient with CF, but she requires tight glycaemic control, particularly since she is contemplating pregnancy. It is unlikely that this could be achieved without insulin, and a basal bolus regimen would be preferred. As more CF patients reach adulthood in a healthier state than could be achieved previously, it is likely that diabetologists will increasingly be involved in managing CFRD, and that pregnancy, diabetes and CF will have to be managed concurrently more frequently.

Further Reading

1   Yankaskas JR, Marshall BC, Sufian B, Simon RH, Rodman D. Cystic fibrosis adult care: consensus conference report. *Chest* 2004; **125**: 1S–39S.

2   Mackie ADR, Thornton SJ, Edenborough FP. Cystic fibrosis-related diabetes. *Diabet Med* 2003; **20**: 425–36.

3   Yung B, Noormohamed FH, Kemp M, Hooper J, Lant AF, Hodson ME. Cystic fibrosis-related diabetes: the role of peripheral insulin resistance and beta-cell dysfunction. *Diabet Med* 2002; **19**: 221–6.

4   Marshall BC, Butler SM, Stoddard M, Moran AM, Liou TG, Morgan WJ. Epidemiology of cystic fibrosis-related diabetes. *J Pediatr* 2005; **146**: 681–7.

5   Boyd JM, Mehta A, Murphy DJ. Fertility and pregnancy outcomes in men and women with cystic fibrosis in the United Kingdom. *Hum Reprod* 2004; **19**: 2238–43.

6   Gilljam M, Ellis L, Corey M, Zielenski J, Durie P, Tullis DE. Clinical manifestations of cystic fibrosis among patients with diagnosis in adulthood. *Chest* 2004; **126**: 1215–24.

52 Diabetes and Dialysis

Case History

A 54-year-old accounts clerk with insulin-treated type 2 diabetes has been on chronic ambulatory peritoneal dialysis for four years. She has persistent problems with erratic blood sugars—finding it particularly difficult to adjust her treatment when she adjusts the glucose content of her dialysis fluid.

What practical advice can you offer?

How should her insulin management be approached?

Background

Between 20% and 30% of patients entering dialysis programmes in industrial nations have diabetes. A lack of suitable kidney donors means that patients may spend many years receiving renal replacement by dialysis—either haemodialysis or peritoneal dialysis.

Continuous ambulatory peritoneal dialysis (CAPD) requires four or five daily 'exchanges' of 1500–3000 ml lactate, electrolyte and glucose solution. Dialysis fluid is infused via a catheter into the abdominal cavity where it will 'dwell' for 4–5 hours. Acid–base correction, electrolyte equilibration and water removal takes place across the peritoneal membrane. There are a significant number of difficulties faced by patients with diabetes requiring dialysis.

Dialysis fluids

The glucose content of peritoneal dialysis fluid, the dwell time and the efficiency of the peritoneal membrane determine how much water is removed. Generally, three strengths of dialysis fluid are available—'strong' (3.86% glucose solution), 'medium' (2.27% glucose) and 'weak' (1.36% glucose). The 'stronger' the bag, the more water is removed by ultrafiltration across the peritoneal membrane. The dialysis prescription generally uses deviation from 'dry' weight as a major determinant of the strength of bag to be used. A standard 'medium' bag (1500 ml, 2.27% glucose) contains 22.7 g/l or approximately 35 g glucose in total. The glucose content of dialysis fluid means that patients may absorb 180 g or so of glucose per day—up to one-third of daily energy requirements.[1]

Where there is particularly high peritoneal glucose transfer, significant hyperglycaemia may occur. Rapid equalization of plasma and peritoneal glucose impairs water ultrafiltration. Higher strength bags, used to increase ultrafiltration of water, then exacerbate the problem of hyperglycaemia. If this occurs—or conversely, if there is loss of glucose efficacy—the large molecular weight glucose polymer, icodextrin, may be used in place of glucose in dialysis fluid. This preserves CAPD as a dialysis option and has the advantage that glucose absorption is eliminated. However, icodextrin is more inflammatory than glucose and may shorten the time that peritoneal dialysis is available as an option for renal replacement.

Effects on glycosylated haemoglobin (HbA1c)

- HbA1c measurement may be falsely lowered due to erythropoeisis in response to exogenous erythropoietin, iron deficiency, reduced red cell lifespan and red cell transfusion.

- Carbamylation of haemoglobin in the presence of urea interferes with some HbA1c assays.

Hypoglycaemic treatment

Changes in pharmacokinetics with renal failure should prompt active adjustment of all hypoglycaemic therapies.

- Uraemia is an insulin-resistant state which dialysis significantly reverses.

- Reduced renal clearance of insulin increases the duration of action of both exogenous and endogenous insulin.

- Sulphonylureas must be selected with care:

- chlorpropamide is mainly excreted renally and should be avoided;

- active metabolites of glibenclamide (glyburide), glimepiride, gliclazide, tolbutamide and glipizide accumulate in renal failure;

- generally, all sulphonylureas should be avoided, but glipizide has a short half-life and is the agent least likely to cause problematic hypoglycaemia;

- biguanides are contraindicated because accumulation of metabolites increases the risk of lactic acidosis;

- thiazolidinediones do not accumulate in renal failure. As they are contraindicated in heart failure, a decision to use thiazolidinediones must be balanced against the risk of accumulation of oedema.

CAPD makes possible intraperitoneal insulin delivery. This route is a physiologically more normal route, delivering insulin via the hepatic portal vein to the liver.[2] There are advantages and disadvantages to using intraperitoneal insulin.[3]

- Intraperitoneal insulin is more effective then subcutaneous insulin in suppressing hepatic glucose output, however glucose absorption—particularly with stronger bags—may be enhanced.

- Accessing dialysis bags to add insulin may increase the risk of contamination and peritonitis.

- Insulin is a trophic hormone that stimulates peritoneal fibroblast proliferation.

Patient on CAPD with erratic glycaemic control

Dialysis related

- Increased insulin resistance
- High glucose absorption from dialysis fluid – consider icodextrin
- Maltose interference from icodextrin-containing CAPD fluid
- Altered pharmacokinetics of insulin/sulphonylurea
- Appetite and calorie intake

Non-dialysis related

- ong-standing poor glycaemic control
- Autonomic dysfunction with abnormal gastric emptying

Fig. 52.1 Appoach to glycaemic control in patient using CAPD.

- Exchanges must take place close to mealtimes so that the peritoneal insulin dose can be adjusted for carbohydrate intake.

Patient-related problems

- Glycaemic control prior to renal failure is frequently poor because of difficulties adhering to principles central to good glycaemic control.

- Uraemic symptoms from inadequate dialysis may impair appetite and require reduction in hypoglycaemic therapy to avoid hypoglycaemia.

- Diabetic autonomic neuropathy may cause unpredictable gastric emptying.

Recent Developments

1   In 2002, icodextrin was approved by the Food and Drug Administration for use in place of glucose in dialysis fluid. Icodextrin (Extraneal®) is absorbed into the systemic circulation and metabolized to maltose. Maltose is not digested to glucose because the peripheral circulation lacks maltase. Maltose interferes with glucose meters that use glucose dehydrogenase-based measurement with the coenzyme pyrroloquinoline quinone. Falsely elevated glucose readings are associated with significant clinical problems.[4] This interaction is important when selecting blood glucose meters for individual patients and for bedside use in institutions where patients with diabetes may undergo peritoneal dialysis.

Conclusion

In most cases, diabetes will have been diagnosed 10 to 20 years previously. Whether good glycaemic control influences the progression of other microvascular complications once end-stage renal failure is established is uncertain, but it seems reasonable to strive for as good control as possible. However, established patterns of behaviour relating to control of blood glucose are often difficult to influence. It is important to clarify whether good over-all glucose control has always been difficult to achieve or whether there has been a recent deterioration. Occult infection, particularly peritoneal or foot, should be actively excluded.

As the problem in this case seems to be associated with adjustments that she is making to the strength of her dialysis bags, the dialysis prescription and agreed oral fluid intake should be reviewed with her nephrologist. In particular, regularizing both bag strength and the timing of exchanges 30 minutes or so before a meal will simplify insulin adjust-ment and make the pattern of hyperglycaemia more apparent. The accuracy of her finger-prick glucose meter, particularly in the light of problems with icodextrin/maltose, should also be assessed.

Insulin can be given as twice-daily pre-mixed injections or as a basal bolus regimen. A basal bolus regimen allows greater flexibility in insulin adjustment, particularly if rapid-acting insulin analogues are used at exchange/mealtimes. Though extra injections are an inconvenience, the rapid onset of action and short half-life of analogues mean that sup-plementary injections can be given to control hyperglycaemia—particularly if gastro-paresis is a contributory problem. Intraperitoneal insulin is not advocated because of the risk of peritonitis.

Further Reading

1 Grodstein GP, Blumenkrantz MJ, Kopple JD, Moran JK, Coburn JW. Glucose absorption during continuous ambulatory peritoneal dialysis. *Kidney Int* 1981; **19**: 564–7.

2 Schade D, Eaton R, Friedman N, Spencer W, Standefer J. Five-day programmed intraperitoneal insulin delivery in insulin-dependent diabetic man. *J Clin Endocrinol Metab* 1981; **52**: 1165–70.

3 Quellhorst E. Insulin therapy during peritoneal dialysis: pros and cons of various forms of administration. *J Am Soc Nephrol* 2002; **13**: S92–6.

4 Riley SG, Chess J, Donovan KL, Williams JD. Spurious hyperglycaemia and icodextrin in peritoneal dialysis fluid. *BMJ* 2003; **327**: 608–9.

53 Diabetes and Coeliac Disease

Case History

A 17-year-old girl who has had type 1 diabetes since the age of 8 years has difficulty in gaining weight. Her body mass index is 19 kg/m². She has no bowel symptoms unless she eats a very-high-carbohydrate meal. A cousin has coeliac disease and she has read that this may be associated with diabetes. She has always been careful with her diabetes but control has deteriorated in the past year (glycosylated haemoglobin [HbA1c] 8.9%).

Why are type 1 diabetes and coeliac disease associated?

Should patients with type 1 diabetes be screened for coeliac disease?

What should be the dietary management of patients who have both conditions?

Would the presence of coeliac disease alter your approach to the management of diabetes?

Background

Coeliac disease is probably the best understood of all the autoimmune diseases.[1] The disease is caused by sensitivity to α-gliadin, which is the principal protein in wheat. Similar proteins are also present in rye and barley, and to a lesser degree in oats. Gliadin contains a 33 amino acid peptide that is resistant to enzymatic digestion in the gut, and which includes three overlapping peptide sequences, each of which contains glutamine. Susceptible individuals are positive for the HLA-DQ2 or HLA-DQ8 antigens. These human leucocyte antigen (HLA) alleles are present in over 95% of patients with coeliac disease but in less than 30% of the general population. Deamidation of the gliadin peptides by the enzyme transglutaminase 2 renders them negatively charged and enhances their interaction with the relevant class II histocompatibility molecules. Subsequent presentation of the peptides to CD4+ T lymphocytes leads to activation, cytokine release and tissue damage. The result is the characteristic histological appearance with inflammation, villous atrophy and crypt hypertrophy.

The classic symptoms of coeliac disease are abdominal pain, failure to thrive (children), diarrhoea and abdominal distension. The symptoms are exacerbated by intake of wheat and wheat products and are absent when the individual adheres to a gluten-free diet. Many adults with coeliac disease have no, or minimal, gastrointestinal symptoms but may complain of non-specific symptoms and general ill health. Coeliac disease is associated with a variety of other manifestations including anaemia (deficiency of iron, folate and sometimes vitamin B12), liver abnormalities, osteoporosis, infertility, neurological problems (neuropathy, ataxia) and dermatitis herpetiformis. It is also associated with other auto-immune diseases including type 1 diabetes. Coeliac disease is present in up to 1% of populations of Northern European descent, the majority of whom are asymptomatic. Typically, around 5% of patients with type 1 diabetes have coeliac disease, and vice versa.

Tissue damage in patients developing coeliac disease is associated with expression of immunoglobulin A antibodies to gliadin, transglutaminase (transglutaminase 2) and endomysium. Measurement of these antibodies in serum provides a useful screening tool. Antibodies to gliadin are the least sensitive and specific. Anti-endomysial antibodies are the most widely used for clinical screening at present. These are measured by indirect immunofluorescence. The test is, therefore, qualitative or, at best, semi-quantitative. The antigen to which anti-endomysial antibodies are directed is now recognized to be transglutaminase 2. Quantification of antibodies to this enzyme by enzyme-linked immunosorbent assay (ELISA) is now acknowledged to be the gold-standard screening tool for coeliac disease. However, over 10% of patients with type 1 diabetes are positive for these antibodies, and not all have coeliac disease. Those who are antibody-positive should have the diagnosis of coeliac disease confirmed by endoscopic duodenal biopsy.

Type 1 diabetes and coeliac disease coexist in many individuals because of an overlapping genetic susceptibility.[2] The genetics of type 1 diabetes are now well understood but are complex, with at least 18 susceptibility loci identified. The most important of these is the HLA locus on the short arm of chromosome 6 (6p), which accounts for at least 50% of the tendency for the disease to aggregate in families. The best-known HLA association with type 1 diabetes is the increased risk conferred by the HLA-DR3 and HLA-DR4 genotypes. Between 30% and 50% of patients with type 1 diabetes are DR3/DR4 heterozygotes. DR3 or DR4 homozygosity appears to confer a slightly lower risk. It is now recognized that the DQ2 and DQ8 haplotypes are even better markers for type 1 diabetes, with 90% prevalence in patients with type 1 diabetes compared with 40% in the general population. Coeliac disease is 70% concordant in monozygotic twins and has a prevalence of 10% in first-degree relatives. Genetic predisposition is, therefore, of major importance. Over 90% of patients with coeliac disease possess the DQA1*0501 and DQB1*0201 alleles, conferring the HLA-DQ2 haplotype. Most of the remainder carry the DQ8 haplotype (DQA1*0301, DQB1*0302). DR3 and DR4 are in linkage disequilibrium with DQ2 and DQ8, respectively. In spite of the strong association of coeliac disease with HLA alleles, it is not currently thought to be useful to use HLA typing as a screening tool for coeliac disease.[3]

The issues around screening for coeliac disease in patients with type 1 diabetes are not clear cut.[4] The prevalence of coeliac disease in children and young adults with type 1 diabetes is around ten times that of the general population. Classic coeliac disease is not difficult to diagnose, and there is no argument that gluten-free diet (GFD) is a highly effective intervention for most of these patients. The major concerns about undiagnosed coeliac disease in younger people centre on the possible relationship with growth failure, osteopenia and hypoglycaemia, and the long-term risk of gastrointestinal malignancies including lymphoma. The growth of children of school age is routinely monitored and, while growth arrest or delay should certainly prompt consideration of coeliac disease as a possible cause, there does not appear to be a justification on this score for routine screening for coeliac disease. Osteopenia arises from vitamin D deficiency, leading to mild hypocalcaemia, and consequent secondary hyperparathyroidism. Bone mineral density should certainly be monitored in those with active coeliac disease, but the balance of evidence in asymptomatic individuals is that bone density is not compromised in children or young adults. Hypoglycaemia due to poor or erratic absorption of nutrients appears to be limited largely to the months before, and following, the diagnosis of coeliac disease. Development of unexplained hypoglycaemia in a patient with type 1 diabetes should prompt screening for coeliac disease. The increased risk of gastrointestinal malignancy appears to be limited to those with prolonged active coeliac disease. In summary, universal screening for coeliac disease, including in patients with type 1 diabetes, is not routinely recommended at present. The benefits of GFD are probably confined to those who have active symptoms of coeliac disease.

Individuals with coeliac disease need to avoid foods with wheat, barley and rye flours. It is not entirely clear whether oats are permissible. A variety of flours can be used including rice, potato, tapioca, sago, arrowroot, maize and cornflour. Care must be taken to avoid products that have seasonings and thickenings incorporating wheat and other flours containing pathogenic peptides. In recent years, it has become much easier to adhere to a GFD because of more ready access to appropriate support and advice, as well as a broader range of gluten-free products becoming available. However, the combination of gluten-free and diabetes diets represents a considerable challenge. Sensitivity to gluten-containing prod-

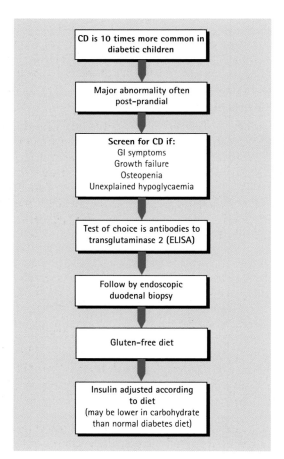

Fig. 53.1 Diabetes and coeliac disease (CD). GI = gastrointestinal.

ucts varies widely amongst individuals who are diagnosed as having coeliac disease. Loss of taste and texture of foods associated with a coeliac diet may make compliance difficult. Also, the dietary recommendations for coeliac disease, along with the tendency to restrict carbohydrate, run somewhat contrary to the normal diet recommendations for people who either have or are at risk of developing diabetes.

Recent Developments

1   The association of coeliac disease and diabetes, as well as their common genetic predisposition, has long been recognized. Several important epidemiological studies have appeared recently. If a temporal relationship between the appearances of the two diseases could be established, a firmer opinion about screening might emerge. Recent evidence is conflicting, with a French study[5] suggesting that coeliac disease generally preceded the diagnosis of diabetes, while in a large Italian series[6] the reverse seemed to hold true. The latter study also suggested that female gender, the presence of thyroid autoimmunity and earlier age of diabetes onset were all associated with increased risk of coeliac disease. Adults with type 1 diabetes have a lower prevalence of undiagnosed coeliac disease than do children, amounting to around 2.5%.[7]

2   Initiation of a GFD in children suffering from diabetes and coeliac disease both improves growth and leads to improved metabolic control of diabetes.[8,9] Decreased carbohydrate content of the diet may be at least partially responsible for the improved glycaemic control. It is equally possible that coexistence of the two conditions improves patients' compliance, and also that the increased dietetic and medical follow-up of patients with both conditions leads to tighter glycaemic control.

3   The link between coeliac disease and type 1 diabetes may not be just through common genetic susceptibility. In animal models of diabetes, exposure to soy protein or wheat gluten enhances the risk of developing diabetes. Exposure to gluten has also been linked with human diabetes. Intestinal inflammation and increased gut permeability have been demonstrated in patients with type 1 diabetes. A recent Italian study[10] has not only demonstrated mucosal inflammation in children with diabetes, but has also shown enhanced lymphocyte responses to gliadin in subjects who had diabetes but no serological or clinical evidence of coeliac disease.

Conclusion

Coeliac disease and type 1 diabetes share a common genetic predisposition, and are thus associated diseases. Furthermore, recent studies suggest that the gut may show an increased inflammatory response to gliadin in patients with type 1 diabetes. At this stage, screening for coeliac disease amongst patients with type 1 diabetes is not routinely advocated. However, coeliac disease should be suspected if there is growth or developmental delay, osteopenia or unexplained hypoglycaemia, or even in the presence of non-specific ill health. There is a strong familial predisposition and the disease should certainly be considered in the above patient.

GFD is a major undertaking at the best of times. The restrictions it places on a patient with type 1 diabetes may lead to decreased overall carbohydrate intake, and increased intake of less complex carbohydrate leading to more rapid absorption and, therefore, hyperglycaemia. If diabetic control is difficult, a basal bolus insulin regimen with short-acting analogue insulin might be considered. The dietary considerations with the two diseases combined are complex and often necessitate frequent review.

Further Reading

1 Alaedini A, Green PHR. Narrative review: celiac disease: understanding a complex autoimmune disorder. *Ann Intern Med* 2005; **142**: 289–98.

2 Ide A, Eisenbarth GS. Genetic susceptibility in type 1 diabetes and its associated autoimmune disorders. *Rev Endocr Metab Disord* 2003; **4**: 243–53.

3 Doolan A, Donaghue K, Fairchild J, Wong M, Williams AJ. Use of HLA typing in diagnosing celiac disease in patients with type 1 diabetes. *Diabetes Care* 2005; **28**: 806–9.

4 Freemark M, Levitsky LL. Screening for celiac disease in children with type 1 diabetes: two views of the controversy. *Diabetes Care* 2003; **26**: 1932–9.

5 Peretti N, Bienvenu F, Bouvet C, Fabien N, Tixier F, Thivolet C, Levy E, Chatelain PG, Lachaux A, Nicolino M. The temporal relationship between the onset of type 1 diabetes and celiac disease: a study based on immunoglobulin a antitransglutaminase screening. *Pediatrics* 2004; **113**: e418–22.

6 Cerutti F, Bruno G, Chiarelli F, Lorini R, Meschi F, Sacchetti C. Younger age at onset and sex predict celiac disease in children and adolescents with type 1 diabetes: an Italian multicenter study. *Diabetes Care* 2004; **27**: 1294–8.

7 Buysschaert M, Tomasi JP, Hermans MP. Prospective screening for biopsy proven coeliac disease, autoimmunity and malabsorption markers in Belgian subjects with Type 1 diabetes. *Diabet Med* 2005; **22**: 889–92.

8 Saadah OI, Zacharin M, O'Callaghan A, Oliver MR, Catto SAG. Effect of gluten-free diet and adherence on growth and diabetic control in diabetics with coeliac disease. *Arch Dis Child* 2004; **89**: 871–6.

9 Kaspers S, Kordonouri O, Schober E, Grabert M, Hauffa BP, Holl RW. Anthropometry, metabolic control, and thyroid autoimmunity in type 1 diabetes with celiac disease: a multicenter survey. *J Pediatr* 2004; **145**: 790–5.

10 Auricchio R, Paparo F, Maglio M, Franzese A, Lombardi F, Valerio G, Nardone G, Percopo S, Greco L, Troncone R. In vitro-deranged intestinal immune response to gliadin in type 1 diabetes. *Diabetes* 2004; **53**: 1680–3.

Index

4S (Scandinavian Simvastatin
Survival Study) 134, 192, 204

A
ABCD (Appropriate Blood Pressure
Control in Diabetes) trial 141,
192
abdominal obesity *see* central
obesity
acanthosis nigricans 22
acarbose 95
value in prevention of type 2
diabetes 6
ACAS (Asymptomatic Carotid
Atherosclerosis Study) 205
ACE (angiotensin-converting
enzyme) inhibitors 11, 141,
142, 159, 160–2
avoidance in pre-eclampsia 117
effect on atherosclerosis
progression 194
and pregnancy 108
in prevention of retinopathy
168–9
and renal artery stenosis 195
stroke reduction 204
value in advancing renal failure
164
value in ischaemic heart disease
188, 190
value in microalbuminuria
155–6, 157
ACHOIS (Australian Carbohydrate
Intolerance Study in Pregnant
Women) 106
acipimox 126
acromegaly 22, 146
acupuncture, value in DPN 151
acute (Charcot) neuroarthropathy
56
acute myocardial infarction *see*
myocardial infarction
acute stroke *see* stroke
adiponectin gene polymorphisms
19
adiponectin levels, effect of
thiazolidinediones 82
adolescent diabetes 69–71

adrenal adenomas 145–6
adrenaline, secretion in
hypoglycaemia 35
adrenergic symptoms,
hypoglycaemia 36
adult diabetes services, transition to
69, 71
adult respiratory distress syndrome
33
African-American women, insulin
sensitivity 10
age-related macular degeneration
(AMD) 175–6
risk factors for 177
albumin-creatinine ratio (ACR)
155
value in cystic fibrosis-related
diabetes 213
albumin excretion rate (AER) 155
albuminuria 130
as predictor of stroke 44
see also microalbuminuria
alcohol binges, as cause of diabetic
ketoacidosis 26
alcohol consumption
as cause of hypertriglyceridaemia
126
and pregnancy 110
aldose reductase inhibitors 157
aldosterone antagonists 147, 157
ALLHAT (Antihypertensive and
Lipid-Lowering treatment to
prevent Heart ATtack) 141
allodynia 150
alpha-glucosidase inhibitors, use by
elderly people 95
alpha-blockers 142
ALLHAT 141
contraindication to PDE-5
inhibitors 112
alpha-lipoic acid, value in DPN 152
alprostadil, intracavernosal
injection 113
alteplase, value after acute stroke 44
amantadine, value in DPN 151
ambulatory blood pressure
monitoring (ABPM) 144, 147
American Diabetes Association
recommendations on aspirin
usage 138

screening protocol for gestational
diabetes 104
American Heart Association
recommendations on aspirin
usage 138
reduction of triglyceride levels
126
amino acid supplementation, elderly
people 96
aminoguanidine 157
amiodarone, as cause of autonomic
neuropathy 178
amitriptyline, value in DPN 150,
152
amoxicillin/clavulinic acid 57
amputation rates
foot ulcers 199, 202
intermittent claudication 47
amylin 79
amyloidosis, as cause of autonomic
neuropathy 178
anaemia, association with coeliac
disease 220
anaerobic infections 57
analogue insulins
use in diabetic ketoacidosis 28, 29
use during pregnancy 110
use in elderly people 95
angina 187–90
angiogenic growth factors, value in
peripheral arterial disease
193–4
angioplasty, for peripheral arterial
disease 48
angiopoietin-1 (ANG-1) 173
angiotensin II receptor blockers 11,
141, 142, 160
avoidance in pre-eclampsia 117
in prevention of retinopathy 169
and renal artery stenosis 195
value in advancing renal failure
164
value in microalbuminuria 156,
157
anion gap, in diabetic ketoacidosis
26
ankle-brachial pressure index
(ABPI) 48, 192

antenatal surveillance, type 1 diabetes 109
anti-endomysial antibodies 221
anti-insulin antibodies 22
Anti-Platelet Trialists (APT) 137
antibiotic resistance 58–9
antibiotic therapy, infected foot 57–8, 59, 200
anticonvulsants, value in DPN 151, 152, 153
antidopaminergic medications, as cause of erectile dysfunction 112
antihypertensive therapy 11
  in advancing renal failure 164
  choice of agent 142–3
  effect on peripheral arterial disease 192
  in microalbuminuria 155
  in pre-eclampsia 117
  in prevention of retinopathy 168–9, 177
  RAS blockade 159–62
  stroke prevention 204, 206
antioxidant vitamins
  and age-related macular degeneration 176
  in HPS 134
antiplatelet drugs 139, 203
  in peripheral arterial disease 192
  value in microalbuminuria 157
  see also aspirin
antithrombotic therapy 203
aortic coarctation 146
aorto-bifemoral bypass 49
Apligraf 202
apnoea-hypopnoea index 208
apolipoprotein C-II deficiency 126
apomorphine, sublingual 113
appetite, effect of cannabinoids 91
aromatase inhibitors, use in polycystic ovarian syndrome 100
arterial blood sampling 26
arteriography, diagnosis of renal artery stenosis 196
aspirin 11, 137–9
  effect on risk of pre-eclampsia 118
  in retinopathy prevention 169, 173
  in stroke prevention 203
  value in advancing renal failure 164
  value in ischaemic stroke 44, 46
  value in microalbuminuria 157

value in peripheral arterial disease 192
ASTRAL (Angioplasty and Stent for Renal Artery Lesions) trial 145, 197–8
atenolol
  in hypertension management 11
  see also beta-blockers
atherosclerosis progression, effect of ACE inhibitors 194
Atkins diet 72
atorvastatin
  CARDS 204
  combination with torcetrapib 135
  TNT study 130
  see also statins
atrial fibrillation
  antithrombotic therapy 203
  stroke risk 44
atrial overpacing 180
atypical diabetes 29
autoantibodies, to insulin receptor 22
autoimmune diabetes, in elderly people 93
autoimmune disease, association with coeliac disease 221
autoimmunity, role in type 1 diabetes 3
autonomic impairment, multiple sclerosis 36
autonomic neuropathy 178–81
  as cause of diabetic ketoacidosis 26
  as cause of sleep disordered breathing 208
  role in Charcot foot 182
  role in ulceration 58
  stroke risk 44

B
background retinopathy 167, 169–70
Baltimore Longitudinal Study of Aging 19
BARI (Bypass Angioplasty Revascularization Investigation) trial 188
bariatric surgery 91, 92
becaplermin 202
beta-blockers 141, 142
  as cause of erectile dysfunction 112
  as cause of weight gain 89
  in hypertension management 11

oxprenolol, use in pre-eclampsia 117
  use in peripheral arterial disease 192
beta cell function assessment 2
bezafibrate 126
bicarbonate, levels in hyperosmolar hyperglycaemic state 31
bicarbonate infusion, diabetic ketoacidosis 29
biguanides see metformin
bisphosphonates, value in neuroarthropathy 183, 185
black patients, antihypertensive treatment 141
bladder dysfunction 178
blindness 167
  causes 175–6
blood pressure
  effect of subutramine 91
  orthostatic hypotension 178, 179–80
  see also hypertension
blood pressure control 141
  effect on microalbuminuria progression 155
  effect on peripheral arterial disease 192
  effect on retinopathy progression 168–9, 177
  effect on stroke risk 204, 206
  see also antihypertensive therapy; hypertension
blue vision, as side effect of sildenafil 114
body mass index (BMI) 89
bone mineral density, in coeliac disease 221–2
bowel habit, altered 178
breast-feeding, effect on risk of type 1 diabetes 2–3, 4
British Hypertension Society AB/CD guideline 204
brittle diabetes 69
Buerger's test 48
bupropion, value in smoking cessation 122–3

C
cachexia 94
Caesarean section 110
  in pre-eclampsia 117
calcitonin gene-related peptide 184
calcium channel blockers 141, 142
  stroke prevention 204
CALM (Candesartan And Lisinopril Microalbuminuria) study 161

candesartan
    CALM study 161
    DIRECT 169
cannabinoids, effect on appetite 91
capillary blood glucose, value in
        screening 19, 20
CAPRIE (Clopidogrel versus Aspirin
        in Patients at Risk of Ischaemic
        Events) 192
capsaicin, value in DPN 151
carbamazepine, value in DPN 151,
        152
carbohydrate
    excessive consumption 72–3
    requirements during exercise 66,
        67
carbohydrate content, enteral feeds
        86
cardiac autonomic neuropathy 179
cardiovascular disease risk
    association with pre-eclampsia
        118
    effect of aspirin 137–9
    estimation of 136, 140
    impact of diabetes 10
    management after menopause
        10–12
    in microalbuminuria 157
    in obstructive sleep apnoea 208
    in peripheral arterial disease
        47–8
    polycystic ovarian syndrome 102
    relationship to IGT and IFG 19
    in type 1 diabetes 129–30
    value of blood pressure reduction
        141
cardiovascular risk assessment 8
cardiovascular risk factors
    effect of aggressive treatment 142
    relationship to diabetes risk 127
cardiovascular risk management,
        peri-menopausal 9–12
CARDS (Collaborative Atorvastatin
        Diabetes Study) 204
CARE (Cholesterol and Recurrent
        Events) study 134
carotid artery stenosis 180–1
carotid artery stenting 205
carotid endarterectomy 205
cataract extraction 173
CBI receptor blockade 91
central line insertion, indication in
        diabetic ketoacidosis 26
central obesity 10, 11
    effect on lipid profile 133
    insulin resistance 21
    stroke risk 44

cerebral oedema
    avoidance in hyperosmolar
        hyperglycaemic state 33
    in diabetic ketoacidosis 26
CETP (cholesteryl ester transfer
        protein) inhibition 135
Charcot neuroarthropathy 56,
        182–5
CHHIPS (Controlling Hypertension
        and Hypotension Immediately
        Post-Stroke) pilot trial 45
childhood type 1 diabetes,
        prevention 2–4
children
    coeliac disease 221, 223
    see also adolescent diabetes
chlorpropamide 77, 94
    avoidance in renal failure 217
chlorthalidone, ALLHAT 141
cholinergic symptoms,
        hypoglycaemia 36
chylomicronaemia 126
cilostazol 139
    value in peripheral arterial disease
        192, 194
cimetidine, as cause of erectile
        dysfunction 112
ciprofibrate 126
ciprofloxacin 57, 58
clindamycin 57, 58
clinically significant macular
        oedema (CSMO) 173
clomiphene citrate 100
clonidine, value in smoking
        cessation 123
clopidogrel 139
    stroke prevention 203, 206
    value in peripheral arterial disease
        192
coarctation of aorta 146
Cochrane Tobacco Addiction
        Review 122
Cockcroft-Gault formula 164
cod liver oil, effect on risk of type 1
        diabetes 3, 4
coeliac disease 220–4
cognitive function 36
    effect of diabetes 37, 38, 94
collateral circulation, improvement
        in peripheral arterial disease
        192, 193–4
colour vision, loss of 175
combination lipid-lowering therapy
        134
combination oral hypoglycaemic
        therapy 82

combined hyperlipidaemia, familial
        126
compliance with treatment 144
    elderly people 94
complications
    of gestational diabetes 103
    of laser photocoagulation 172–3
    of PEG feeding 87
    of pre-eclampsia 116
congenital malformations, type 1
        diabetes 107–8
connective tissue glycation 182
Conn's syndrome 145–6
constipation 178
consultations, common agenda
        69–70
continuous ambulatory peritoneal
        dialysis (CAPD) 216–19
continuous subcutaneous infusion
        of insulin (CSII) 61–4
coronary angiography, indications
        188
coronary artery bypass grafting
        (CABG) 188, 189–90
coronary heart disease risk, in type 1
        diabetes 129–30
cortisol 35
    24 hour measurement 145
costs of treatment, CSII 62
cows' milk exposure, effect on risk of
        type 1 diabetes 3
CPAP (continuous positive airway
        pressure), in management of
        sleep apnoea 210, 211
creatinine clearance 164
creatinine levels, raised in RAS
        blockade 160–1, 164, 196
critical limb ischaemia 47–50, 58
Cushing's syndrome 145
cyclophosphamide, use in insulin
        resistance syndrome 22, 23
cystic fibrosis-related diabetes
        (CFRD) 212–15
cystic fibrosis transmembrane
        conductance regulator gene
        212

D
dalfopristin resistance 59
daptomycin resistance 59
dawn phenomenon 62
DCCT (Diabetes Control and
        Complications Trial) 108
    cognitive function 37
    CSII 62
    hypoglycaemic episodes 35
    prevention of retinopathy 168

DCCT/EDIC (Diabetes Control and Complications Trial/Epidemiology of Diabetes Intervention and Complications) 163
deafness, MIDD (maternally inherited diabetes and deafness) 15
death, diabetes as cause 94
debridement, foot ulcers 200
Dermagraft 202
dermatitis herpetiformis 221
detemir insulin, use during pregnancy 110
dexamethasone, use with clomiphene citrate 100
dexamethasone suppression test 145
dextrose infusion
  in diabetic ketoacidosis 26–8
  in hyperosmolar hyperglycaemic state 32
diabetes
  diagnostic criteria 17, 18
  see also type 1 diabetes; type 2 diabetes
Diabetes Prevention Trial-Type 1 3–4
diabetic amyotrophy 93–4
diabetic ketoacidosis (DKA) 25–6
  biochemical abnormalities 31
  management 26–9
diabetic maculopathy (DMa) 175–7
Diabetic Retinopathy Study (DRS) 169, 171
Diabetic Retinopathy Vitrectomy Study 173
diagnosis, of diabetic ketoacidosis 26
diagnostic criteria
  critical limb ischaemia 48
  diabetes 17, 18
  hyperosmolar hyperglycaemic state 31
  impaired fasting glucose 18
  impaired glucose tolerance 18
  insulin resistance state 21
  pre-eclampsia 116
dialysis 216–19
dialysis fluids 216–17
diarrhoea, as cause of diabetic ketoacidosis 26
diet
  as cause of hypertriglyceridaemia 126
  in cystic fibrosis 213

effect on risk of type 2 diabetes 7–8
enteral feeding 86–8
in gestational diabetes 104
interaction with genes 127
low-carbohydrate 72–6
low glycaemic index diets 74
risk factors for type 1 diabetes 2–3, 4
whole-grain consumption 74–5
see also lifestyle intervention
DIGAMI (Diabetes and Insulin-Glucose Infusion in Acute Myocardial Infarction) studies 41, 45
dipyridamole
  value in peripheral arterial disease 192
  value in stroke prevention 203
DIRECT (DIabetic REtinopathy Candesartan Trial) 169
distal sensory peripheral neuropathy (DPN) 149–54
DPP (Diabetes Prevention Program) 5–6, 19
  capillary blood glucose, value in screening 19
DPP-IV (dipeptidyl peptidase IV) inhibitors 80
DPS (Diabetes Prevention Study) 6, 7, 19
drug-eluting stents 190
drugs
  as cause of diabetic ketoacidosis 26
  as cause of hyperosmolar hyperglycaemic state 30
dry age-related macular degeneration (AMD) 176
dual ACE inhibitor and ARB therapy 161, 164
duplex ultrasound scanning, investigation of renal impairment 196
duration of diabetes, relationship to cardiovascular disease risk 129
dysbetalipoproteinaemia, familial 126
dyslipidaemia
  as cause of erectile dysfunction 112
  stroke risk 44

E
ECG, indications for coronary angiography 188

eclampsia 116
  use of magnesium 117–18
economic analysis, CSII 62
ECST (European Carotid Surgery Trial) 205
educational input, insulin pump therapy 63–4
educational interventions, adolescent diabetes 70–1
elderly people 93–6
embolectomy, limbs 48–9
ENDIT (European Nicotinamide Diabetes Intervention Trial) 3
endomysium antibodies, coeliac disease 221
endothelial function, effect of statins 194
endurance running 65–8
enteral feeding 85–8
enteroviruses, as risk factor for type 1 diabetes 3
environmental factors in type 1 diabetes 2
ephedrine, value in orthostatic hypotension 179, 180
epidemiology, cystic fibrosis-related diabetes 214–15
eplerenone 157
erectile dysfunction 111–15, 141, 178
ertiprotafib 83
erythropoietin, use in autonomic neuropathy 180, 181
essential amino acid supplementation, elderly people 96
ETDRS (Early Treatment Diabetic Retinopathy Study) 138, 169, 171, 172, 173
EUCLID (EURODIAB Controlled Trial of Lisinopril in Insulin-Dependent Diabetes Mellitus) study 155–6, 168–9
euglycaemic insulin clamp technique 22
EURODIAB study, risk factors for autonomic neuropathy 180
exenatide 38, 80
exercise
  as aid to smoking cessation 122
  effect on autonomic responses 35
  effect on glucose tolerance 7
  lack of, as cause of hypertriglyceridaemia 126
  and type 1 diabetes 65–8
  see also lifestyle intervention

exercise ECG 188, 190
exercise programmes, peripheral
    arterial disease 192
ezetimibe 134

F
familial causes,
    hypertriglyceridaemia 126
family history
    MODY 13, 14
    of type 1 diabetes 1, 2, 4
    of type 2 diabetes 5
femoral artery revascularization
    procedures 49–50
fetus
    complications of gestational
        diabetes 103, 105, 106
    effect of ACE inhibitors 108
fibrates 126, 134
fibre, addition to enteral feeds 86
fibrinogen, levels in insulin
    resistance syndrome 22
fibroblasts, abnormalities in diabetic
    ulcers 199
finger-prick blood tests, value in
    screening 19, 20
fish consumption 126
flash pulmonary oedema 196
flucloxacillin 57, 58
fludrocortisone, value in orthostatic
    hypotension 179, 180, 181
fluid intake, in orthostatic
    hypotension 180
fluid replacement
    in diabetic ketoacidosis 26–8
    in hyperosmolar hyperglycaemic
        state 31–3, 34
fluid retention, as side effect of
    thiazolidinediones 82
fluoxetine 150
folic acid supplementation,
    pregnancy 108, 110
FOOD (Feed Or Ordinary Diet)
    trials 87
foot
    Charcot neuroarthropathy 182–5
    critical ischaemia 47–50
    hot 55–9
foot ulceration 199–202
    predictors of risk 150
footwear
    aiding ulcer healing 58, 59, 201
    Charcot foot 183, 185
foreign bodies, in foot 55, 56
fractures, of foot 55, 56, 182, 184–5
Framingham Study 125

G
GABA (gamm-aminobutyric acid),
    as target for smoking cessation
    therapies 124
gabapentin, value in DPN 151, 152,
    153
gamma-linoleic acid, value in DPN
    152–3
gangrene, lower limb 48
gastric banding 92
gastric paresis 178
gastrointestinal malignancy, risk in
    coeliac disease 222
gastrointestinal side effects
    of aspirin 138
    of metformin 81
    of orlistat 90
gemfibrozil 126, 134, 204
gender differences
    cardiovascular disease risk 10,
        137
    intima-media thickness,
        teenagers 130
    risk of type 1 diabetes 4
gene therapy 4
gene transfer, VGEF 193–4
general anaesthesia, glycaemic
    control 52
genetic factors
    in coeliac disease 221
    in diabetic nephropathy 161
    in hypertriglyceridaemia 126
    in insulin resistance 135
    in MODY 14
    in smoking behaviour 124
    in type 1 diabetes 2, 3–4, 221
    in type 2 diabetes 19
gestational diabetes 103–6
gestational hypertension 116
glargine insulin, use during
    pregnancy 110
gliadin, enhanced lymphocyte
    responses in diabetes 223
gliadin sensitivity, coeliac disease
    220, 221
glibenclamide 77, 94
    use in gestational diabetes 105
    use in renal failure 217
glicazide 75, 77
    glicazide MR 94
    use in renal failure 217
    value in MODY 15
glimepiride 77, 94, 217
glipizide 217
glitazones 80, 82, 84
    in prevention of type 2 diabetes 6

use by elderly people 95
use in cystic fibrosis-related
    diabetes 213
use in polycystic ovarian
    syndrome 102
use in renal failure 217
glomerular epithelial cells,
    abnormalities in albuminuria
    157
glomerular filtration rate (GFR)
    164
glucagon 35, 36
glucagon-like peptide-1 (GLP-1)
    80, 91, 96
glucokinase genes, defect in MODY
    2 14
gluconeogenesis 65, 67
glucose content, dialysis fluids 216
glucose insulin potassium (GIK)
    infusion
    after acute myocardial infarction
        41, 42
    after acute stroke 45
glucose metabolism, NMR
    spectroscopy 67
glucose meters, interference from
    maltose 218
glucose tolerance
    effect of exercise 7
    effect of weight reduction 89
GLUT4 73, 135
glutamate receptors, as target for
    smoking cessation therapies
    124
gluten-free diet 221, 222–3, 223–4
glycaemic control
    CSII 61–4
    in cystic fibrosis-related diabetes
        213
    during pregnancy 104–5, 108,
        110
    effect on advancing renal failure
        164
    effect on DPN 150
    effect of GFD in coeliac disease
        223
    effect on lipid profile 133
    effect of low-carbohydrate diet
        73
    effect on macrovascular disease
        188
    effect on microalbuminuria
        progression 155, 156–7, 163
    effect on peripheral arterial
        disease 193
    in peritoneal dialysis 218, 219

glycaemic control (*cont.*)
  in prevention of retinopathy 168,
  171
  relationship to stroke risk 44
  risk of hypoglycaemia 35
  targets in elderly people 94
glycaemic index 7–8
glycaemic load 74
glycaemic vascular injury,
  pathophysiology 194
glycation of connective tissue 182
glyceryl trinitrate, value in DPN 151
glycogenolysis 65, 67
glycoprotein IIb/IIIa antagonists
  139
gonadotrophin treatment,
  polycystic ovarian syndrome
  100–1
gram-positive infections, antibiotic
  choice 57
granulocyte colony-stimulating
  factor (G-CSF) 59
growth, effect of coeliac disease 221
growth hormone 35, 146
gum, nicotine 122
gustatory sweating 178

H
haemodialysis 166
haemoglobin carbamylation 217
haemoglobin levels, effect of
  thiazolidinediones 82
haemorrhage, risk from aspirin
  therapy 138
HAIR-AN syndrome 22
HbA1c
  effect of CSII 62
  in peritoneal dialysis 217
  value in perioperative
  management 52
  value in screening 19
HDL-cholesterol 133
  effect of raising levels 204–5
  effect of torcetrapib 135
  in insulin resistance syndrome 22
headache, after laser
  photocoagulation 172–3
healing process, abnormalities in
  foot ulcers 199–200
heart disease, use of sibutramine 91
helical CT 145
HELLP (Haemolysis, Elevated Liver
  enzymes, Low Platelets)
  syndrome 116
Helsinki Heart Study 125, 134

heparin, use in hyperosmolar
  hyperglycaemic state 33
hepatic lipase deficiency 126
hepatic nuclear factor genes, defects
  in MODY 14
hepatic transaminase levels,
  prediction of type 2 diabetes
  127
HERS (Hormone Estrogen-
  Progestin Replacement Study)
  10
high-protein diets 73
HIV therapy, interaction with PDE-
  5 inhibitors 112
HLA associations
  coeliac disease 220
  type 1 diabetes 221
homocysteine, levels in insulin
  resistance syndrome 22
Honolulu Heart Programme 125
HOPE (Heart Outcome Protection
  Evaluation) study 6–7, 159,
  192, 204
hot foot 55–9
HOT (Hypertension Optimal
  Treatment) trial 140–1
HPS (Heart Protection Study) 130,
  134
  effect on GFR decline 165
  peripheral arterial disease 192
  stroke reduction 204
HRT (hormone replacement
  therapy) 10, 11
  as cause of hypertriglyceridaemia
  126
human chorionic gonadotrophin,
  use in polycystic ovarian
  syndrome 100
human recombinant IGF-1, value in
  insulin resistance syndrome
  22, 23–4
hunger 73
hydralazine, use in pre-eclampsia
  117
hyperaesthesia 150
hyperaldosteronism 145–6, 147
hyperandrogenism 22
hypercatabolic states, enteral feeding
  86
hypercoagulable state 137
hyperfiltration 155
hyperglycaemia
  chronic, risk of cognitive
  impairment 37
  as complication of PEG feeding
  87

in diabetic ketoacidosis 26
  effect on healing process 199
  hyperosmolar hyperglycaemic
  state 30–4
  insulin resistance syndrome 21–4
  management after acute
  myocardial infarction 40–2
  perioperative 52
  in peritoneal dialysis 216–17
hyperinsulinaemia, stroke risk 44
hyperkalaemia 29
  in RAS blockade 160
hyperlipidaemia
  in type 1 diabetes 129–32
  in type 2 diabetes 133–6
  see also hypertriglyceridaemia
hyperlipoproteinaemia, type I 126
hypernatraemia, in hyperosmolar
  hyperglycaemic state 31, 33
hyperosmolar hyperglycaemic state
  (HHS) 30–1
  biochemical abnormalities 31
  management 31–4
hyperparathyroidism, in coeliac
  disease 221
hyperprolactinaemia, as cause of
  erectile dysfunction 112
hypertension 140–2
  association with obstructive sleep
  apnoea 208, 210
  as cause of erectile dysfunction
  112
  choice of hypotensive agent
  141–2
  gestational 116
  intervention threshold 140–1
  in microalbuminuria 155
  in obstructive sleep apnoea 147
  resistance to therapy 143–4
  as risk factor for retinopathy
  168–9
  secondary 144–6
  after stroke 45
  stroke risk 44, 204
  see also antihypertensive therapy;
  blood pressure; pre-eclampsia
hypertriglyceridaemia 125–8
  pathogenesis 133
hypocalcaemia, in coeliac disease
  221
hypoglycaemia
  coeliac disease as cause 222
  during pregnancy 108
  exercise-induced 67, 68
  perioperative 52
  recurrent 34–9

as side effect of sulphonylureas 77
susceptibility in MODY 15
hypoglycaemia associated autonomic failure (HAAF) 35, 37
hypoglycaemic awareness 35, 36, 37–8, 179
during pregnancy 108
hypokalaemia, risk in diabetic ketoacidosis 28, 29
hypophosphataemia
diabetic ketoacidosis 28
in hyperosmolar hyperglycaemic state 33
hypotension
avoidance of PDE-5 inhibitors 114
orthostatic 178, 179–80, 181
hypothyroidism
as cause of erectile dysfunction 112
as cause of hypertriglyceridaemia 126

I
123I-metaiodobenzylguanidine imaging 180
icodextrin, in dialysis fluid 217, 218
iliac artery stenting 50
imaging techniques
Charcot foot 183
renal artery stenosis 196
immobilization, in treatment of neuroarthropathy 183, 185
immunisation, effect on risk of type 1 diabetes 3, 4
immunosuppression, preventive value 2
immunosuppressive treatment in insulin resistance 22, 23, 24
impaired fasting glucose (IFG) 19
diagnostic criteria 18
impaired glucose tolerance (IGT) 19–20
diagnostic criteria 18
prevention of type 2 diabetes 5–8
stroke risk 44
incretin-like molecules 38
infection
as cause of diabetic ketoacidosis 26
as cause of hyperosmolar hyperglycaemic state 30
hot foot 55–9
infection control, foot ulcers 200

infectious diseases, as risk factor for type 1 diabetes 3
inflammatory markers, prediction of type 2 diabetes 11
infratentorial infarcts 44
injection site prior to exercise 66
insoles 201
insulin
combination therapy with thiazolidinediones 82
intraperitoneal delivery 217–18
perioperative intravenous regimen 54
insulin error, as cause of diabetic ketoacidosis 26
Insulin in Intensive Care Study 41
insulin-like growth factor-1 (IGF-1) 22, 146
human recombinant, use in insulin resistance 22, 23–4
IGF-1 receptor affinity, insulin analogues 110
insulin promoter factor gene defect, MODY 14
insulin pump therapy 61–4
insulin receptor substrate-1 polymorphisms 79
insulin resistance 11, 19
association with obstructive sleep apnoea 208
association with raised tissue triglyceride levels 127
association with smoking 124
effect on lipid profile 133
effect of tissue lipid accumulation 134–5
increase with age 93
stroke risk 44
Insulin Resistance Atherosclerosis Study 127
insulin resistance state (IRS) 21–4
insulin secretagogues 77–80
see also nateglinide; repaglinide; sulphonylureas
insulin sensitivity
effect of low-carbohydrate diet 73
effect of whole-grain foods 74–5
racial differences 10
insulin sensitizers
in management of sleep apnoea 211
use in insulin resistance syndrome 22
see also metformin; thiazolidinediones

insulin treatment
adjustment for exercise 66–7, 68
after acute myocardial infarction 41–2
after acute stroke 45, 46
in coeliac disease 224
in cystic fibrosis-related diabetes 213
in diabetic ketoacidosis 28
in elderly people 95–6
in enteral feeding 86–7
in gestational diabetes 105
in hyperosmolar hyperglycaemic state 33
introduction in type 2 diabetes 79, 80
in MODY 15
perioperative adjustments 52, 53
in peritoneal dialysis 217–18, 219
during pregnancy 110
in recurrent hypoglycaemia 36–7, 38–9
intensive glycaemic control, effect on retinopathy 168
intensive insulin therapy, value after stroke 45
interleukin-6, increased levels in pre-eclampsia 118
interleukin-6 gene polymorphisms 19
intermittent claudication 47, 191–4
intervention threshold, hypertension 140–1
intima-media thickness, teenagers 130
intracavernosal alprostadil 113
intrauterine fetal death, incidence in type 1 diabetes 109
intrauterine growth retardation in pre-eclampsia 117
intravenous insulin regimen, perioperative 54
iron stores 11
ischaemic heart disease 187–90
avoidance of PDE-5 inhibitors 114
use of sibutramine 91
ischaemic ulcers 200–1
islet cell antibodies 2
isosorbide dinitrate (ISDN), value in DPN 153

K
K+ channels, role in hyopglycaemic awareness 37–8
kappa B kinase-, inhibitor 84
ketoacidosis see diabetic ketoacidosis

ketoconazole, interaction with PDE-5 inhibitors 112
ketone bodies 73
ketonuria/ ketonaemia, in diabetic ketoacidosis 26

L

labetalol, use in pre-eclampsia 117
lactic acidosis, as side effect of metformin 81
lacunar strokes 44, 45
laser photocoagulation 171–3, 174
   for age-related macular degeneration 176
late onset cystic fibrosis 215
LDL-cholesterol 133
   effect of torcetrapib 135
   in insulin resistance syndrome 22
left ventricular dysfunction 141
leg, critical ischaemia 47–50
LIFE (Losartan Intervention For Endpoint reduction in hypertension) study 159
lifestyle intervention
   benefit in MODY 14
   in elderly people 94
   in hypertriglyceridaemia 126, 128
   in obesity 89
   in peripheral arterial disease 192, 193, 194
   in polycystic ovarian syndrome 100, 102
   in prevention of type 2 diabetes 5–6, 7, 8, 19
linezolid resistance 58–9
linloeic acids, conjugated 135
lipid accumulation, effect on tissue insulin resistance 134–5
LIPID (Long-term Intervention with Pravastatin in Ischaemic Disease) study 134, 204
lipid-lowering drugs, preventive value 6
lipid-lowering therapy, value in peripheral arterial disease 192
lipid profile
   dietary factors 135
   effect of low-carbohydrate diet 73
   effect of poor glycaemic control 133
   effect of ragaglitazar 83
   effect of thiazolidinediones 82–3
   in insulin resistance syndrome 22
   in type 1 diabetes 129
lipohypertrophy 22

lipoprotein lipase deficiency 126
liraglutide 80
Lisfranc dislocation 183
lisinopril
   CALM study 161
   EUCLID study 155–6, 168–9
lispro insulin, use during pregnancy 110
liver, lipid accumulation 127
liver X receptor 134–5
Liverpool Diabetic Eye Study 175
loop diuretics 156
low-carbohydrate diets 72–6
low-carbohydrate feed, enteral nutrition 87
low glycaemic diet 7–8
lung function abnormalities, association with diabetes 210–11
lutein 176

M

macroalbuminuria 130, 163–6
macrosomia
   in gestational diabetes 103, 105, 106
   in type 1 diabetes 107
macrovascular complications
   angina in type 2 diabetes 187–90
   foot ulceration 199–202
   peripheral arterial disease 191–4
   prevention in elderly people 94
   renal artery stenosis 195–8
   transient ischaemic attack 203–6
macrovascular complications risk, relationship to plasma glucose 18
macular disease 175–7
macular oedema (MO) 167, 173
   vitreal triamcinolone acetonide 174
magnesium
   use in eclampsia 117–18
   value after acute stroke 45
magnesium deficiency 94
magnesium levels 8, 11
magnetic resonance angiography (MRA) 145, 147, 196, 198
maltose, interference with glucose meters 218
maternal complications, gestational diabetes 103
maternal death, pre-eclampsia as cause 116
maturity-onset diabetes of youth (MODY) 13–16

maxepa 126
menopause 9–12
metabolic abnormalities, during PEG feeding 87
metabolic acidosis, in diabetic ketoacidosis 26, 28
metabolic syndrome 19, 20, 84, 89
   association with obstructive sleep apnoea 208
   effect of oestrogen 10
   effects of aspirin 139
   hypertriglyceridaemia 125–8
   nutritional management 96
   stroke risk 44
metanephrine, plasma levels 146
metatarsal fractures 182, 184–5
metformin 80, 81–2, 84
   avoidance in renal failure 217
   and cystic fibrosis-related diabetes 213
   in MODY 15
   in polycystic ovarian syndrome 100
   in prevention of type 2 diabetes 5–6, 8
   and surgery 52
   use by elderly people 94–5
   use in cardiovascular disease 41
   use during pregnancy 101, 102
   use with insulin 95
   use with orlistat 92
   use with sibutramine 91
methyldopa, use in pre-eclampsia 117
metronidazole 58
mexiletine, value in DPN 151
microalbuminuria 130, 154–8, 159
   ACE inhibitor therapy 159–62
   effect of glycaemic control 163
   risk of autonomic neuropathy 180
microbiology, foot infections 57, 200
micronutrient status, relationship to risk of type 2 diabetes 11
microvascular complications
   advancing renal failure 163–6
   association with IGT 19–20
   autonomic neuropathy 178–81
   background retinopathy 167–70
   Charcot foot 182–5
   in cystic fibrosis-related diabetes 213
   macular disease 175–7
   microalbuminuria 130, 154–8
   painful neuropathy 149–54

proliferative and pre-proliferative retinopathy 171–4
risk in MODY 14, 15
value of blood pressure reduction 141
MIDD (maternally inherited diabetes and deafness) 15
midrodine 180
miglitol 95
mitochondrial diabetes syndromes 15
Modification of Diet in Renal Disease (MDRD) study 164
moisturising of skin 58
MONICA surveys 208
morphine, value in DPN 153
mortality benefits, ACE inhibitors 161
motor neuropathy 58
MRFIT (Multiple Risk Factor Intervention Trial) 7, 140–1
MRI scanning, osteomyelitis 57
MRSA (methicillin-resistant Staphylococcus aureus) infections 57, 58
mucosal insulin, Diabetes Prevention trial-Type 1 3–4
multiple sclerosis 36
muscle cells, fuel supply 65
muscular imbalance 58
mycophenolate, value in insulin resistance syndrome 23
myocardial infarction 40–2
avoidance of PDE-5 inhibitors 114
as cause of hyperosmolar hyperglycaemic state 30
secondary prevention, value of aspirin 137
smoking cessation 122

N
NASCET (North American Symptomatic Carotid Endarterectomy Trial) 205
nasogastric feeding, indication after stroke 87
nateglinide 15, 78
use by elderly people 95
National Cholesterol Education Programme, triglyceride levels classification 125
neonatal care, type 1 diabetes 110
nephropathy 130, 154–5, 159
advancing renal failure 163–6

microalbuminuria 155–8
natural history 157
slowing of progression 141
nephrotic syndrome, as cause of hypertriglyceridaemia 126
nerve growth factor (NGF), value in DPN 153
nerve stimulation, value in DPN 151
neural tube defects 108
neuroarthropathy 182–5
neuroglycopaenic symptoms 36
neuropathy
autonomic 178–81
painful 149–54
neuropathy-modifying drugs 152–3
neuroprotectant drugs, value after stroke 44–5
neurosurgery, after acute stroke 44
NHANES (National Health and Nutrition Evaluation Study) III 93, 210
niacin (vitamin B3), effect on risk of type 1 diabetes 3
Niaspan 126
NICE (National Institute for Health and Clinical Excellence), economic analysis of CSII 62
nicotinamide, ENDIT (European Nicotinamide Diabetes Intervention Trial) 3
nicotine replacement therapy (NRT) 122, 123
nicotinic acid derivatives, value in hypertriglyceridaemia 126, 128, 134
nifedipine, use in pre-eclampsia 117
nimodipine, value after subarachnoid haemorrhage 45
nitrate treatment, contraindication to PDE-5 inhibitors 112
nitric oxide synthesis, impaired, role in DPN 153
nitroso compounds, effect on risk of type 1 diabetes 3
NMR (nuclear magnetic resonance) spectroscopy 67
non-adherence to treatment 94, 144
non-arteritic optic ischaemic neuropathy (NAOIN), association with sildenafil 114
'non-dipping' nocturnal blood pressure 204
non-proliferative diabetic retinopathy 168

non-steroidal anti-inflammatory drugs, effect on efficacy of aspirin 137
noradrenaline, secretion in hypoglycaemia 35
nortriptylline, value in smoking cessation 123
Norwegian Childhood Diabetes Study Group 3
Nurses' Health Study 10–11
nutritional requirements, cystic fibrosis 213

O
obesity 89–92
association with obstructive sleep apnoea 208
as cause of hypertriglyceridaemia 126
management in elderly people 96
risk of age-related macular degeneration 177
sarcopoenic 93
treatment 6
see also central obesity
obstetric surveillance, type 1 diabetes 109
obstructive sleep apnoea (OSA) 147, 207–10, 211
octreotide 180
oestrogen, effect on insulin sensitivity 10
oestrogen replacement 10, 11
as cause of hypertriglyceridaemia 126
office (white coat) hypertension 144, 147
offloading
in treatment of foot ulcers 201
in treatment of neuroarthropathy 183, 185
oligohydramnios in pre-eclampsia 117
oligomeric feeds 86
Omacor 126
omega-3 fatty acids 126, 128, 134
ophthalmology referral, criteria for 170, 171
oral glucose tolerance test (oGTT) 18, 19, 20
screening after gestational diabetes 105, 106
screening for gestational diabetes 104, 106
oral hypoglycaemic drugs
improvement of insulin resistance 81–4

oral hypoglycaemic drugs (*cont.*)
    insulin secretagogues 77–80
    use with enteral feeding 87
    see also metformin;
        sulphonylureas;
        thiazolidinediones
oral insulin, Diabetes Prevention
    trial-Type 1 3–4
orlistat 89, 90, 92
    XENDOS study 6
orthostatic hypotension 178,
    179–80
    and carotid artery stenosis 180–1
osteomyelitis 57, 58, 183, 200
osteopenia in coeliac disease 221
otitis externa 94
ovarian drilling 101
overt nephropathy 155
oxprenolol, use in pre-eclampsia
    117

P
paclitaxel-eluting stents 190
painful neuropathy 149–54
pamidronate, value in
    neuroarthropathy 183
pancreatitis, as cause of
    hyperosmolar hyperglycaemic
    state 30
panretinal photocoagulation 172
paraneoplastic syndrome, as cause
    of autonomic neuropathy 178
paroxetine, value in DPN 150
PARP (poly-ADP-ribose
    polymerase) 3
PDE (phosphodiesterase)-5
    inhibitors 112, 114
PEG (percutaneous endoscopic
    gastrostomy) feeding 85, 86–7
penile prostheses 114
percutaneous coronary intervention
    (PCI) 188–9
    restenosis 190
peri-menopause 10
perindopril, PROGRESS 204
perioperative management of
    diabetes 51–4
peripheral arterial disease (PAD)
    47–8, 191–4
    as cause of foot ulcers 200–1
    critical limb ischaemia 48–50
peripheral neuropathy 58
    Charcot foot 182–5
    painful 149–54
peritoneal dialysis 216–19
pH, in hyperosmolar
    hyperglycaemic state 31

phaeochromocytoma 146
phosphate replacement
    in diabetic ketoacidosis 28
    in hyperosmolar hyperglycaemic
        state 33
photocoagulation 171–3, 173
    for age-related macular
        degeneration 176
photodynamic therapy 176
pigment epithelial-derived factor
    (PEDF) 173
pioglitazone
    effect on lipid profile 82–3
    use by elderly people 95
    use in polycystic ovarian
        syndrome 102
placental abruption 116, 117
placental vascular insufficiency, role
    in pre-eclampsia 118
plasma osmolality, in hyperosmolar
    hyperglycaemic state 30, 31, 33
plasmapheresis, use in insulin
    resistance 22
plasminogen activator inhibitor-1,
    levels in insulin resistance
    syndrome 22
platelet-derived growth factor
    (PDGF), value in foot ulcers
    200, 202
platelet function, effect of smoking
    cessation 123
podocytes, abnormalities in
    albuminuria 157
polycystic ovarian syndrome
    (PCOS) 99–102
polymeric feeds 86
polymicrobial infections 57
polysomnography 147, 208
polyunsaturated fatty acids,
    interaction with PPAR-Á gene
    polymorphism 127
potassium excretion, effect of RAS
    blockade 160
potassium levels, hyperosmolar
    hyperglycaemic state 33
potassium regimen, diabetic
    ketoacidosis 28
PPAR-· gene polymorphism 135
PPAR-· agonists 126, 134
    combined PPAR-· and PPAR-Á
        agonists 83
PPAR-Á 82
PPAR-Á gene polymorphism,
    interaction with
    polyunsaturated fatty acids
    127

pramlintide 79–80
pravastatin
    LIPID study 134, 204
    see also statins
pre-diabetic phase, type 1 diabetes 2
pre-eclampsia 115–18
    in type 1 diabetes 107
pre-term deliveries, type 1 diabetes
    107, 118
pregabalin, value in DPN 151, 152
pregnancy 71
    as cause of hypertriglyceridaemia
        126
    complications of poor glycaemic
        control 100
    effect on retinopathy 169
    gestational diabetes 103–6
    outlook in cystic fibrosis 215
    pre-eclampsia 115–18
    type 1 diabetes 107–10
    use of metformin 101
preparation for exercise 66–7
preparation for pregnancy, type 1
    diabetes 108
preservatives, effect on risk of type 1
    diabetes 3
prevalence
    of MODY 14
    of type 1 diabetes 2
prevention
    of retinopathy 168–9
    of stroke 137, 203–6
    of type 1 diabetes 1–4
    of type 2 diabetes 5–8, 90
        effect of RAS blockade 161
priapism, as side effect of alprostadil
    113
primary hyperaldosteronism
    145–6, 147
primary prevention, value of aspirin
    137–8
Primary Prevention Project (PPP)
    138, 139
PROGRESS (Perindopril
    pROtection aGainst REcurrent
    Stroke Study) 204
proliferative retinopathy 168, 171–4
proprioceptive loss 182
prostacyclin infusion, value in
    critical limb ischaemia 49
prostaglandin E1, intracavernosal
    injection 113
protease inhibitors, interaction with
    PDE-5 inhibitors 112
protein kinase C (PKC), role in
    retinopathy 173

protein kinase C-, inhibitor
(ruboxistaurin) 157, 165, 169
pseudoacromegaly 22
psychological factors, insulin pump
therapy 63
psychological interventions,
adolescent diabetes 70–1

Q
QT interval, effect of vardenafil 112
quinupristin resistance 59

R
racial differences, insulin sensitivity
10
radionuclide scanning, investigation
of renal impairment 196
ragaglitazar 83
ramipril, HOPE study 192, 204
RANKL/osteoprotogerin signalling
pathway 184
recombinant tissue plasminogen
activator (rTPA)
use after acute stroke 44
use in critical limb ischaemia 49
recurrence rate, foot ulcers 201
recurrent hypoglycaemia 34–9
refeeding syndrome 87
Regranex gel 202
renal artery stenosis 144–5, 147,
195–8
avoidance of RAS blockade 161
renal disease
assessment 165
effect of statins 130
see also microalbuminuria;
nephropathy
renal failure 163–6
hypoglycaemic treatment 217
renal function monitoring, ACE
inhibitor therapy 160–1, 162
renal glucose threshold, age-related
changes 93
renal papillary necrosis 94
renin-angiotensin system (RAS)
blockade 159–62
effect on microalbuminuria
progression 155–6, 157
effect in renal artery stenosis 195
in prevention of retinopathy
168–9
preventive value 6
stroke reduction 204
value in advancing renal failure
164

repaglinide 15, 78
use by elderly people 95
resistant hypertension, causes
144–6
respiratory disease 207–11
restenosis after PCI 190
retinopathy 165, 167
classification 168
criteria for ophthalmology
referral 170
effect of pregnancy 108–9
prevention 168–9
proliferative 171–4
safety of aspirin 138
stroke risk 44
value of blood pressure reduction
141
revascularization
in carotid artery stenosis 205
coronary artery disease 188–90
in critical limb ischaemia 49–50
foot ulcers 200–1
in renal artery stenosis 196–8
rhabdomyolysis, as side effect of
fibrates 126, 134
RIO (Rimonabant In Obesity) trial
91
risk factors
for age-related macular
degeneration 177
for autonomic neuropathy 180
for coeliac disease 223
for stroke 43, 44
for surgery 51
for type 1 diabetes 2–4
rituximab, value in insulin resistance
syndrome 23
'rocker-bottom' foot 183
rosiglitazone
effect on lipid profile 82–3
use by elderly people 95
use in polycystic ovarian
syndrome 102
rubella vaccination 3
ruboxistaurin 157, 165, 169

S
St Vincent declaration 107
sarcopoenic obesity 93
Scandinavian Simvastatin Survival
Study (4S) 134, 192, 204
screening
for coeliac disease 221, 222, 223
for diabetes 18–19, 20
after gestational diabetes 105,
106

cystic fibrosis patients 213
for gestational diabetes 103–4,
106
for distal sensory peripheral
neuropathy 150
for retinopathy 169
for secondary hypertension 147
secondary hypertension 144–6, 147
secondary prevention, value of
aspirin 137, 138
self-management of diabetes
adolescents 69–71
perioperative 52
self-monitoring of blood glucose,
during pregnancy 104–5, 108
sensory loss 150
in Charcot foot 182
sertraline, value in DPN 150
sex-hormone binding globulin,
levels in insulin resistance
syndrome 22
SHHS (Sleep Heart Health Study)
208, 210
shoulder problems 94
sibutramine 89, 90–1, 92
value in DPN 151
side effects
of amitriptyline 150
of aspirin 138
of fibrates 126, 134
of metformin 81
of nicotinic acid 126
of orlistat 90
of PDE-5 inhibitors 112, 114
of sibutramine 91
of sublingual apomorphine 113
of sulphonylureas 77
of thiazolidinediones 82
sildenafil 112
sudden deaths 114
silent myocardial infarction 40
silent phase, diabetic nephropathy
155
simvastatin 134
stroke reduction 204
value in peripheral arterial disease
192
see also statins
sirolimus-eluting stents 190
skin, dryness 58
skin substitutes 202
sleep apnoea 147, 207–10, 211
sleep disordered breathing (SDB)
208
sleep disturbance, association with
type 2 diabetes 208

'sliding scale' insulin replacement
      regimen 28
small-molecule insulino-mimetic
      drugs 84
smoking 7, 8, 47, 121–2
   as cause of hypertriglyceridaemia
      126
   and pregnancy 110
   risk of age-related macular
      degeneration 177
smoking cessation 122–4
snoring, sleep apnoea 208
sodium levels
   in hyperosmolar hyperglycaemic
      state 31, 33
   in PEG feeding 87
sodium valproate, value in DPN
      152
somatostatin analogues 180
specialist care, value in diabetic
      ketoacidosis 26
spinal cord stimulation, value in
      DPN 151
spironolactone, as cause of erectile
      dysfunction 112
statins 126, 134
   effect on endothelial function
      194
   stroke prevention 204
   use in type 1 diabetes 129–30,
      131, 132
   value in advancing renal failure
      164, 165
   value in microalbuminuria 157
   value in peripheral arterial disease
      192
Steno Trial 190
stenting 188–9
   of carotid artery 205
   restenosis rates 190
steroids, use in insulin resistance 22
STOP-NIDDM (Study to Prevent
      Non-Insulin-Dependent
      Diabetes Mellitus) 6
stress hyperglycaemia, stroke risk
      44
stress imaging 188
stroke 44–6
   as cause of hyperosmolar
      hyperglycaemic state 30
   nutritional support 85, 87–8
   secondary prevention, value of
      aspirin 137
stroke prevention 203–6
stroke risk 43, 44
structured consultations 69–70

subarachnoid haemorrhage 44, 45
sublingual apomorphine 113
sudden death, risk in autonomic
      neuropathy 179
sulodexide 165
sulphonylureas 77, 80
   secondary treatment failure 7–9
   and surgery 53
   use by elderly people 94
   use in cardiovascular disease 40
   use in cystic fibrosis-related
      diabetes 213
   use in renal failure 217
   value in MODY 15
   value in prevention of type 2
      diabetes 6
surgery
   after acute stroke 44
   bariatric 91, 92
   carotid endarterectomy 205
   for critical limb ischaemia 48–50
   for foot ulcers 200–1
   perioperative management of
      diabetes 51–4
   role in neuroarthropathy 183
SWAN (Study of Women's health
      Across the Nation) 10
sweating, abnormalities in
      autonomic neuropathy 178
Swedish Obese Subjects Study 91
sympathectomy, in critical limb
      ischaemia 49
symptoms of diabetes, in elderly
      people 93–4
symptoms of hypoglycaemia 35, 36
systolic hypertension, stroke risk
      204

T
tadalafil 112
target levels, antihypertensive
      therapy 142, 144
   in advancing renal failure 166
   in microalbuminuria 155
teenagers
   adolescent diabetes 69–71
   intima-media thickness 130
testosterone, levels in insulin
      resistance syndrome 22
testosterone deficiency, as cause of
      erectile dysfunction 112
thiazide diuretics, as cause of erectile
      dysfunction 112, 141
thiazolidinediones 80, 82, 84
   in prevention of type 2 diabetes 6
   use by elderly people 95

   use in cystic fibrosis-related
      diabetes 213
   use in polycystic ovarian
      syndrome 102
   use in renal failure 217
thirst mechanism, age-related
      changes 93
thrombocytopenia, in pre-eclampsia
      117
thrombolysis 40
   after acute stroke 44
thrombosis risk, use in
      hyperosmolar hyperglycaemic
      state 33
thromboxane 137
thyroid autoimmunity, association
      with coeliac disease 223
TNT (Treating to New Target) study
      130
toes, clawing 58
tolbutamide 77
   use in renal failure 217
topiramate, use for weight reduction
      91
torcetrapib 135
total contact casting (TCC) 201
tramadol, value in DPN 151
transaminase levels, in
      thiazolidinedione treatment
      82
transdermal nicotine replacement
      therapy 122
transglutaminase 2 antibodies 221
transient ischaemic attack 203–6
transurethral alprostadil 113
trauma, as cause of hyperosmolar
      hyperglycaemic state 30
trazodone, value in DPN 150
treatment failure, insulin
      secretagogues 78–9, 80
triamcinolone acetonide, vitreal
      injection 174
tricyclic antidepressants, value in
      DPN 150, 152, 153–4
triggers for hyperosmolar
      hyperglycaemic state 30
triggers for hypoglycaemia 35
triglycerides 125
   levels in insulin resistance
      syndrome 22
   see also hypertriglyceridaemia
troglitazone, in prevention of type 2
      diabetes 6
tumour necrosis factor-· (TNF-·)
      gene polymorphisms 19

type 1 diabetes
  ACE inhibitor treatment 159–62
  association with coeliac disease
    221, 223
  exercise 65–8
  hyperlipidaemia 129–32 107–10
    pre-eclampsia 115–18
  prevention 1–4
type 2 diabetes
  angina 187–90
  association with sleep disturbance
    208
  diabetic ketoacidosis 29
  hyperlipidaemia 133–6
  introduction of insulin treatment
    79, 80
  prevention 5–8, 90
  protective role of RAS inhibition
    159
type A and type B insulin resistance
    syndrome 21–4

U
UKPDS (United Kingdom
    Prospective Diabetes Studies)
  hypertension 44, 140–1, 204
  oral hypoglycaemics, use in
    cardiovascular disease 40–1
  peripheral arterial disease 192
  retinopathy 167, 168, 177
  risk engine 136
  stroke, mortality 44
  value of metformin 81–2
ulceration of foot 48, 55–9, 199–202
ultrasound, investigation of renal
    impairment 196
undernutrition 85
uraemic symptoms, effect on
    appetite 218
urinalysis, limitations in MODY 15
urinary free-cortisol measurement
    145
urine testing, value in screening 19,
    20

V
VA-HIT (Veterans Affairs High-
    Density Lipoprotein
    Intervention Trial) 134, 204
vaccination, effect on risk of type 1
    diabetes 3, 4
vacuum tumescence 114
Valsalva manoeuvre 179
vanadium compounds 84
vancomycin resistance 58–9
vardenafil 112
vascular endothelial growth factor
    (VGEF) therapy, peripheral
    arterial disease 193–4
vascular endothelium, effect of
    smoking 122
vascular reconstructive surgery,
    critical limb ischaemia 49–50
vincristine, as cause of autonomic
    neuropathy 178
viral infections, as risk factor for
    type 1 diabetes 3
visceral obesity see central obesity
vision, side effect of sildenafil 14,
    112
vitamin B3 (niacin), effect on risk of
    type 1 diabetes 3
vitamin D deficiency, coeliac disease
    221
vitamin D status, effect on risk of
    type 1 diabetes 3, 4
vitamins
  and age-related macular
    degeneration 176
  antioxidant HPS 134
vitreal injection, triamcinolone
    acetonide 174
vitrectomy 173
VLDL (very-low density
    lipoprotein) 133
vomiting, as cause of diabetic
    ketoacidosis 26

W
walking programmes, peripheral
    arterial disease 192
walnuts, effect on lipid profile 135
warfarin, stroke prevention 203
weight gain
  effect on risk of type 1 diabetes 3,
    4
  effect of sulphonylureas 77
  effect of thiazolidinediones 82
  perimenopausal 10
  as side effect of medication 89
weight reduction 89–92
  effect on glucose tolerance 89
  effect on lipid profile 133–4
  in management of polycystic
    ovarian syndrome 100
  in management of sleep apnoea
    210
  value of low-carbohydrate diet
    73, 75
  XENDOS study 6
wet age-related macular
    degeneration (AMD) 176
WHI (Women's Health Initiative)
    10
white coat hypertension 144, 147
whole-grain consumption 74–5
WOSCOPS (West of Scotland
    Coronary Prevention Study)
    127
wound debridement, foot ulcers
    200

X
X-ray findings, Charcot foot 183
XENDOS (XENical in the
    prevention of Diabetes in
    Obese Subjects) study 6, 90

Z
zeaxanthin 176
zinc deficiency 94